Respiratory Medicine
Lecture Notes

Respiratory Medicine
Lecture Notes

Stephen J. Bourke

Consultant Physician
Royal Victoria Infirmary
Newcastle upon Tyne;
Honorary Senior Lecturer
Newcastle University

Graham P. Burns

Consultant Physician
Royal Victoria Infirmary
Newcastle upon Tyne;
Honorary Senior Lecturer
Newcastle University

Eighth Edition

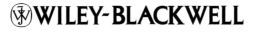

A John Wiley & Sons, Ltd., Publication

This edition first published 2011 © 2011 by John Wiley & Sons, Ltd.

Wiley-Blackwell is an imprint of John Wiley & Sons, formed by the merger of Wiley's global Scientific, Technical and Medical business with Blackwell Publishing.

Registered office: John Wiley & Sons, Ltd, The Atrium, Southern Gate, Chichester, West Sussex, PO19 8SQ, UK

Editorial offices: 9600 Garsington Road, Oxford, OX4 2DQ, UK
The Atrium, Southern Gate, Chichester, West Sussex, PO19 8SQ, UK
111 River Street, Hoboken, NJ 07030-5774, USA

For details of our global editorial offices, for customer services and for information about how to apply for permission to reuse the copyright material in this book please see our website at www.wiley.com/wiley-blackwell

Library of Congress Cataloging-in-Publication Data

Bourke, S. J.
  Lecture Notes: Respiratory Medicine / Stephen J. Bourke, Graham P. Burns. – 8th ed.
      p. ; cm.
  Respiratory medicine
  Includes bibliographical references and index.
  ISBN 978-0-4706-5442-2 (pbk. : alk. paper) 1. Respiratory organs–
Diseases–Outlines, syllabi, etc. I. Burns, Graham P. II. Title. III. Title:
Respiratory medicine.
  [DNLM: 1. Respiratory Tract Diseases. WF 140]
  RC731.B69 2011
  616.2–dc22

                                                        2010047390

A catalogue record for this book is available from the British Library.

Set in 8.5pt/11pt Utopia font by Thomson Digital, Noida, India.
Printed and bound in Malaysia by Vivar Printing Sdn Bhd

1   2011

Contents

Preface, vii

Part 1 Structure and Function

1 Anatomy and physiology of the lungs, 1

Part 2 History Taking, Examination and Investigations

2 History taking and examination, 13
3 Pulmonary function tests, 23
4 Radiology of the chest, 37

Part 3 Respiratory Diseases

5 Upper respiratory tract infections and influenza, 46
6 Pneumonia, 52

7 Tuberculosis, 68
8 Bronchiectasis and lung abscess, 78
9 Cystic fibrosis, 87
10 Asthma, 98
11 Chronic obstructive pulmonary disease, 115
12 Carcinoma of the lung, 130
13 Interstitial lung disease, 142
14 Occupational lung disease, 151
15 Pulmonary vascular disease, 160
16 Pneumothorax and pleural effusion, 169
17 Acute respiratory distress syndrome, 179
18 Sleep-related breathing disorders, 185
19 Lung transplantation, 192

Part 4 Self-assessment

Multiple choice questions, 197
Answers to multiple choice questions, 207

Index, 215

Preface

It is now more than 35 years since the first edition of *Lecture Notes: Respiratory Medicine* was written by our predecessor and colleague, Dr Alistair Brewis. It rapidly became a classic textbook that opened the eyes of generations of students to the special fascinations of the subject such that many were attracted into the specialty. Thus, students became teachers, and continued to learn by teaching. Subsequent editions show how respiratory medicine has developed over the years to become such a major specialty in hospitals and in the community, treating a wide range of diseases from cystic fibrosis to lung cancer, asthma to tuberculosis, sleep disorders to occupational lung diseases.

In the eighth edition the text has been revised and expanded to provide a concise up-to-date summary of respiratory medicine for undergraduate students and junior doctors preparing for postgraduate examinations. Dr Graham Burns who has a particular interest in the teaching of respiratory physiology and who was also a student of Dr Alistair Brewis joins the authorship. A particular feature of respiratory medicine in recent years has been multidisciplinary teamwork, focusing the skills from a variety of disciplines in providing the best care for patients with respiratory diseases, and this book should be useful to colleagues such as physiotherapists, lung function technicians and respiratory nurse specialists. Some of Dr Alistair Brewis' original drawings and diagrams have been retained. The emphasis of *Respiratory Medicine: Lecture Notes* has always been on information that is useful and relevant to everyday clinical medicine, and the eight edition remains a patient-based book to be read before and after visits to the wards and clinics where clinical medicine is learnt and practised. As *Respiratory Medicine: Lecture Notes* develops over time, we remain grateful to our teachers and their teachers, and we pass on our evolving knowledge of respiratory medicine to our students and their students.

S. J. Bourke
G. P. Burns

Anatomy and physiology of the lungs

The anatomy and physiology of the respiratory system are designed in such a way as to bring air from the atmosphere and blood from the circulation into close proximity across the alveolar capillary membrane in order to facilitate the exchange of oxygen and carbon dioxide.

Clinical anatomy

Bronchial tree and alveoli

The **trachea** has cartilaginous horseshoe-shaped 'rings' supporting its anterior and lateral walls. The posterior wall is flaccid and bulges forward during coughing. The trachea divides into the right and left main bronchi at the level of the sternal angle (angle of Louis). The **left main bronchus** is longer than the right and leaves the trachea at a more abrupt angle. The **right main bronchus** is more directly in line with the trachea so that inhaled material tends to enter the right lung more readily than the left. The main bronchi divide into **lobar bronchi** (upper, middle and lower on the right; upper and lower on the left) and then **segmental bronchi** as shown in Fig. 1.1. The position of the lungs in relation to external landmarks is shown in Fig. 1.2. **Bronchi** are airways with cartilage in their walls, and there are about 10 divisions of bronchi beyond the tracheal bifurcation. Smaller airways without cartilage in their walls are referred to as **bronchioles**. **Respiratory bronchioles** are peripheral bronchioles with alveoli in their walls. Bronchioles immediately proximal to alveoli are known as **terminal bronchioles**. In the bronchi, smooth muscle is arranged in a spiral fashion internal to the cartilaginous plates. The muscle coat becomes more complete distally as the cartilaginous plates become more fragmentary. The epithelial lining is ciliated and includes goblet cells. The cilia beat with a whip-like action, and waves of contraction pass in an organised fashion from cell to cell so that material trapped in the sticky mucus layer above the cilia is moved upwards and out of the lung. This mucociliary escalator is an important part of the lung's defences. Larger bronchi also have acinar mucus-secreting glands in the submucosa that are hypertrophied in chronic bronchitis. **Alveoli** are about 0.1–0.2 mm in diameter and are lined by a thin layer of cells of which there are two types: type I pneumocytes have flattened processes that extend to cover most of the internal surface of the alveoli; type II pneumocytes are less numerous and contain lamellated structures that are concerned with the production of surfactant (Fig. 1.3). There is a potential space between the alveolar cells and the capillary basement membrane that

Respiratory Medicine Lecture Notes, Eighth Edition. Stephen J. Bourke and Graham P. Burns.
© 2011 John Wiley & Sons, Ltd. Published 2011 by John Wiley & Sons, Ltd.

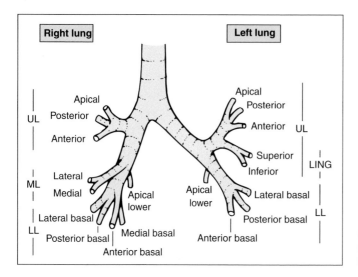

Figure 1.1 Diagram of bronchopulmonary segments. LING, lingula; LL, lower lobe; ML, middle lobe; UL, upper lobe.

is only apparent in disease states when it may contain fluid, fibrous tissue or a cellular infiltrate.

Lung perfusion

The lungs receive a blood supply from both the pulmonary and systemic circulations. The **pulmonary artery** arises from the right ventricle and divides into left and right pulmonary arteries, which further divide into branches accompanying the bronchial tree. The pulmonary capillary network in the alveolar walls is very dense and provides a very large surface area for gas exchange. The pulmonary venules drain laterally to the periphery of lung lobules and then pass centrally in the interlobular and intersegmental septa, ultimately

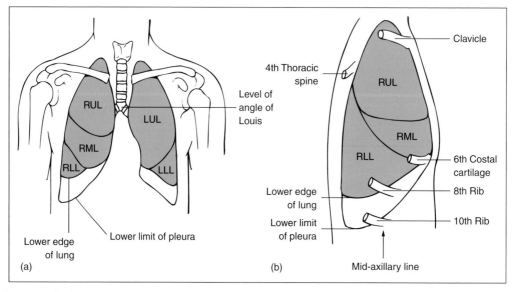

Figure 1.2 Surface anatomy. (a) Anterior view of the lungs. (b) Lateral view of the right side of chest at resting end-expiratory position. LLL, left lower lobe; LUL, left upper lobe; RLL, right lower lobe; RML, right middle lobe; RUL, right upper lobe.

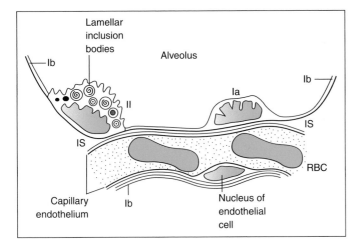

Figure 1.3 Structure of the alveolar wall as revealed by electron microscopy. Ia, type I pneumocyte; Ib, flattened extension of type I pneumocyte covering most of the internal surface of the alveolus; II, type II pneumocyte with lamellar inclusion bodies that are probably the site of surfactant formation; IS, interstitial space; RBC, red blood corpuscle. Pneumocytes and endothelial cells rest upon thin continuous basement membranes that are not shown.

joining to form the four main pulmonary veins that empty into the left atrium. Several small **bronchial arteries** usually arise from the descending aorta and travel in the outer layers of the bronchi and bronchioles supplying the tissues of the airways down to the level of the respiratory bronchiole. Most of the blood drains into radicles of the pulmonary vein contributing a small amount of desaturated blood that accounts for part of the 'physiological shunt' (blood passing through the lungs without being oxygenated) observed in normal individuals. The bronchial arteries may undergo hypertrophy when there is chronic pulmonary inflammation, and major haemoptysis in diseases such as bronchiectasis or aspergilloma usually arises from the bronchial rather than the pulmonary arteries and may be treated by therapeutic bronchial artery embolisation. The pulmonary circulation normally offers a much lower resistance and operates at a lower perfusion pressure than the systemic circulation. The pulmonary capillaries may be compressed as they pass through the alveolar walls if alveolar pressure rises above capillary pressure.

Physiology

The core business of the lungs is to bring oxygen into the body and to take carbon dioxide out.

This is brought about by a process best considered in two steps:

1 moving air in and out of the lungs (between the outside world and the alveoli);

2 gas exchange: the exchange of oxygen and carbon dioxide between the airspace of the alveoli and the blood.

This process continues throughout life largely unconsciously, coordinated by a centre in the brain stem. The factors that regulate the process, 'the control of breathing' will also be considered here.

Moving air in and out of the lungs

To understand this process we need to consider the muscles that 'drive the pump' and the resistive forces they have to overcome. These forces include the inherent elastic property of the lungs and the resistance to airflow through the bronchi (airway resistance).

The muscles that drive the pump

Inspiration requires muscular work. The diaphragm is the principal muscle of inspiration. At the end of the previous expiration the diaphragm sits in a soft, domed position high in the thorax (Fig. 1.4). To inspire, the strong muscular sheet contracts, it stiffens and tends to push the abdominal contents down. There is variable resistance to this downward pressure by the abdomen; which means that to accommodate the new shape of the diaphragm the lower ribs (to which it is attached) also move upwards and outwards. The degree of resistance the abdomen presents can be voluntarily increased by contracting the abdominal muscles, inspiration then leads to a visible expansion of the thorax. The resistance may also be increased by abdominal obesity. In such circumstances there

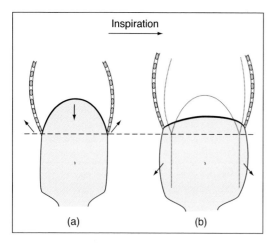

Inspiration

(a)   (b)

Figure 1.4 Effect of diaphragmatic contraction. Diagram of the ribcage, abdominal cavity and diaphragm showing the position at the end of resting expiration (a). As the diaphragm contracts it pushes the abdominal contents down (the abdominal wall moves outwards) and reduces pressure with the thorax which 'sucks' air in through the mouth (inspiration). As the diaphragm shortens and descends it also stiffens. The diaphragm meets a variable degree of resistance to downward discursion that forces the lower ribs to move up and outward to accommodate its new position (b).

is an involuntary limitation to the downward excursion of the diaphragm and, as the potential for upward movement of the ribs is limited, the capacity for full inspiration is diminished. This inability to fully inflate the lungs is an example of a **restrictive ventilatory defect** (see Chapter 3).

Other muscles are also involved in inspiration. The scalene muscles elevate the upper ribs and sternum. These are active even in quiet breathing although they were once considered, along with the sternocleidomastoids, as '**accessory muscles of respiration**', only brought into play during the exaggerated ventilatory effort of acute respiratory distress.

The intercostal muscles bind the ribs to ensure the integrity of the chest wall. They therefore transfer the effects of actions on the upper or lower ribs to the whole rib cage. They also brace the chest wall, resisting the bulging or indrawing effect of changes in pleural pressure during breathing. This bracing effect can be overcome to some extent by the exaggerated pressure changes seen during periods of more extreme respiratory effort, and in slim individuals **intercostal recession** may be observed as a sign of respiratory distress.

Whereas inspiration is the result of active muscular effort, quiet expiration is a more passive process. The inspiratory muscles steadily release their contraction and the elastic recoil of the lungs brings the tidal breathing cycle back to its start point. Forced expiration however, either volitional or as in coughing for example, requires muscular effort. The abdominal musculature is the principal agent in this.

The inherent elastic property of the lungs

Lung tissue has a natural elasticity. Left to its own devices a lung would tend to shrink to little more than the size of a fist. This can sometimes be observed radiographically in the context of a complete **pneumothorax** (Chapter 16). The lung's tendency to contract is counteracted by the semi-rigid chest wall that has a tendency to spring outward from its usual position. At the end of a normal tidal expiration the two opposing forces are nicely balanced and no muscular effort is required to hold this 'neutral' position. Breathing close to this lung volume (normal tidal breathing) is therefore relatively efficient and minimises the work of breathing. Unfortunately in some diseases (asthma, chronic obstructive pulmonary disease (COPD)) tidal ventilation is obliged to occur at higher lung volumes (see Chapter 3). This increases the work of breathing, a factor that contributes to the sensation of breathlessness. Test this yourself; take a good breath in and try to breathe normally at this high lung volume for a minute.

The opposing forces from the lung and chest wall generate a negative pressure within the pleural space. This negative pressure maintains the lung in its stretched state. Clearly at higher lung volumes the lung is at greater stretch and a more negative pleural pressure is required to hold it in position. The relationship between pleural pressure (the force on the lung) and lung volume can be plotted graphically (Fig. 1.5). The lung, however, does not behave as a perfect spring. You may recall the length of a spring is proportional to the force applied to it (Hooke's law). In the case of the lung, as its volume increases, greater and greater force is needed to achieve the same additional increase in volume i.e. the lung becomes less 'compliant' as its volume increases. **Lung compliance** is defined as: 'the change in lung volume brought about by a unit change in transpulmonary (intrapleural) pressure'.

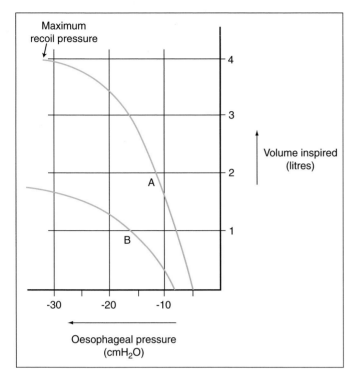

Figure 1.5 Graph of (static) lung volume against intrapleural pressure. In both subjects A and B, we see that **lung compliance** – the change in lung volume per unit change in intrapleural pressure (or slope of the curve) is reduced at higher lung volumes. A: normal individual. B: individual with reduced lung compliance e.g. lung fibrosis.

Airway resistance

In addition to overcoming the elastic properties of the lungs and the chest wall, during active breathing the muscles of respiration also have to overcome the frictional forces opposing flow up and down the airways.

Site of maximal resistance

It is generally understood that resistance to flow in a tube increases sharply as luminal radius (r) decreases (with laminar flow, resistance is inversely proportional to r^4). It may be surprising to learn therefore that in a healthy individual the greater part of total airway resistance is situated in the large airways (larynx, trachea and main bronchi). This is in part due to the fact that the flow velocity is greatest and flow more turbulent here but also due to the much greater *total* cross-sectional area in the later generations of airway that effectively function in parallel (Fig. 1.6). Conditions may be different in disease states. Asthma and COPD, diseases which affect airway calibre, tend to have a greater proportionate effect on smaller generations of airways. The reduced calibre of the smaller airways then becomes

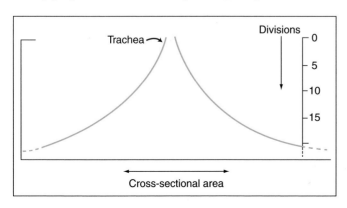

Figure 1.6 Diagrammatic representation of the increase in total cross-sectional area of the airways at successive divisions.

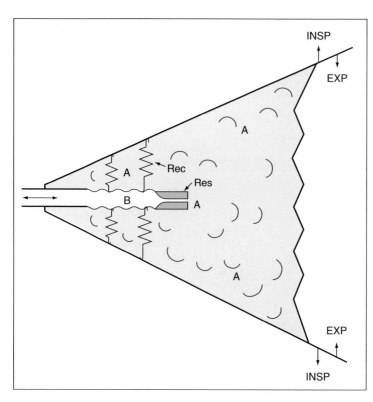

Figure 1.7 Model of the lung to demonstrate the flow limiting mechanism (see text). The chest is represented as a bellows. The airways of the lungs are represented collectively as having a distal resistive segment (Res) and a more proximal collapsible or 'floppy' segment. The walls of the floppy segment are kept apart by the retractive force of lung recoil (Rec). EXP, expiration; INSP, inspiration.

overwhelmingly important and the site of principal resistance moves distally.

Consider the model of the lung represented in Fig. 1.7. Here the tube represents a route through generations of airways from the alveoli to the mouth. The smaller generations of airways, without cartilaginous support, are represented by the 'floppy' segment (B). Airways are embedded within the lung and are attached externally to lung tissue whose elastic recoil and ultimate connection to the chest wall supports the floppy segments. This recoil force is represented by the springs. During expiration a positive pressure is generated in the alveolar space (A). Air flows from A along the airway, past point B where the pressure is lower (it must be otherwise the air would not have flowed in this direction) and on to the mouth where the pressure is nominally 'zero'. The pressure difference across the walls of the floppy segment (A minus B) would tend to cause this part of the airway to collapse. It is prevented from doing so by the tension within the springs.

The flow-limiting mechanism

During expiration the extent of the pressure drop between A and B is proportional to the flow rate. Clearly with increased effort, flow rate will be increased…up to a point. Eventually a critical flow rate will be reached where the pressure gradient between A and B will be sufficient to overcome the retractive force of the lung, the airway wall will collapse and airflow will cease. The pressure inside the airway at point B will rise and almost immediately equal that at A. The retractive force of the lung will then open the airway again and flow will recommence. The cycle thus starts again. It will be apparent that this mechanism determines a maximum flow rate along the airway. As each route out of the lung will similarly have a maximal possible flow rate, the expiratory flow from the lung as a whole will have an absolute limit. It can be seen that this limit is set by the internal mechanics of the lung, not by muscular effort (above a certain level of effort). If that were not the case then **peak expiratory flow rate** (PEFR), for example, would not be a lung function test; it would be a test of muscular strength.

The effects of disease on maximum flow rate

In asthma (Chapter 10) airway narrowing occurs leading to a greater resistance between the alveolus

(A) and point B. The pressure drop, A to B, for any given flow rate will therefore be greater than in the healthy lung. The critical (maximal) flow rate (when the pressure difference between A and B is just enough to overcome the retractive force of the lung) will therefore be lower. You may have known for some time that peak expiratory flow is reduced in asthma but now you understand why. In COPD (Chapter 11) the loss of alveolar walls (emphysema) reduces the elastic recoil of the lung. There is therefore less protective retractive force on the airway wall and the critical pressure drop along the airway required to cause airway collapse will occur at a lower flow rate. Thus maximum expiratory flow is also reduced in COPD.

Airway resistance and lung volume

It can easily be seen in the model that as lung volume decreases, lung elastic recoil (tension within the springs) diminishes and so provides less and less support for the floppy airway. It is clear therefore that the maximum flow rate achievable is dependant on lung volume and is reduced as lung volume is reduced. For any given lung volume there will be a maximum expiratory flow that cannot be exceeded no matter what the effort. A true PEFR can therefore only be achieved by beginning expiration at full inspiration. You can confirm this by inspecting the shape of a flow loop (Chapter 3). Although I would suggest you have been aware of this fact for longer than you realise. Immediately prior to blowing the candles out on your second birthday cake you probably took a big breath in, instinctively understanding the relationship between lung volume and the power of your puff.

Lung volume and site of maximal airway resistance

As discussed above (in health) the greater part of airway resistance resides in the central airways. These airways are well supported by cartilage so generally maintain their calibre even at low lung volumes. The calibre of the small airways, without cartilaginous support, are heavily dependant on lung volume. As lung volume diminishes resistance in the smaller generations of airway increases substantially. During expiration therefore as lung volume is diminished, the site of principal resistance moves from the central airways to the peripheral airways. The PEFR (Chapter 3) tests expiratory flow at high lung volume. The **forced expiratory volume in one second**, FEV_1 (Chapter 3) is also heavily influenced by the central airway

(though not as much as PEFR). Specialised lung function tests that measure expiratory flow at lower lung volumes (e.g. $\mathbf{FEF_{25-75}}$ **and** $\mathbf{\dot{V}_{max50}}$ see Chapter 3) are believed to provide more information about the smaller airways.

Gas exchange

The lung is ventilated by air and perfused by blood; for gas exchange to occur these two elements must come into intimate contact.

Where does the air go?

An inspired breath brings air into the lung. That air, however, does not distribute itself evenly. Some parts of the lung are more compliant than others and are therefore more accommodating. This variability in compliance occurs on a gross scale across the lungs (upper zones verses lower zones) and also on a very small scale in a more random pattern. At the gross level, the lungs can be imagined as 'hanging' inside the thorax, the effect of gravity means that the upper parts of the lungs are under considerable stretch whereas the bases sit relatively compressed on the diaphragm. During inspiration, as the upper parts of the lung are already stretched it is difficult for them to accommodate more air, the bases, on the other hand, are ripe for inflation. Therefore far more of each inspired breath will go to the lower zones then the upper zones. On a small scale adjacent lobules or even alveoli may not have the same compliance, airway anatomy is not precisely uniform either and airway resistance between individual lung units will vary. It can be seen therefore that ventilation will vary in an apparently random fashion on a small scale throughout the lung. This phenomenon may be rather modest in health but is likely to be exaggerated in many lung diseases in which airway resistance or lung compliance is affected.

Where does the blood go?

The pulmonary circulation operates under much lower pressure than the systemic circulation. At rest, the driving pressure is only in the order of 15 mmHg. In the upright posture therefore there is barely enough pressure to fill the upper parts of the system and the apices of the lung receive very little perfusion at all from the pulmonary circulation. The relative overperfusion of the bases mirrors the pattern seen with ventilation (which is fortunate if our aim is to bring blood and air into contact) but the disparity is even greater in the case of perfusion. Thus, at the bases of the lungs perfusion exceeds ventilation, at the apices ventilation exceeds perfusion. The distribution of perfusion is also heavily influenced by another factor – hypoxia. By a mechanism we do not fully understand low oxygen levels in a region of the lung have a direct vasoconstrictor effect on the pulmonary artery supplying it. This has the beneficial effect of diverting blood away from the areas of lung that are poorly ventilated towards the well-ventilated areas. This 'automatic' **ventilation/perfusion (V/Q) matching system** aims to maximise the contact between air and blood and is critically important to gas exchange.

Relationship between P_{O_2} and P_{CO_2}

During steady-state conditions the relationship between the amount of carbon dioxide produced by the body and the amount of oxygen absorbed depends upon the metabolic activity of the body and is referred to as the respiratory quotient (RQ).

$$RQ = \frac{CO_2 \text{ produced}}{O_2 \text{ absorbed}}$$

The actual value varies from 0.7 during pure fat metabolism to 1.0 during pure carbohydrate metabolism. The RQ is usually about 0.8 but it is often assumed to be 1.0 to make calculations easier.

Carbon dioxide

If carbon dioxide is being produced by the body at a constant rate the P_{CO_2} of alveolar air depends only upon the amount of outside air that the carbon dioxide is mixed with in the alveoli, i.e. it depends only upon alveolar ventilation. If alveolar ventilation increases the P_{CO_2} will fall. If alveolar ventilation decreases P_{CO_2} will rise. Alveolar P_{CO_2} (indeed arterial P_{CO_2} likewise) is a sensitive index of alveolar ventilation.

Oxygen

The level of alveolar P_{O_2} also varies with alveolar ventilation. If alveolar ventilation were increased greatly the P_{O_2} would rise and begin to approach the P_{O_2} in the inspired air. If alveolar ventilation were reduced P_{O_2} would be reduced. Whilst arterial P_{O_2} would also vary with alveolar ventilation (in the same direction as alveolar P_{O_2}) it is not a reliable index of alveolar ventilation as it is profoundly affected by regional changes in ventilation/perfusion (V/Q) matching (see below).

The possible combinations of P_{CO_2} and P_{O_2} are shown in Fig. 1.8. Moist atmospheric air at 37°C has

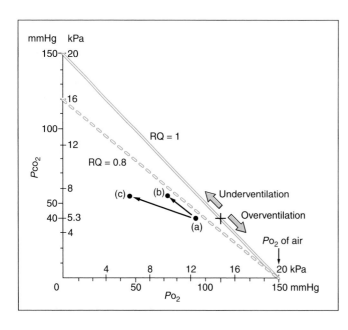

Figure 1.8 Oxygen–carbon dioxide diagram. The continuous and interrupted lines describe the possible combinations of P_{CO_2} and P_{O_2} in alveolar air when the RQ is 1 and 0.8, respectively. (a) A hypothetical sample of arterial blood. (b) Progressive underventilation. (c) P_{O_2} lower than can be accounted for by underventilation alone.

a P_{O_2} of about 20 kPa. In this model, oxygen could be exchanged with carbon dioxide in the alveoli to produce any combination of P_{O_2} and P_{CO_2} described by the oblique line that joins P_{O_2} 20 kPa and P_{CO_2} 20 kPa. The position of the cross on this line represents the composition of a hypothetical sample of alveolar air. A fall in alveolar ventilation would result in an upward movement of this point along the line and conversely an increase in alveolar ventilation would result in a downward movement of the point.

In practice RQ is not 1.0 but closer to 0.8. In other words:

$$\text{alveolar } P_{O_2} + (\text{alveolar } P_{CO_2}/0.8) = 20 \text{ kPa}$$

This is represented by the dotted line in the figure.

Point (a) represents the P_{CO_2} and P_{O_2} of arterial blood (it lies a little to the left of the RQ 0.8 line because of the small normal alveolar–arterial oxygen tension difference). Point (b) represents the arterial gas tension after a period of underventilation. If the arterial P_{CO_2} and P_{O_2} were those represented by point (c) this would imply that the fall in P_{O_2} was more than could be accounted for by reduced alveolar ventilation alone.

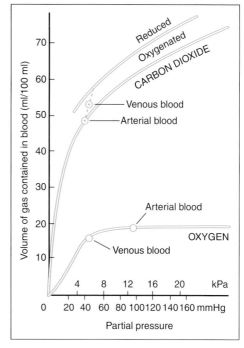

Figure 1.9 The blood oxygen and carbon dioxide dissociation curves drawn to the same scale.

The carriage of CO_2 and O_2 by blood

The quantity of gas carried by blood when exposed to different partial pressures of the gas is described by the dissociation curve. The dissociation curves for oxygen and carbon dioxide are very different and are shown together on the same scale in Fig. 1.9. Over the range normally encountered the amount of carbon dioxide carried by the blood is roughly proportional to the P_{CO_2}. However, the quantity of oxygen carried is roughly proportional to the P_{O_2} only over a very limited range of about 3–7 kPa (22–52 mmHg). Above 13.3 kPa (100 mmHg) the haemoglobin is fully saturated and hardly any additional oxygen is carried.

Effect of local differences in VQ

In the normal lung the vast majority of alveoli receive ventilation and perfusion in about the right proportion ((a) in Fig. 1.10). In diffuse disease of the lung however, it is usual for ventilation and perfusion to be irregularly distributed so that a

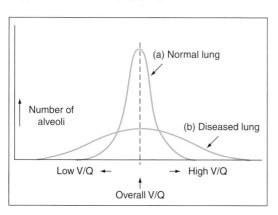

Figure 1.10 Distribution of ventilation/perfusion relationships within the lungs. Although the overall ventilation/perfusion (V/Q) ratio is the same in the two examples shown, the increased spread of V/Q ratios within the diseased lung (b) will result in a lower arterial oxygen tension and content than in the normal lung (a). Arterial P_{CO_2} will be similar in both cases.

greater scatter of V/Q ratios is encountered ((b) in Fig. 1.10). Even if the overall V/Q remains normal there is wide local variation in V/Q. Looking at Fig. 1.10 it is tempting to suppose the effects of the alveoli with low V/Q might be nicely balanced by the alveoli with high V/Q. In fact this is not the case;

the increased range of V/Q within the lung affects the transport of CO_2 and O_2 differently.

In Figure 1.11 (b) and (c) are regions of low and high V/Q respectively and the result of mixing blood from these two regions is shown at (d) where the arterial CO_2 and O_2 contents are represented.

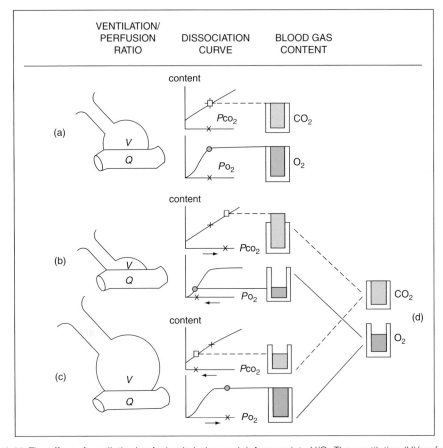

Figure 1.11 The effect of ventilation/perfusion imbalance. (a) Appropriate V/Q. The ventilation (V)/perfusion (Q) ratio is shown diagrammatically on the left. When ventilation is appropriately matched to perfusion in an alveolus or in the lung as a whole, the Pco_2 is about 5.3 kPa (40 mmHg) and the Po_2 is about 12.6 kPa (95 mmHg). The dissociation curves shown in the centre of the diagram describe the relationship between the blood gas tension and the amount of gas carried by the blood. The normal blood gas contents are represented very diagrammatically on the right. (b) Low V/Q. Reduced ventilation relative to blood flow results in a rise in Pco_2 and a fall in Po_2. Reference to the dissociation curves shows that this produces a rise in arterial CO_2 content and a fall in O_2 content. (c) High V/Q. Increased ventilation relative to blood flow results in a fall in Pco_2 and a rise in Po_2. Reference to the dissociation curves shows that this results in a fall in CO_2 content below the normal level but in the case of O_2 there is no increase in content. In health, the vast majority of alveoli have an appropriate balance of ventilation and perfusion and the arterial blood has a normal CO_2 and O_2 content as shown in (a). In many disease states the V/Q ratio varies widely between areas. Such variation always results in a disturbance of blood gas content. The effects of areas of low V/Q are not corrected by areas of high V/Q. The result of mixing blood from areas of low and high V/Q is shown diagrammatically on the extreme right of the diagram (d). It will be seen that with respect to CO_2 content, the high content of the blood from underventilated areas is balanced by the low content from the overventilated areas. However in the case of O_2, the low content of the blood from underventilated areas cannot be compensated for by an equivalent increase in the O_2 content of blood from overventilated areas. *Arterial hypoxaemia is inevitable if there are areas of low V/Q (relative underventilation or overperfusion).*

Effect on arterial CO_2 content

Blood with a high CO_2 content returning from low V/Q areas mixes with blood with a low CO_2 content returning from high V/Q areas and the net CO_2 content of arterial blood may be near normal, as the two balance out.

Effect on arterial O_2 content

Here the situation is different. Blood returning from low V/Q areas has a low Po_2 and low O_2 content but there is a limit to which this deficit can be made good by mixture with blood returning from high V/Q areas; which although it has a high Po_2 cannot carry more than the 'normal' quantity of oxygen as its O_2 content limited by saturation of the haemoglobin.

- Areas of low V/Q result in a rise in arterial CO_2 and a fall in arterial O_2 content.
- Increased ventilation in the areas of high V/Q may balance the effect on CO_2 content but will only partially correct the reduction in O_2 content of arterial blood; a degree of hypoxaemia is inevitable.
- It follows that where arterial oxygen levels are lower than would be expected from consideration of Pco_2 (overall ventilation alone), then there must be a disturbance to the normal V/Q matching system in the lung i.e. there is likely to be an intrinsic problem with the lung or its vasculature.

When looking at arterial blood gas results, how can we distinguish a low oxygen level due to underventilation from a level caused by intrinsic lung disease? Answer: *The alveolar gas equation.*

The alveolar gas equation

An understanding of the relationship between P_aco_2 and P_ao_2 is critical to the interpretation of blood gases (Chapter 3). The relationship can be summarised in an equation known as 'the alveolar gas equation'.

- Pure underventilation leads to an increase in Pco_2 and a 'proportionate' fall in Po_2. This is known as **type 2 respiratory failure**.
- A disturbance of VQ matching leads to a fall in Po_2 but no change in Pco_2. This is known as a **type 1 respiratory failure**.
- These two problems can, of course, occur simultaneously. The alveolar gas equation is then needed to determine if the fall in Po_2 can be accounted for by underventilation alone or whether there is also an intrinsic problem with the lungs.

Rather than merely memorising the alveolar gas equation, spend just a moment here understanding its derivation (this is NOT a rigorous mathematical derivation, merely an attempt to impart some insight into its meaning).

Imagine a lung, disconnected from the circulation, being ventilated. Clearly, in a short space of time the **alveolar** partial pressure of P_Ao_2 would come to equal the partial pressure of oxygen in the inspired air:

$$P_Ao_2 = P_Io_2$$

A pulmonary circulation does exist of course and it is continuously removing O_2 from the alveoli. The alveolar partial pressure of O_2 is therefore equal to the partial pressure in the inspired air minus the amount removed. If the exchange of oxygen for carbon dioxide were a 1:1 swap then the amount of O_2 removed would equal the amount of CO_2 added to the alveoli and the equation would become:

$$P_Ao_2 = P_Io_2 - P_Aco_2$$

The $CO_2 : O_2$ exchange, as discussed above is, however, not usually 1:1. The RQ is usually taken to be 0.8.

Thus:

$$P_Ao_2 = P_Io_2 - (P_Aco_2/0.8)$$

As CO_2 is a very soluble gas the **alveolar** partial pressure (P_Aco_2) is virtually the same as the **arterial** partial pressure (P_aco_2). The arterial partial pressure of CO_2 (available in the blood gas analysis) can therefore be used in the equation in its place:

$$P_Ao_2 = P_Io_2 - (P_aco_2/0.8)$$

This is (the simplified version of) the alveolar gas equation. If the inspired pressure of oxygen is known then the P_Ao_2 can be calculated.

Unlike in the case of CO_2, there is normally a difference between alveolar and arterial Po_2 (which should be the greater?). The difference $P_Ao_2 - P_ao_2$ is often written: $P_{A-a}o_2$ and is known as the **alveolar–arterial (A–a) gradient**. In healthy young adults this gradient is small and would be expected to be comfortably less than 2 kPa. If the gradient is greater than this then the abnormality in the blood gas result cannot be accounted for by a change in ventilation alone; there must be an abnormality intrinsic to the lung or its vasculature causing a disturbance of VQ matching.

For examples see the multiple choice questions at the end of the book.

The control of breathing

To understand this we first have to remember why we breathe. Although oxygen is an essential requirement for life; to survive we do not need the high level of oxygenation usually seen in health. We operate with a substantial margin of safety. This safety margin allows us to vary our ventilation (sometimes at the expense of a normal oxygen level) in order to precisely regulate the CO_2 content of the blood. CO_2 is intimately linked with pH. Although it is possible to live for years with low oxygen levels, we cannot survive long at all with pH outside of the normal range. Keeping pH in the normal range is therefore a priority and CO_2 rather than O_2 is the principal driver of ventilation.

In health P_{CO_2} is maintained very close to 5.3 kPa (40 mmHg). Any increase above this level provokes hyperventilation, any dip leads to hypoventilation. In practice, P_{CO_2} is so exquisitely tightly regulated that such fluctuations are not observable. Even when substantial demands are placed on the respiratory system, such as hard physical exercise, with its dramatic increase in O_2 utilisation and CO_2 production, the arterial P_{CO_2} will barely budge.

Like any finely tuned sensor however, if it is exposed to levels it is not designed to deal with for long enough, it will tend to break. In some patients with chronic lung disease (commonly COPD) the CO_2 sensor begins to fail. Underventilation then occurs and over time, P_{CO_2} drifts upward. In addition P_{O_2} will, of course, fall although initially the respiratory centre remains blissfully unconcerned. Only when a P_{O_2} level of around 8 kPa (60 mmHg) is reached does a previously dormant sensor, the hypoxic sensor, wake up and declare that 'enough is enough!' Prepared to put up with a certain degree of hypoxia, it springs into action when the P_{O_2} reaches this important threshold. Hypoxia then takes up the reins as the driver to ventilation and prevents what would have been a progressive decline to death. Once an individual is dependent on this '**hypoxic drive**' they need a certain level of hypoxia to keep breathing. This is not always appreciated. At times a 'high flow' oxygen mask may be applied to a patient by a well-meaning doctor, which may abolish the hypoxia. The result can be catastrophic underventilation which, if not dealt with properly, can be fatal. When treating hypoxic patients who may have chronic lung disease, until their ventilatory drive is known (from arterial blood gas analysis) oxygen should be judiciously controlled to achieve an oxygen saturation (based on pulse oxymetry) between 88% and 92%. At this level the patient will not die of hypoxia, nor is ventilation likely to be depressed to any significant degree.

 KEY POINTS

- The essential function of the lungs is the exchange of oxygen and carbon dioxide between the blood and the atmosphere.
- Ventilation is the process of moving air in and out of the lungs, and it depends on the tidal volume, respiratory rate, resistance of the airways and the compliance of the lungs. A fall in ventilation leads to a rise in P_{CO_2} and a fall in P_{O_2}; type 2 respiratory failure.
- Derangement in the matching of ventilation and perfusion in the lungs (which may be caused by any disease intrinsic to the lung or its vasculature) leads to a fall in P_{O_2}; type 1 respiratory failure.
- The respiratory centre in the brain stem is responsible for the control of breathing, pH and P_{CO_2} are the primary stimuli to ventilation. Hypoxia only acts as a stimulant when P_{O_2} is less than about 8 kPa.

 FURTHER READING

Brewis RAL, White FE. Anatomy of the thorax. In: Gibson GJ, Geddes DM, Costabel U, Sterk PJ, Corrin B, eds. *Respiratory Medicine*. Edinburgh: Elsevier Science, 2003: 3–33.

Cotes JE. *Lung Function: Assessment and Application in Medicine*. Oxford: Blackwell Science, 1993.

Gibson GJ. *Clinical Tests of Respiratory Function*. Oxford: Chapman and Hall, 2009.

West JB. *Pulmonary Pathophysiology – The Essentials*. Baltimore, MD: Williams and Wilkins, 1987.

History taking and examination

History taking

History taking is of paramount importance in the assessment of a patient with respiratory disease. Difficult diagnostic problems are more often solved by a carefully taken history than by laboratory tests. It is during history taking that the doctor also gets to know the patient and the patient's fears and concerns. The relationship of trust thus established forms the basis of the therapeutic partnership. Start by asking the patient to describe the symptoms in his or her own words. Listening to the patient's account of the symptoms is an active process in which the doctor is seeking clues to underlying processes, judging which items require further exploration and noting the patient's attitude and anxieties. By carefully posed questions the skilled clinician directs the patient to focus on pertinent points, to clarify crucial details and to explore areas of possible importance. History-taking skills develop with experience and with a greater knowledge of respiratory disease.

It is important to appreciate the differences between **symptoms**, which are a patient's subjective description of a change in the body or its functions that may indicate disease, **signs**, which are abnormal features noted by the doctor on examination and **tests**, which are objective measurements undertaken at the bedside or in the diagnostic laboratories. Thus, for example, a patient might complain of pain on breathing, the doctor might elicit tenderness on pressing on the chest and an X-ray might show a fractured rib.

Symptoms (Table 2.1)

Dyspnoea

This is an unpleasant sensation of **being unable to breathe easily** (i.e. breathlessness). Analysis of this symptom requires an assessment of the speed of onset, progression, periodicity and precipitating and relieving factors. The severity of dyspnoea is graded according to the patient's exercise tolerance (e.g. dyspnoeic on climbing a flight of stairs; dyspnoeic at rest). Onset may be sudden as in the case of a pneumothorax, or gradual and progressive as in chronic obstructive pulmonary disease (COPD). An episodic dyspnoea pattern is characteristic of asthma with symptoms typically being precipitated by cold air or exercise. **Orthopnoea** is dyspnoea that occurs when lying flat and is relieved by sitting upright. It is a characteristic feature of pulmonary oedema or diaphragm

Respiratory Medicine Lecture Notes, Eighth Edition. Stephen J. Bourke and Graham P. Burns.
© 2011 John Wiley & Sons, Ltd. Published 2011 by John Wiley & Sons, Ltd.

Table 2.1 Main respiratory symptoms

- Dyspnoea
- Wheeze
- Cough
- Sputum
- Haemoptysis
- Chest pain

paralysis but is also found in many respiratory diseases. **Paroxysmal nocturnal dyspnoea** (PND) refers to the phenomenon of the patient waking up breathless at night. It is most commonly associated with pulmonary oedema but must be distinguished from the nocturnal wheeze and the sleep disturbance of asthma. It is important to note what words the patient uses to describe the symptoms: 'tightness in the chest' may indicate breathlessness or angina. Dyspnoea is not a symptom that is specific to respiratory disease and it may be associated with various cardiac diseases, anxiety, anaemia and metabolic states such as ketoacidosis.

Wheeze

This is a whistling or sighing noise that is characteristic of air passing through a narrow tube. The sound of wheeze can be mimicked by breathing out almost to residual volume and then giving a further sharp forced expiration. Wheeze is a characteristic feature of airways obstruction caused by asthma or COPD but can also occur in pulmonary oedema. In asthma, wheeze is characteristically worse on waking in the morning and may be precipitated by exercise or cold air. Wheeze that improves at weekends or on holidays away from work and deteriorates on return to the work environment is suggestive of occupational asthma. In asthma and COPD wheezing is more prominent in expiration. An inspiratory wheeze – **stridor** – is a feature of disease of the central airways (e.g. obstruction of the trachea by a carcinoma).

Cough and sputum

Cough is a forceful expiratory blast produced by contraction of the abdominal muscles with bracing by the intercostal muscles and sudden opening of the glottis. It is a protective reflex that removes secretions or inhaled solid material, and it is provoked by physical or chemical stimulation of irritant receptors in the larynx, trachea or bronchial tree. Cough may be dry or associated with sputum production. The duration and nature of the cough should be assessed, and precipitating and relieving factors explored. It is important to examine any **sputum** produced, noting whether it is mucoid, purulent or bloodstained, for example. Cough occurring on exercise or disturbing sleep at night is a feature of asthma. A transient cough productive of purulent sputum is very common in respiratory tract infections. A weak ineffective cough that fails to clear secretions from the airways is a feature of bulbar palsy or expiratory muscle weakness, and predisposes the patient to aspiration pneumonia. Cough is often triggered by the accumulation of sputum in the respiratory tract. Chronic bronchitis is defined as cough productive of sputum on most days for at least 3 months of 2 consecutive years. Bronchiectasis is characterised by the production of copious amounts of purulent sputum. A chronic cough may also be caused by gastro-oesophageal reflux with aspiration, sinusitis with post-nasal drip and occasionally by drugs (e.g. lisinopril). Violent coughing can generate sufficient force to produce a '**cough fracture**' of a rib or to impede venous return and cerebral perfusion causing '**cough syncope**'. Patients with alveolar cell carcinoma sometimes produce very large volumes of watery sputum: **bronchorrhoea**. Patients with coalworker's pneumoconiosis will occasionally cough up black material: **melanoptysis**.

Haemoptysis

This is the **coughing up of blood**. It is a very important symptom that requires investigation. In particular, it may be the first clue to the presence of bronchial carcinoma, and early investigation may detect the tumour at a stage when curative surgery can be performed. All patients with haemoptysis should have a chest X-ray performed, and further investigations such as bronchoscopy, computed tomography (CT), sputum cytology and microbiology may be indicated depending on the circumstances. The most important causes of haemoptysis are bronchial carcinoma, lung infections (pneumonia, bronchiectasis, tuberculosis), chronic bronchitis, pulmonary infarction, pulmonary oedema and pulmonary vasculitis (Table 2.2). In some cases no cause is found and the origin of the blood may have been in the upper airway (e.g. nose (epistaxis), pharynx or gums).

Table 2.2 Major causes of haemoptysis

Tumours
- Bronchial carcinoma
- Laryngeal carcinoma

Infections
- Tuberculosis
- Pneumonia
- Bronchiectasis
- Infective bronchitis

Infarction
- Pulmonary embolism

Pulmonary oedema
- Left ventricular failure
- Mitral stenosis

Pulmonary vasculitis
- Goodpasture's syndrome
- Wegener's granulomatosis

Chest pain

Pain that is aggravated by inspiration or coughing is described as **pleuritic pain**, and the patient can often be seen to wince when breathing in, as the pain 'catches'. Irritation of the pleura may result from inflammation (pleurisy), infection (pneumonia), infarction of underlying lung (pulmonary embolism) or tumour (malignant pleural effusion). Chest wall pain resulting from injury to the intercostal muscles or fractured ribs, for example, is also aggravated by inspiration or coughing and is associated with tenderness at the point of injury.

In addition to these major respiratory symptoms it is important to consider other associated symptoms. For example, **anorexia** and **weight loss** are features of malignancy or chronic lung infections (e.g. lung abscess). **Pyrexia** and **sweating** are features of acute (e.g. pneumonia) and chronic infections (e.g. tuberculosis). **Lethargy**, malaise and confusion may be features of hypoxaemia. **Headaches**, particularly on awakening in the morning, may be a symptom of hypercapnia. **Oedema** may indicate cor pulmonale. **Snoring** and daytime **somnolence** may indicate obstructive sleep apnoea syndrome. **Hoarseness** of the voice may indicate damage to the recurrent laryngeal nerve by a tumour.

Many respiratory diseases have their roots in previous **childhood lung disease** or in the **patient's environment** so that it is crucial to make specific enquiries concerning these points during history taking.

History

Past medical history

Did the patient suffer any major illness in childhood? Did the patient have frequent absences from school? Was the patient able to play games at school? Did any abnormalities declare themselves at a pre-employment medical examination or on chest X-ray? Has the patient ever been admitted to hospital with chest disease? A long history of childhood 'bronchitis' may in fact indicate asthma. Severe whooping cough or measles in childhood may cause bronchiectasis. Tuberculosis acquired early in life may reactivate many years later.

General medical history

Has the patient any systemic illness that may involve the lungs (e.g. rheumatoid arthritis)? Is the patient taking any medications that might affect the lungs (e.g. amiodarone), which can cause interstitial lung disease, or β-blockers (e.g. atenolol), which may provoke bronchospasm? What effect will the patient's lung disease have on other illnesses (e.g. fitness for surgery?).

Family history

Is there any history of lung disease in the family? An increased prevalence of lung disease in a family may result from 'shared genes', that is inherited traits such as cystic fibrosis, α_1-anti-trypsin deficiency, asthmatic tendency; or from 'shared environment' (e.g. tuberculosis).

Social history

Does the patient smoke, or have they ever smoked? Is the patient exposed to passive smoking at home? It is important to obtain a clear account of total smoking exposure over the years so as to assess the patient's risk for diseases such as lung cancer or COPD. Does the patient keep any pets or participate in any sports (e.g. diving) or hobbies (e.g. pigeon racing) that may be important in assessing the lung disease?

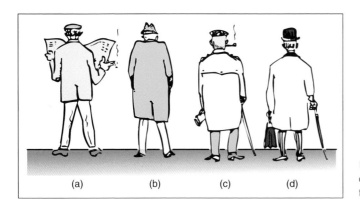

Figure 2.1 Which man has airways obstruction? (Answer at foot of this page.)

Occupational history

What occupations has the patient had over the years, what tasks were performed and what materials used? Did symptoms show a direct relationship to the work environment as in the case of occupational asthma improving away from work and deteriorating on return to work? Has the patient been exposed to substances that may give rise to disease many years later as in the case of mesothelioma arising from exposure to asbestos 20–40 years previously?

Examination

Examination of the respiratory system is, of course, integrated into the general examination of the patient as a whole, but outlining the different stages in the assessment of the respiratory system is useful in focusing attention on the features of particular importance to be sought. Powers of observation are developed by training; and knowing what to look for and how to look for it are learned by experience.

General examination

Be alert to clues to respiratory disease that may be evident from the moment the patient is first seen (Fig. 2.1) or that become apparent during history taking. These include the rate and **character of breathing**, signs of respiratory distress such as **use of accessory muscles** of respiration (e.g. sternocleidomastoids), the **shape of the chest**, spine and shoulders and the character of any **cough**. **Hoarseness** of the voice may be a clue to recurrent laryngeal nerve damage by a carcinoma. **Stridor** or

wheeze may be audible. Count the **respiratory rate** over a period of 30 seconds. The respiratory rate is best counted surreptitiously, perhaps while feeling the pulse, as patients tend to breath faster if they are aware that you are focusing on their breathing. Avoid proceeding directly to examination of the chest but first pause to look for signs in the hands such as **clubbing**, **tar staining** or **features of rheumatoid arthritis**. Signs of carbon dioxide retention include peripheral **vasodilatation** and **asterixis**, a flapping tremor detected by asking the patient to spread his or her fingers and cock the wrists back. It may be accentuated by applying gentle pressure against the patient's hands in this position. Count the **pulse rate** over 30 seconds and note any abnormalities in rhythm (e.g. atrial fibrillation) or character (e.g. a bounding pulse of carbon dioxide retention). Next examine the head and neck, particularly seeking signs of **cyanosis**, **anaemia** (pallor of conjunctiva), elevation of **jugular venous pressure** or **lymph node enlargement**. Be alert for uncommon signs such as **Horner's syndrome** (ptosis, meiosis, enophthalmos, anhydrosis) indicating damage to the sympathetic nerves by a tumour situated at the lung apex (see Chapter 12).

Clubbing

This is increased curvature of the nail with loss of the angle between the nail and nail bed (Fig. 2.2). It is a very important sign that is associated with a number of diseases (Table 2.3), most notably bronchial carcinoma and fibrotic lung disease, such as idiopathic pulmonary fibrosis and asbestosis. Advanced clubbing is sometimes associated

Answer to question in Fig. 2.1: (b) has airways obstruction – note the high position of the shoulders.

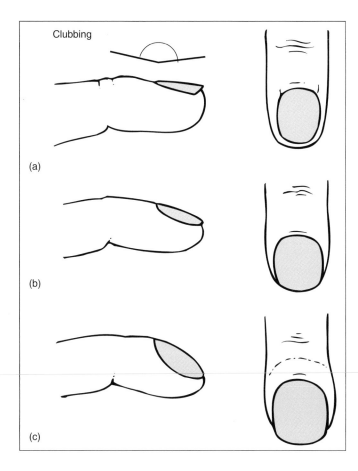

Clubbing

(a)

(b)

(c)

Figure 2.2 Clubbing. (a) Normal, showing the 'angle'. (b) Early clubbing; the angle is absent. (c) Advanced clubbing. The nail shows increased curvature in all directions, the angle is absent, the base of the nail is raised up by spongy tissue and the end of the digit is expanded.

with hypertrophic pulmonary osteoarthropathy in which there is new bone formation in the subperiosteal region of the long bones of the arms and legs that is detectable on X-ray and is associated with pain and tenderness.

Cyanosis

This is a bluish discolouration of the skin and mucous membranes as a result of an excessive amount of reduced haemoglobin (usually >5 g/dL). **Central cyanosis** is best seen on the tip of the tongue and is the cardinal sign of hypoxaemia, although it is not a sensitive sign because it is not usually detectable until the oxygen saturation has fallen to well below 85%, corresponding to a Po_2 of <8 kPa (60 mmHg). Cyanosis is more difficult to detect if the patient is anaemic or has dark-coloured skin. Because of the poor sensitivity of cyanosis it is essential to measure oxygenation by oximetry or arterial blood gas sampling in patients at risk for hypoxaemia. **Peripheral cyanosis** may be caused

by local circulatory slowing in the peripheries resulting in more complete extraction of oxygen from the blood (e.g. blue hands and ears in cold weather).

Jugular veins

Jugular veins are examined with the patient in a semi-reclining position with the trunk at an angle of about 45° from the horizontal. The head is turned slightly to the opposite side and fully supported so that the sternocleidomastoid muscles are relaxed. The jugular venous pulse is seen as a diffuse superficial pulsation of multiple wave form that is distinct from the carotid arterial pulse. The height of the pulse wave is measured from the top of the oscillating column of blood vertically to the sternal angle. The jugular venous pressure normally falls during inspiration. It is elevated in right heart failure, which may occur as a result of pulmonary embolism or cor pulmonale in COPD, for example. Other signs of right heart failure such

Table 2.3 **Causes of clubbing**

Respiratory
- Neoplastic
  - Bronchial carcinoma
  - Mesothelioma
- Infections
  - Bronchiectasis
  - Cystic fibrosis
  - Chronic empyema
  - Lung abscess
- Fibrosis
  - Idiopathic pulmonary fibrosis
  - Asbestosis

Cardiac
- Bacterial endocarditis
- Cyanotic congenital heart disease
- Atrial myxoma

Gastrointestinal
- Hepatic cirrhosis
- Crohn's disease
- Coeliac disease

Congenital
- Idiopathic familial clubbing

as hepatomegaly and peripheral oedema may also be present.

Chest examination

Ask the patient to undress to the waist, and proceed to examine the chest in a methodical way using the techniques of inspection, palpation, percussion and auscultation.

Inspection

Look at the chest from the front, back and sides noting the overall **shape** and any **asymmetry**, **scars** or **skeletal abnormality**. The normal chest is flattened anteroposteriorly whereas the hyperinflated chest of COPD is barrel-shaped with an increased anteroposterior diameter. Watch the **movement** of the chest carefully as the patient breathes in and out. Diminished movement of one side of the chest is a clue to disease on that side. Overall movement is reduced if the lungs are hyperinflated (e.g. emphysema) or have reduced compliance (e.g. fibrosis). The costal margins normally move upwards and outwards in inspiration as the chest expands. In a chest that is already severely over-inflated (e.g. COPD) there is sometimes paradoxical movement of the costal margins such that they are drawn inwards during inspiration: **costal margin paradox** (Fig. 2.3). The abdominal wall normally moves outwards on inspiration as the diaphragm descends. **Abdominal paradox**, in which the abdominal wall moves inwards during inspiration when the patient is supine, is a sign of diaphragm weakness.

Palpation

Chest movements during respiration may be more easily appreciated by placing the hands exactly symmetrically on either side of the upper sternum with the thumbs in the midline. The relative movement of the two hands and the separation of the thumbs reflect the overall movement of the chest and any asymmetry between the two sides. The position of the mediastinum is assessed by locating the **tracheal position** and the cardiac **apex beat**. Inserting a finger between the trachea and the sternocleidomastoid muscle on each side is a useful way of detecting any tracheal deviation. Running a finger gently up and down the trachea from the cricoid cartilage to the sternal notch may indicate the direction of the trachea as it enters the chest. Reduction in the **crico-sternal distance** is a sign of a hyperinflated chest. The apex beat is the most inferior and lateral point at which the cardiac impulse can be felt. The intercostal space in which the apex beat is felt should be counted down from the second intercostal space, which is just below the sternal angle, and its location should also be related to landmarks such as the mid-clavicular or anterior axillary lines. It is normally located in the fifth left intercostal space in the mid-clavicular line. The mediastinum may be deviated towards or away from the side of disease. For example, fibrosis of the apex of the lung caused by previous tuberculosis may *pull* the trachea to that side, whereas a large pleural effusion or tension pneumothorax may *push* the trachea and apex beat away from the side of the lesion. **Tactile fremitus** refers to the ability to palpate vibrations set up by the voice in the large airways and transmitted to the chest wall. Ask the patient to say '99' or '1, 1, 1'

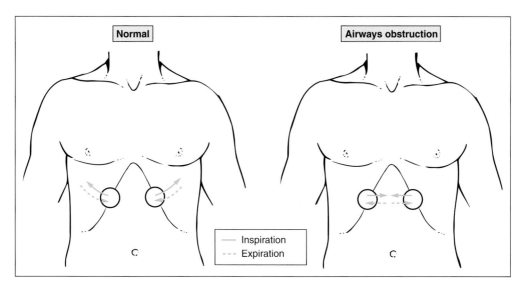

Figure 2.3 Movement of the costal margin. The arrows indicate the direction of movement in normal individuals and in those with airways obstruction (see text).

and palpate the vibrations, which are reduced in conditions such as pleural effusion or pleural thickening that muffle the transmission of the vibrations from the lung to the chest wall (Fig. 2.4). Consolidation of the lung may sometimes enhance transmission of the vibration.

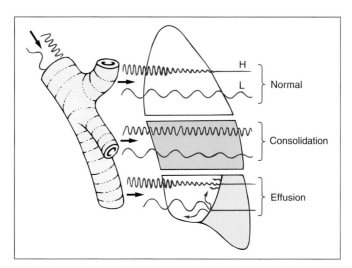

Figure 2.4 Summary of sound transmission in the lung. Sound is generated either by turbulence in the larynx and large airways or by the voice. Both sources are a mixture of high- (H) and low- (L) pitched components. *Normal aerated lung* filters off the high-pitched component but transmits the low-pitched component quite well. This results in soft low-pitched breath sounds, well-conducted vocal resonance and easily palpable very-low-pitched sound (vocal fremitus). *Consolidated lung* transmits high-pitched sound well and filters off some of the lower pitched sound. This results in loud high-pitched breath sounds (bronchial breathing), high-pitched bleating vocal resonance (aegophony) and easy transmission of high-pitched consonants of speech (whispering pectoriloquy). *Pleural effusion* causes reduction in the transmission of all sound – probably because of reflection of sound waves at the air–fluid interface. Breath sounds are absent, vocal resonance much reduced and vocal fremitus is absent.

Percussion

Percussion over normal air-filled lung produces a **resonant note** whereas percussion over solid organs such as the liver or heart produces a **dull note**. Abnormal dullness is found over areas of lung consolidation (e.g. lobar pneumonia) or fluid (e.g. pleural effusion). **Hyper-resonance** may be present in emphysema or over the area of a pneumothorax, although it is rarely a reliable sign. Percussion technique is important and requires practice. The resting finger should be placed flat against the chest wall in an intercostal space. The percussing finger should strike the dorsal surface of the middle phalanx and should be lifted clear after each percussion stroke. All areas should be percussed, paying particular attention to comparison between the two sides. When percussing the back of the chest it is helpful to ask the patient to rotate his or her arms such that one elbow is placed on top of the other in order to bring the scapulae forward and out of the way.

Auscultation

Listen with the diaphragm or bell of the stethoscope to the **intensity** and **character** of the **breath sounds**, comparing both sides symmetrically, and note any **added sounds** (e.g. wheeze, crackles, pleural rub). The sources of audible sound in the lungs are turbulent airflow in the larynx and central airways and the voice. Reduction in the intensity of breath sounds (sometimes loosely referred to as reduced 'air entry') over an area of lung is an important sign that may, for example, indicate obstruction of a large bronchus preventing air from entering a lobe of the lung, or the presence of a pleural effusion reducing transmission of sound to the stethoscope. In normal individuals the **inspiratory phase** of respiration is usually longer than the **expiratory phase**. Prolongation of the expiratory phase is a feature of airways obstruction and this is often accompanied by **wheeze (rhonchi)** – a high-pitched whistling or sighing sound. Diffuse wheeze is a feature of asthma or COPD. Wheeze localised to one side, or one area of the lung, suggests obstruction of a bronchus by a carcinoma or foreign body (e.g. inhaled peanut). **Crackles (crepitations)** may be loud and coarse or fine and high pitched, and may occur early or late in inspiration. It is thought that crackles are produced by the opening of previously closed bronchioles. The 'crackling' noise may be imitated by rolling a few hairs together close to the ear. Early crackles are sometimes heard at the beginning of inspiration in patients with COPD but these usually disappear when the patient is asked to cough. Persistent pan-inspiratory or late-inspiratory crackles are a feature of pulmonary oedema, lung fibrosis (e.g. idiopathic pulmonary fibrosis) or bronchiectasis. During inspiration, areas of lung open up in sequence according to their compliance (distensibility). In airways obstruction there may be terminal airway closure during expiration, particularly in relatively compliant (floppy) parts of the lung damaged by emphysema. During inspiration air initially enters these areas more readily and crackles are probably produced by the opening of these airways early in inspiration. Coarse late-inspiratory crackles are particularly associated with diseases where there is reduced lung compliance (increased stiffness), which is to some extent patchily distributed. During inspiration, air first enters the more compliant parts of the lung and then enters the stiffer parts later in inspiration as elastic recoil forces build up in the stretching lung. **Pleural rubs** are 'creaking' sounds that are often quite localised and indicate roughening of the normally slippery pleural surfaces.

Vocal resonance is assessed by listening over the chest with the stethoscope as the patient says '99' or '1, 1, 1' in much the same way as vocal fremitus is palpated. Normal aerated lung transmits the booming low-pitched components of speech and attenuates the high frequencies. Consolidated lung, however, filters off the low frequencies and transmits the higher frequencies so that speech takes on a bleating quality, **aegophony**. The facilitated transmission of high frequencies can be demonstrated by the clear transmission of whispering over consolidated lung, **whispering pectoriloquy**. The term '**bronchial breathing**' refers to the harsher breath sounds normally heard over the trachea and main bronchi. It is also heard over areas of consolidated lung that conduct the higher frequency 'hiss' component from the larger airways.

Signs

See Fig. 2.5 for signs of localised lung disease. It is important to realise that major disease of the lungs may be present without any detectable physical signs and it is therefore essential to obtain a chest X-ray where there is good reason to suspect localised lung disease.

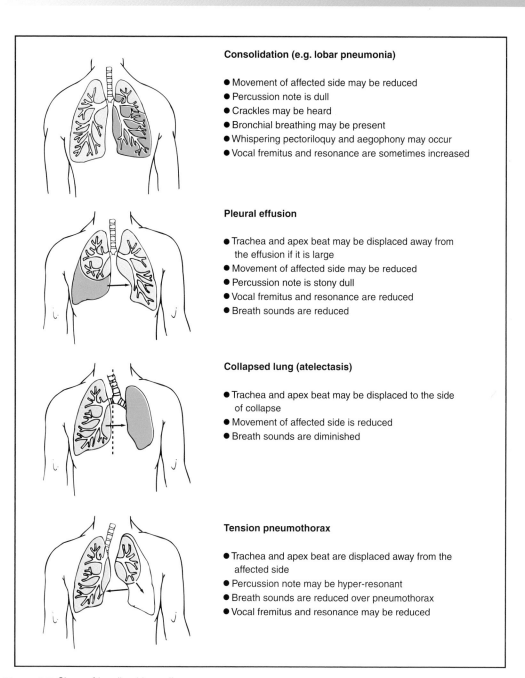

Consolidation (e.g. lobar pneumonia)

- Movement of affected side may be reduced
- Percussion note is dull
- Crackles may be heard
- Bronchial breathing may be present
- Whispering pectoriloquy and aegophony may occur
- Vocal fremitus and resonance are sometimes increased

Pleural effusion

- Trachea and apex beat may be displaced away from the effusion if it is large
- Movement of affected side may be reduced
- Percussion note is stony dull
- Vocal fremitus and resonance are reduced
- Breath sounds are reduced

Collapsed lung (atelectasis)

- Trachea and apex beat may be displaced to the side of collapse
- Movement of affected side is reduced
- Breath sounds are diminished

Tension pneumothorax

- Trachea and apex beat are displaced away from the affected side
- Percussion note may be hyper-resonant
- Breath sounds are reduced over pneumothorax
- Vocal fremitus and resonance may be reduced

Figure 2.5 Signs of localised lung disease.

KEY POINTS

- The main respiratory symptoms are breath-lessness, wheeze, cough, sputum, haemopty-sis and chest pain.
- Haemoptysis is an important symptom which requires investigation as it may indicate lung cancer, laryngeal cancer, bronchitis or tuberculosis etc.
- Diminished movement of one side of the chest on inspiration is a clue to disease on that side.
- Major disease of the chest may be present without detectable signs, and tests (e.g. chest X-ray) are required where there is suspicion of lung disease.

 FURTHER READING

Alverti A, Quaranta M, Chakrabarti B, Albuquerque ALP, Calverley PM. Paradoxical movement of the lower rib cage at rest and during exercise in COPD patients. *Eur Respir J* 2009; **33**: 49–60.

Douglas G, Nicol F, Robertson C. *Macleod's Clinical Examination*. Churchill Livingston Elsevier, 2009.

Morice AH, McGarvey L, Pavord I, British Thoracic Society guideline. Recommendations for the management of cough in adults. *Thorax* 2006; **61** (suppl 1): 1–24.

Spiteri M, Cook D, Clarke S. Reliability of eliciting physical signs in examination of the chest. *Lancet* 1988; **1**: 873–5.

Vyshedsky A, Alhashem RM, Paciej R, et al. Mechanism of inspiratory and expiratory crackles. *Chest* 2009; **135**: 156–64.

Pulmonary function tests

Despite the bewildering array of sophisticated tests and investigations now available a few, fairly basic, tests of lung function remain central to clinical practice. Together with a good history, clinical examination and a chest X-ray these tests provide most of the information needed for diagnosis, quantification of severity and monitoring of disease.

This chapter covers all you will probably ever need to know about lung function. The tests are not difficult to understand, yet despite their simplicity, they are all too often misinterpreted or even misunderstood. Master the next few pages and you may find you acquire the status of 'expert' in whatever medical circle you move in.

being only 1.5 standard deviations from the mean, many normal individuals (of the same age and size) with no apparent lung disease will have values lower than this. The same result could have been expressed as 75% of the predicted mean, however an injudicious interpretation of this may have led to the mistaken assumption that there was a 25% 'disability'.

Pulmonary function tests should not be interpreted in isolation and should be considered in the context of all additional information concerning the patient.

In this chapter we will look at: simple tests of ventilatory function, transfer factor and arterial blood gases.

Normal values

Ventilatory performance varies greatly with the patient's height, age and sex. Tables and prediction equations are available for determining a patient's 'predicted normal value'. The patient's test result may be compared with the mean reference value and the standard deviation of results obtained in the healthy population or (more commonly, though less usefully) expressed as a percentage of the population's mean reference value. For example: the standard deviation for vital capacity (VC) is about 500 ml. So, if a medium-sized adult has a VC 750 ml below the predicted value, that may be the result of respiratory disease; on the other hand,

Simple tests of ventilatory function

Ventilation refers to the process of moving air in and out of the lungs.

Lung volumes (Fig. 3.1)

Tidal volume is the volume of air that enters and leaves the lungs during normal breathing. The volume of gas within the lungs at the end of a normal expiration is the **functional residual capacity**. The volume of gas in the lungs after a full inspiration is the **total lung capacity**. After a full expiration there is still some gas remaining in

Respiratory Medicine Lecture Notes, Eighth Edition. Stephen J. Bourke and Graham P. Burns.
© 2011 John Wiley & Sons, Ltd. Published 2011 by John Wiley & Sons, Ltd.

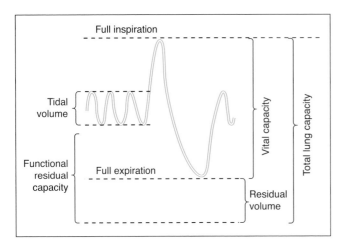

Figure 3.1 Total lung capacity and its subdivisions.

the lungs: the **residual volume**. **Vital capacity** (VC) VC is the volume of air expelled by a full expiration from a position of full inspiration. VC and its subdivisions can be measured directly by spirometry, whereas measurements of residual volume and total lung capacity require the use of gas dilution or plethysmography methods.

Spirometry

Spirometry is the most commonly used test of pulmonary function. It is the measurement of the amount (volume) and/or speed (flow) of air that can be exhaled. Traditionally, the result of this test is represented graphically as a plot of the volume of air exhaled against time during a forced expiratory manoeuvre: the **forced expiratory spirogram** (Fig. 3.2).

Vital capacity

This is the **volume of air expelled by a full expiration from a position of full inspiration**. The patient is usually encouraged to exhale with maximum effort, in which case it is referred to as the **forced vital capacity** (FVC). It may also be measured by a slow exhalation and this is sometimes referred to as the **'slow' VC**. In normal individuals, slow VC and FVC are very similar but in patients with airways obstruction, air trapping occurs during forced expiration so that the FVC may be significantly smaller than the slow VC. VC may be reduced by any condition that limits the lungs ability to achieve a 'full' inspiration, such as:

- reduced lung compliance (e.g. lung fibrosis, loss of lung volume);
- chest deformity (e.g. kyphoscoliosis, ankylosing spondylitis);

- muscle weakness (e.g. myopathy, myasthenia gravis)

It may also be reduced in chronic obstructive pulmonary disease (COPD) when air trapping causes increased residual volume.

Forced expiratory volume in 1 second (FEV_1) and FEV_1/FVC ratio

FEV_1 is the volume of air expelled in the first second of a maximal forced expiration from a position of full inspiration. It is reduced in any condition that reduces VC but it is particularly reduced when there is diffuse airways obstruction. Normally, during a forced expiratory manoeuvre at least 70% of the air is expelled in the first second. In diffuse airways obstruction the FEV_1 is affected to a greater extent than the FVC and the ratio of **FEV_1/FVC** is reduced to below 0.70. This pattern is referred to as an **obstructive defect** and is most commonly seen in asthma and COPD. When lung volume is restricted (by for example: reduced lung compliance, chest deformity or muscle weakness), the VC is reduced and the FEV_1 is also reduced roughly in proportion so that the FEV_1/FVC ratio is essentially normal. This pattern of ventilatory impairment is referred to as a **restrictive defect**.

Maximal mid-expiratory flow

In addition to FEV_1 and FVC a number of other indices may be calculated from a forced expiratory spirogram. The forced expiratory flow measured over the middle half of expiration (**$FEF_{25-75\%}$**) reflects changes in the **smaller peripheral airways** whereas **peak expiratory flow (PEF)** and FEV_1 are predominantly influenced by diffuse changes of

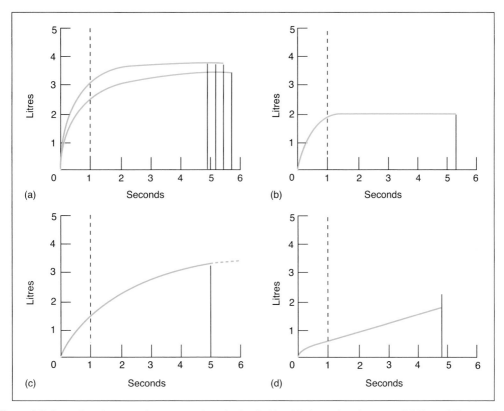

Figure 3.2 Forced expiratory spirogram tracing obtained with a Vitalograph spirometer. (a) *Normal*. Four expirations have been made. Three of these were true maximal forced expirations as indicated by their *reproducibility*. The forced expiratory volume in 1 second (FEV$_1$) is 3.2 L and the forced vital capacity (FVC) is 3.8 L. The forced expiratory ratio (FEV$_1$/FVC) is 84%. (b) *Restrictive ventilatory defect*. Patient with pulmonary fibrosis. The FVC in this case was 2 L less than the predicted value for the patient. The FEV$_1$ is also reduced below the predicted value but it represents a large part of the FVC. The forced expiratory ratio is greater than 90%. (c) *Obstructive ventilatory defect*. The FEV$_1$ is much reduced. The rate of airflow is severely reduced as indicated by the reduced slope of the curve. Note that the forced expiratory time is increased – the patient is still blowing out at 5 seconds. The VC has not been adequately recorded in this case because the patient did not continue the expiration after the chart stopped moving; he or she could have expired further. (This is a common technical error.) (d) *Severe airways obstruction*. The FEV$_1$ is about 0.5 L. FVC is also reduced but not so strikingly as FEV$_1$. Forced expiratory ratio is 23%. Very low expiratory flow rate. This pattern of a very brief initial rapid phase followed by a straight line indicating little change in maximal flow rate with change in lung volume is sometimes associated with severe emphysema. (e) *Airways obstruction and bronchial hyper-reactivity*. Five expirations have been made. FEV$_1$ and FVC become lower with each expiration. Patient with asthma. These features suggest poor control of asthma and liability to severe attacks. (f) *A non-maximal expiration*. Compare with (a). In a true forced expiration the steepest part of the curve always occurs at the beginning of expiration; which is not the case in (f). A falsely low FEV$_1$ and forced expiratory ratio are obtained. Usually the patient has not understood what is required or is unable to coordinate his or her actions. Some patients wish to appear worse than they really are. This pattern is unlikely to be mistaken for a true forced expiration because of its shape and because it cannot be reproduced repeatedly. (g) *Escape of air* from the nose or lips during expiration. (h) *Inability to perform the manoeuvre*. Five attempts have been made. In some the patient has breathed in and out. Other attempts are either not maximal forced expirations or are unfinished. Bizarre patterns such as this are often seen in patients with psychogenic breathlessness and in elderly people and those with dementia. Even with poor cooperation it is often possible to obtain useful information. In the example shown (h), significant airways obstruction can be excluded because of the steep slope of at least two of the expirations that follow an identical course and show appropriate curvature (dotted line) and the FVC can be estimated as not less than 3.2 L. The pattern seen in large airways obstruction is shown in Fig. 3.5.

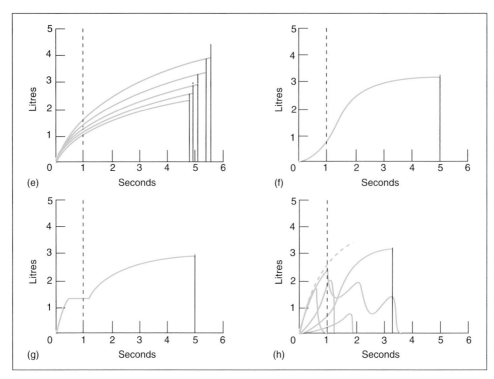

Figure 3.2 (*Continued*)

the medium-sized and larger airways, at least in health (see Chapter 1).

Peak expiratory flow

The PEF is the maximum rate of airflow that can be achieved during a sudden forced expiration from a position of full inspiration. The best of three attempts is usually accepted as the peak flow rate. It is somewhat dependent on effort but is mainly determined by the calibre of the airways and is therefore an index of diffuse airways obstruction. Its principal advantage is derived from its portability and low cost (Fig. 3.3). This allows for multiple measurements performed independently by patients at different times and in different environments. Variability can thus be observed which makes it useful in the diagnosis and monitoring of asthma (see Chapter 10).

Flow–volume loop

The familiar spirogram plots volume against time (Fig. 3.2). Forced expiratory manoeuvres may also be displayed by plotting flow against volume.

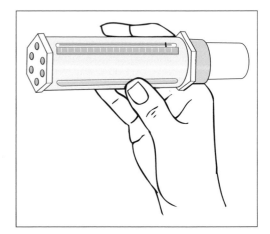

Figure 3.3 Measurement of peak expiratory flow (PEF). The subject takes a *full inspiration*, applies the lips to the mouthpiece and makes a sudden maximal expiratory blast. A piston is pushed down the inside of the cylinder progressively exposing a slot in the top, until a position of rest is reached. The position of the piston is indicated by a marker and PEF read from a scale. It is customary to take the best of three properly performed attempts as the PEF.

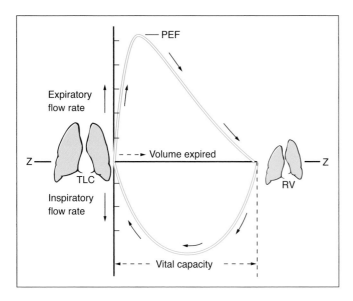

Although the result may be less familiar, it is worth remembering it contains precisely the same information. When an inspiratory manoeuvre is also included the trace returns to its starting point and a Flow–volume loop is formed. A normal flow–volume loop is shown in Fig. 3.4.

By convention the starting point of full inspiration (total lung capacity, TLC) is to the left, expiratory flow appears above the horizontal, inspiratory flow below it. At TLC the airways are at their most stretched (dilated) and airway resistance minimised, so the maximum (peak) expiratory flow is reached quickly after the start of the forced expiration (see Chapter 1). As expiration continues, lung volume progressively diminishes, airway resistance increases and the maximum flow achievable (for the given lung volume) declines. In health this declining portion of the expiratory limb is surprisingly straight. When no further air can be exhaled flow is zero and the loop reaches the horizontal axis. The inspiratory manoeuvre can then begin. This tends to be more effort dependent and therefore less reproducible. Even when perfectly performed, the inspiratory limb is NOT a mirror image of the expiratory limb. Although airway calibre would again favour faster flow nearer TLC, mechanical advantage for the muscles of inspiration means more inspiratory force can be applied nearer RV. The coexistence of these two factors produces a more symmetrical inspiratory portion to the loop, with maximum inspiratory flow being at the mid-point of inspiration. Note too, maximum inspiratory flow is less than maximum expiratory flow.

($FEF_{25-75\%}$) and the maximum flow at specific lung volumes (e.g. $[\dot{V}]_{max50}$, $[\dot{V}]_{max25}$) can be derived from the flow–volume loop.

The flow–volume loop really comes into its own when assessing localised narrowing of the central airways as illustrated in Figs. 3.5 and 3.6. Although the traditional spirogram has a characteristic appearance in this context (Fig. 3.5), the abnormality is not so striking as when observed in the flow–volume loop (Fig. 3.6 (c) and (d)). Without the flow–volume loop large airway obstruction may be overlooked. By comparing the relative effects on the expiratory and inspiratory limbs it is also possible to determine if the large airway obstruction is inside (e.g. tracheal stricture) or outside the thorax (e.g. compression by a goitre in the neck, Fig. 3.7).

Total lung capacity

The measurement of TLC is not considered in detail here, the interested reader is referred to the reading list at the end of the chapter.

Whereas VC and its subdivisions can be measured directly by spirometry, measurement of residual volume and TLC require the use of **helium dilution** or **plethysmography** methods. In the dilution technique a gas of known helium concentration is breathed through a closed circuit and the volume of gas in the lungs is calculated from a measure of the dilution of the helium, which, being

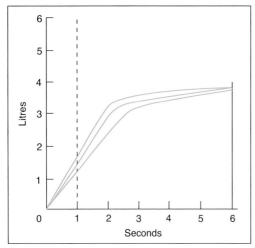

Figure 3.5 Large (central) airways obstruction. Typical tracing obtained with a Vitalograph spirometer. The subject has made three maximal forced expirations. Each shows a strikingly straight section that then changes relatively abruptly, at about the same volume, to follow the expected curve of the forced expiratory spirogram. The straight section is not as reproducible as a normal spirogram. A 'family' of similar tracings is thus obtained, each with straight and curved sections. Explanation: over the straight section, flow is limited by the fixed localised obstruction in a large airway. This is little influenced by lung recoil so the critical flow is similar during expiration and the spirogram appears straight. A lung volume is eventually reached where maximum flow is even lower than that permitted by the central obstruction. The ordinary forced expiratory spirogram is described after this point. In the example shown there must also be an element of diffuse airways obstruction, as forced expiratory time is somewhat prolonged (see Fig. 3.2c).

an inert gas, is neither absorbed nor metabolised. This dilution method measures only gas in communication with the airways and tends to underestimate total lung capacity in patients with severe airways obstruction because of the presence of poorly ventilating bullae. The body plethysmograph is a large airtight box that allows the simultaneous determination of pressure–volume relationships in the thorax of a patient placed inside the box. When the plethysmograph is sealed, changes in lung volume are reflected by a change in pressure within the plethysmograph. Plethysmography tends to overestimate TLC because it measures all intrathoracic gas, including gas in bullae, cysts, stomach and oesophagus. The

chest X-ray can be used to give a rough estimate of TLC. In airways disease, TLC is increased as a manifestation of hyperinflation and as a result of increased lung compliance in emphysema (Chapter 1). TLC is reduced in restrictive lung disease.

Respiratory muscle function tests

Weakness of the respiratory muscles causes a **restrictive ventilatory defect** with reduced TLC and VC. Comparison of the VC in the erect and supine position is useful because the pressure of the abdominal contents on a weak diaphragm typically causes a fall of around 30% in the **supine VC**. Chest X-ray often shows small lung volumes with basal atelectasis and high hemi-diaphragms. **Ultrasound screening** may show paradoxical upward movement of a paralysed diaphragm during inspiration. Global respiratory muscle function may be assessed by measuring **mouth pressures**. Maximum inspiratory mouth pressure, P_I **max**, is measured during maximum inspiratory effort from residual volume against an obstructed airway using a mouthpiece and transducer device. Maximum expiratory mouth pressure, P_E **max**, is measured during a maximal expiratory effort from TLC. When there is severe respiratory muscle weakness ventilatory failure develops with **hypercapnia**.

Transfer factor for carbon monoxide

At one time the rate at which gases diffused across the alveolar–capillary membrane was thought to be the principal factor limiting gas exchange. The term '**diffusing capacity**' was thus coined, defined as: 'The quantity of gas transported across in each minute for every unit of pressure gradient'.

Although the measurement proved to be very useful clinically, it was later realised that it was affected by many other factors as well as diffusion; V/Q matching particularly. It was therefore renamed '**transfer factor**'.

Clearly, it is the transfer of oxygen that is of most interest to clinicians. This is very difficult to measure in practice however as transfer of oxygen into the blood quickly becomes limited by the saturation of haemoglobin. Carbon monoxide is used as a

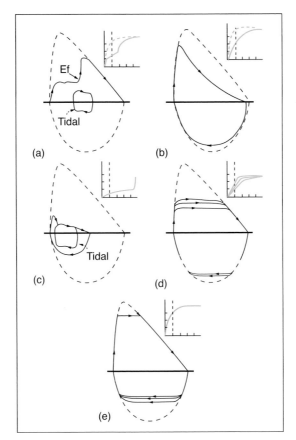

Figure 3.6 Further flow–volume loops. The dotted outline represents a typical normal loop. The small graphs show the appearances of a forced expiration on a Vitalograph spirometer (as in Fig. 3.4). (a) Demonstration of maximum flow. A normal individual makes an unhurried expiration from full inspiration and then about halfway through the vital capacity, a maximal expiratory effort (Ef) is made. The flow–volume tracing rejoins the maximum flow–volume curve that describes the highest flow which can be achieved at that lung volume. Also shown in (a) is the flow–volume loop of typical tidal breathing. At the resting lung volume there is an abundant reserve of both inspiratory and expiratory flow available. (b) Moderate airway obstruction (asthma or chronic obstructive pulmonary disease). Maximum expiratory flow is reduced. The declining portion of the expiratory limb has a characteristic curvilinearity. Inspiration is less severely affected. (c) Very severe airways obstruction. Maximum expiratory flow is very severely reduced. There is a brief peak, followed by an abrupt fall in flow rate (probably caused by airway closure) after which flow falls very slowly. Also shown in (c) is a loop representing quiet tidal breathing. It is clear that every expiration is limited by maximum flow. Expiratory wheezing or purse lip breathing would be expected. The tidal loop has been obliged to move to the left, the patient is ventilating at a higher lung volume. This has obviated, to some degree, the airway narrowing but adds to the work of breathing and contributes to the sensation of breathlessness (see Chapter 1). (d) Intrathoracic large airways obstruction: here the peak inspiratory and expiratory flows have been truncated in a characteristic pattern. Intrathoracic lesions (e.g. tracheal compression by a mediastinal tumour) have a more pronounced effect on the expiratory limb than the inspiratory limb. (e) Extrathoracic obstruction (e.g. tracheal compression by a goitre in the neck) results in inspiratory collapse of the airway below the obstruction (but still outside the thorax) attenuating maximum inspiratory flow rate to a greater degree than maximum expiratory flow rate.

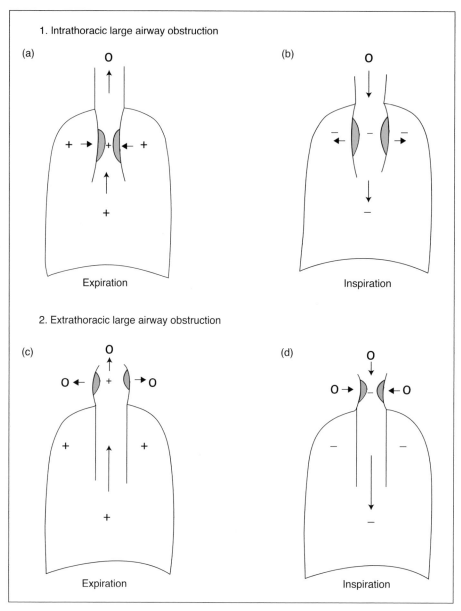

Figure 3.7 The relative effects on expiratory and inspiratory flow of intra- and extrathoracic large airway obstruction. 1 Large airway obstruction within the thorax. (a) Positive intrathoracic (alveolar) pressure generated during expiration acts to compress the airway and further narrow the point of obstruction. (b) Negative intrathoracic pressure during inspiration acts to reduce narrowing at the point of obstruction. Therefore in large airway obstruction within the thorax, expiratory flow is diminished to a greater degree than inspiratory flow (see Fig. 3.6 (d)). 2 Large airway obstruction outside the thorax. (c) Positive pressure within the airway during expiration in relation to atmospheric ('zero') pressure outside, acts to reduce narrowing at the point of obstruction. (d) Negative pressure within the airway during inspiration acts to compress the airway and further narrow the point of obstruction. Therefore in large airway obstruction outside of the thorax, inspiratory flow is diminished to a greater degree than expiratory flow (see Fig. 3.6 (e)).

surrogate for oxygen in this measurement. Very low concentrations are used so that haemoglobin remains avid for the gas as it passes through the alveolar capillaries. The term diffusion capacity ($D_L$co) can still be found in some texts, this is synonymous with transfer factor ($T_L$co).

To measure $T_L$co we need to know:

1 The amount of CO transferred per minute.
2 The pressure gradient across the alveolar membrane (in effect the alveolar partial pressure as the partial pressure in blood is zero)

Single-breath method (Fig. 3.8)

The patient inspires a gas mixture of helium and carbon monoxide, holds the breath for 10 seconds and then breathes out. An initial volume equivalent to the dead space (the part of the respiratory tract not involved in gas exchange) is discarded and then a sample of the expired gas is collected and analysed for alveolar concentrations of helium and carbon monoxide. The change in concentration of helium (which, being an inert gas, is neither absorbed nor metabolised) between the inspired and alveolar sample is the result of gas dilution and gives a measurement of the alveolar gas volume (V_A). The expired concentration of carbon monoxide is also lower than the inspired level but the fall is proportionately greater than in the case of helium because some of the carbon monoxide has been absorbed into the bloodstream. The rate of uptake of carbon monoxide can then be calculated as the uptake per minute per unit of partial pressure of carbon monoxide (mmol/min/kPa).

Many factors influence $T_L$co including:

- V/Q imbalance (disturbed in many diseases affecting lung parenchyma or vasculature);
- the area of the membrane (reduced in emphysema);
- the thickness of the alveolar capillary membrane (increased in fibrotic lung disease);
- the pulmonary capillary blood volume (increased in high cardiac output states);
- the haemoglobin concentration.

Free blood in the lungs from pulmonary haemorrhage will also avidly absorb carbon monoxide and lead to an elevated $T_L$co.

Transfer coefficient (Kco)

Clearly $T_L$co can be reduced by a number of disease processes within the lung, it is also reduced if there is simply 'less lung' (a reduced lung volume) participating in gas transfer (e.g. respiratory muscle weakness causing restriction or after pneumonectomy). It is useful to distinguish between these two very different mechanisms.

Transfer coefficient (Kco) is the transfer factor divided by the alveolar volume (V_A). This tells us about the transfer factor 'per unit lung volume'. Like $T_L$co, Kco is reduced when there is intrinsic lung disease, but unlike $T_L$co, when a healthy lung

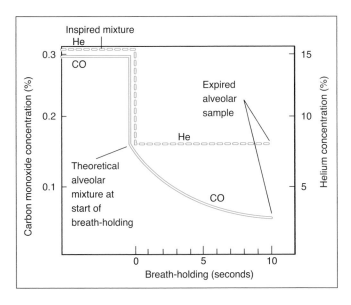

Figure 3.8 Measurement of transfer factor by the single-breath method. Schematic representation of the helium and carbon monoxide concentrations in the inspired mixture and in alveolar air during breath holding.

is reduced in volume by some external factor K_{CO} is not diminished.

Interpretation

In the presence of **normal ventilatory function** (spirometry) a reduced K_{CO} is a strong indicator of intrinsic lung disease (affecting the alveoli or vasculature; consider pulmonary hypertension or a combination of emphysema and fibrosis).

In **restrictive conditions**, a reduced K_{CO} suggests an intrapulmonary cause (e.g. fibrosis). In extrapulmonary causes (e.g. chest wall deformity, respiratory muscle weakness, obesity) the K_{CO} tends to be elevated. This is because the K_{CO} is effectively telling us about the transfer of CO only in the alveoli that are ventilated. The non-ventilated alveoli are discounted because they don't contribute to V_A. As the V/Q matching system will divert blood away from the non-ventilated alveoli, the ventilated alveoli will have more than the normal share of blood. The greater blood volume increases CO absorption and thus gas transfer.

In **obstructive conditions** a reduced K_{CO} suggests COPD (emphysema). In asthma the K_{CO} may be elevated. Asthma does not affect every airway to an identical degree; there is therefore an exaggerated heterogeneity of ventilation. As discussed above K_{CO} is more heavily influenced by the well ventilated areas which, because of V/Q matching, have more than their fair share of perfusion.

Arterial blood gases

Normal values are listed in Table 3.1.

A **sample of arterial blood** may be obtained from any artery but the **radial artery** at the wrist or the **brachial artery** in the antecubital fossa are the sites most commonly used. The blood enters the heparinised needle and syringe under its own pressure with a pulsatile action. The syringe containing the arterial blood is capped, placed in **ice** and analysed in the laboratory within 30 minutes of sampling.

Review of acid–base balance

CO_2 dissolves in H_2O and forms carbonic acid (H_2CO_3) that dissociates into H^+ and HCO_3^- in a constant relationship:

Table 3.1 Normal values for arterial blood gases while breathing normal room air at sea level

Arterial blood gases	Normal values
pH	7.35–7.45
P_{CO_2}	4.5–6.0 kPa (34–45 mmHg)
P_{O_2}	12–14 kPa (90–105 mmHg)
Actual bicarbonate ($aHCO_3^-$)	22–26 mmol/L
Standard bicarbonate ($sHCO_3^-$)	22–26 mmol/L
Base excess	−3 to +3 mmol/L
Oxygen saturation	96–99%

$$K = \frac{[H^+][HCO_3^-]}{[H_2CO_3]}$$

thus:

$$[H^+] \; \alpha \; \frac{[H_2CO_3]}{[HCO_3^-]}$$

As $[H_2CO_3]$ directly relates to the partial pressure of CO_2 then:

$$[H^+] \; \alpha \; \frac{P_{CO_2}}{[HCO_3^-]}$$

In other words, for a given concentration of bicarbonate P_{CO_2} has a direct linear relationship with $[H^+]$ (and thus an inverse relationship with pH that is the negative logarithm of $[H^+]$).

Similarly, for a given P_{CO_2} there is a direct relationship between $[HCO_3^-]$ and pH.

These relationships can be represented graphically (Fig. 3.9).

Bicarbonate concentration

Most blood gas analysers provide two different measurements of bicarbonate: 'actual bicarbonate' and 'standard bicarbonate' and another value; 'base excess'. This can cause confusion, although it need not. The analyser measures the bicarbonate level in the blood sample. This actual measurement is (conveniently) known as the '**actual bicarbonate**' ($aHCO_3^-$). As can be seen in Fig. 3.9, the actual level is directly dependant on the P_{CO_2} (for a given

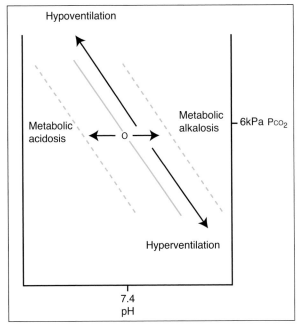

Figure 3.9 In the figure the diagonal lines are bicarbonate isopleths (the bicarbonate level is constant along the line). It can be seen therefore that if the bicarbonate level and P_{CO_2} are known then the pH can be calculated. Indeed, if any two of the three values of: bicarbonate, pH and P_{CO_2} are known then the other value can be calculated. Theses values are yoked together. A change in ventilation will move the arterial point up or down an isopleth as shown, changing pH (bicarbonate level does not change). A pure metabolic disturbance (before any respiratory response) changes the bicarbonate level, moving from one bicarbonate isopleth to another and changing pH.

pH, the higher the P_{CO_2} the higher the $aHCO_3{}^-$, the lower the P_{CO_2} the lower the $aHCO_3{}^-$). If pH and P_{CO_2} are known the bicarbonate level can be calculated. For a given pH the level of bicarbonate can be calculated for a 'standard' P_{CO_2} (5.3 kPa). This calculated value is (conveniently) known as the '**standard bicarbonate**' ($sHCO_3{}^-$). There is little to choose between these two indices but the $sHCO_3{}^-$ takes out the immediate effect of CO_2 on the bicarbonate level and could be loosely regarded as giving a more direct indication of the metabolic activity influencing acid–base balance. The **base excess** takes into account the fact that there are other buffers apart from bicarbonate in the blood. It tells a similar story to the bicarbonate level in terms of acid–base disturbance. Its principal advantage is the ease with which its normal range can be remembered. As one might anticipate from the name, the 'excess' should be zero (normal range is zero +/– 3 mmol/litre). There are not many numbers easier to remember than zero.

Acid–base disturbances

The three variables pH, P_{CO_2} and bicarbonate are yoked together as described above. Analysis of their values provides information on the acid–base balance of the body and the broad nature of its cause. It may also provide information about the chronicity of an abnormality.

Changes in the acid–base status caused by changes in P_{CO_2} (hyper- or hypoventilation) are termed **respiratory**. Changes in acid–base status caused by changes in bicarbonate are termed **metabolic.** A disturbance in one system tends to prompt a compensatory response in the other. When needed, the respiratory system responds promptly and changes are evident within seconds to minutes. The metabolic system, largely regulated via renal excretion, is mush slower; taking between hours and days to equilibrate. In respiratory disturbances therefore, the degree of correction achieved by the metabolic system can tell us something about the duration of the abnormality.

As a general principal **physiological compensatory mechanisms do not overcompensate,** in fact they often stop just short of total correction. This is a useful fact to remember when trying to interpret a blood gas result that displays respiratory and metabolic changes. If the pH is in the normal range, it could be difficult to determine which is the primary abnormality and which the compensatory response. Look again at the pH. If the pH is towards the higher end of the normal range, the primary abnormality was probably an alkalosis, if at the lower end then the primary disturbance was an acidosis.

In reading the following examples of acid–base disturbance refer to Figs. 3.9 and 3.10.

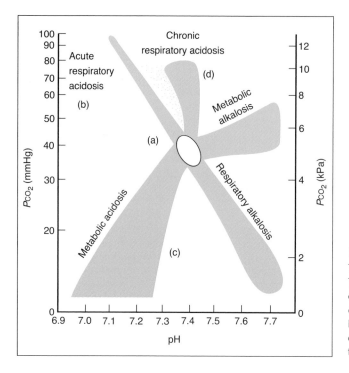

Figure 3.10 **Acid–base disturbances**. The oval indicates the normal position. The shaded areas indicate the direction of observed 'pure' or uncomplicated disturbances of acid–base balance. Bicarbonate levels are omitted for clarity. Letters (a)–(d) are referred to in the text (see Mixed disturbances).

- *Respiratory acidosis (acute)*: **pH reduced, P_{CO_2} raised, bicarbonate normal**. A reduction in alveolar ventilation causes an increase in arterial P_{CO_2}. The pH falls. In the short term there is insufficient time for renal correction so the bicarbonate concentration remains almost unchanged. This pattern is seen where there is a sudden reduction in ventilation, for example obstruction of the airway, overdose of sedative drugs or acute neurological damage.
- *Respiratory acidosis (chronic)*: **pH normal (lower half of normal range), P_{CO_2} raised, bicarbonate high**. If underventilation, from whatever cause, is sustained beyond a few days renal tubular reabsorption of bicarbonate will achieve a significant elevation in plasma bicarbonate level that will correct the acidosis caused by the underventilation. This can be caused by any process that results in sustained hypoventilation – commonly seen in COPD.
- *Respiratory alkalosis* (cases are usually acute as the causes are rarely sustained): **pH raised, P_{CO_2} reduced, bicarbonate normal**. Alveolar hyperventilation causes a fall in P_{CO_2} and a corresponding rise in pH. Bicarbonate concentration is virtually unchanged. This pattern is seen in any form of acute hyperventilation, for example pulmonary embolism, acute severe asthma, anxiety-related hyperventilation, salicylate poisoning.
- *Metabolic acidosis*: **pH reduced, P_{CO_2} reduced, bicarbonate reduced**. The primary disturbance is generally an increase in acid. This has an effect on the equilibrium $H^+ + HCO_3^- \rightleftharpoons H_2O + CO_2$ pushing it to the right. The carbon dioxide produced is removed by increased ventilation and the net result is a lowering of plasma bicarbonate. In practice the fall in pH causes further respiratory stimulation so that carbon dioxide is promptly blown off and the pH changes are therefore much less dramatic than they would have been. The arterial point moves in the direction indicated in Fig. 3.10. This respiratory compensation is an inevitable accompaniment of metabolic acidosis – acute and chronic – unless there is some other factor limiting ventilatory function or responsiveness. This pattern is seen in diabetic ketoacidosis, renal tubular acidosis, acute circulatory failure, sepsis and other forms of lactic acidosis.
- *Metabolic alkalosis*: **pH raised, P_{CO_2} high normal or slightly raised, bicarbonate raised**. An increase in bicarbonate concentration causes a rise in pH. To compensate ventilation is reduced in order to accumulate CO_2. This occurs despite the inevitable fall in P_{O_2}. For this reason however,

scope for correction is limited and the compensatory fall in alveolar ventilation is modest and correction in pH may not be complete. This pattern is seen where there has been administration of excessive alkali, loss of acid through vomiting, or reabsorption of bicarbonate (e.g. in hypokalaemia).

- *Mixed disturbances*: mixed respiratory and metabolic disturbances are common and there are usually a number of possible explanations, therefore it is essential to consider all the clinical details before interpreting the acid–base data. Figure 3.10 shows the situations that may arise in complex acid–base disturbances. For example: point (a) in Fig. 3.10 (low pH, normal $P\text{co}_2$, low bicarbonate) indicates a mixed metabolic and respiratory acidosis. The metabolic disturbance was perhaps obvious, the respiratory component could have been deduced as the $P\text{co}_2$ is higher than might have been suspected had this been a pure metabolic problem. This pattern could arise in a number of different clinical scenarios: a patient with acute severe pulmonary oedema with low cardiac output and ventilatory compromise. The same blood gas result could arise in a patient in renal failure given a narcotic sedative suppressing ventilatory response to acidosis. Blood gas results should be interpreted in light of clinical data. Point (b) could represent the situation soon after a cardiac arrest where severe lactic acidosis exists and ventilation has been insufficient. Point (c) could represent the situation in severe aspirin poisoning where aspirin-induced hyperventilation has been complicated by aspirin-induced metabolic acidosis. Point (d) could represent the situation in an individual with chronic ventilatory failure as a result of COPD who is stimulated to increase ventilation by a pulmonary embolism.

Arterial oxygenation

Arterial oxygen tension ($P_a\text{O}_2$)

In addition to the acid–base balance arterial blood gas analysis provides valuable information on $P_a\text{O}_2$.

Respiratory failure

Respiratory failure is a clinical term used to describe failure to maintain oxygenation (usually taken as an arbitrary cut-off point of $P\text{O}_2$ 8.0 kPa (60 mmHg)).

- Type I respiratory failure is hypoxaemia in the absence of hypercapnia. Overall alveolar ventilation is therefore normal. This pattern of abnormality usually indicates a disturbance of the V/Q matching system within the lung. Such a disturbance can be caused by any intrinsic lung disease affecting the airways, parenchyma or vasculature (e.g. acute asthma, lung fibrosis or pulmonary embolism).
- Type II respiratory failure is hypoxaemia with hypercapnia and indicates alveolar hypoventilation. Note this is NOT merely a severe form of type I respiratory failure, it is brought about by an entirely different mechanism. This may occur from reduced ventilatory drive (e.g. sedative overdose), reduced neuromuscular power (e.g. myopathy) or resetting of the chemoreceptors that drive ventilation in chronic lung disease (e.g. COPD).

Of course, type I and Type II respiratory failure can coexist (and commonly do). These matters are dealt with in more detail in Chapter 1.

Oxygen saturation can be measured non-invasively and continuously using a **pulse oximeter**. Oxygenated blood appears red whereas reduced blood appears blue (clinical sign of cyanosis). An oximeter measures the ratio of oxygenated to total haemoglobin in arterial blood using a probe placed on a finger or ear lobe, which comprises two light-emitting diodes – one red and one infrared – and a detector. The light absorbed varies with each pulse, and measurement of light absorption at two points of the pulse wave allows the oxygen saturation of arterial blood to be determined. The accuracy of measurement is reduced if there is reduced arterial pulsation (e.g. low-output cardiac states) or increased venous pulsation (e.g. tricuspid regurgitation, venous congestion). Skin pigmentation or use of nail varnish may interfere with light transmission. Oximetry is also inaccurate in the presence of carboxyhaemoglobin (e.g. in carbon monoxide poisoning), which the oximeter detects as oxyhaemoglobin. The relationship of $P\text{O}_2$ to oxygen saturation is described by the **oxyhaemoglobin dissociation curve** (see Fig. 1.9). This curve is sigma-shaped so that oxygen saturation is closely related to $P\text{O}_2$ only over a short range of about 3–7 kPa. Above this level the dissociation curve begins to plateau and there is only a small increase in oxygen saturation as the $P\text{O}_2$ rises. Oximetry can reduce the need for arterial puncture, but arterial blood gas analysis is necessary to determine accurately the

P_{O_2} on the plateau part of the oxyhaemoglobin dissociation curve, to measure carbon dioxide level and to assess acid–base status.

A simple algorithm for reviewing blood gas results

Most blood results in medicine are relative easy to make sense of; there is one value and it's either high, low or normal. When faced with the results of an arterial blood gas measurement the clinician usually has six different values that have to be drawn together and interpreted as one. The inexperienced often find their attention skipping from one number to the next, mumbling something about 'not retaining' before becoming utterly confused and giving up. A simple stepwise system for interpreting blood results would help. The following algorithm is easy to follow and will make sense of most of results you will come across in clinical practice.

1 **Look at the pH**. Decide whether this is an acidosis or alkalosis. Once that fact is determined don't be diverted from this essential truth after reviewing the other values. It won't change. If the pH is in the normal range note if it is erring towards one end of the range or another. If there is a compensated abnormality the position of the pH within the range may indicate the nature of the primary disturbance. Remember physiological compensatory mechanisms don't over compensate.
2 **Look at the P_{CO_2}**. Ask if the P_{CO_2} is contributing to or attempting to compensate for the abnormality identified in the pH. That will allow you to know whether the primary disturbance is respiratory or metabolic.
3 **Look at the bicarbonate**. I would suggest either the $sHCO_3^-$ or base excess. In the case of a primary metabolic problem the bicarbonate may hold no surprises. In the case of a primary respiratory problem the bicarbonate may be: normal (suggesting the problem is acute), attempting to correct the respiratory effect on the pH (suggesting the problem is chronic) or compounding the problem (suggesting a mixed disturbance).
4 **Look at the P_{O_2}**. Knowing the inspired partial pressure of oxygen ask whether the P_{O_2} is what

you would expect given the level of ventilation (P_{CO_2}), or lower. This may be difficult to gauge, in which case the alveolar gas equation should be applied (Chapter 1). One can then determine if type I respiratory failure is present.

  KEY POINTS

- A reduced FEV_1/VC ratio indicates airways obstruction, for example asthma, COPD.
- A reduced K_{CO} and $T_{L}CO$ indicates disease of the lung parenchyma or its blood supply for example emphysema, lung fibrosis, pulmonary embolism.
- Type 1 respiratory failure is hypoxia without hypercapnia and may occur in any disease intrinsic to the lung e.g. asthma, pulmonary oedema, pulmonary embolism and lung fibrosis.
- Type 2 respiratory failure is hypoxia with hypercapnia and indicates hypoventilation that occurs in sedative overdose, neuromuscular disease (and moderate to severe COPD where it occurs in conjunction with a type 1 respiratory failure).
- An elevated alveolar–arterial gradient implies a problem intrinsic to the lung.

FEV_1: forced expiratory volume in one second; VC: vital capacity.
$T_{L}CO$: transfer factor for carbon monoxide; K_{CO}: transfer coefficient (= $T_{L}CO$ corrected for lung volume).

  FURTHER READING

Cotes JE. *Lung Function: Assessment and Application in Medicine*. Oxford: Blackwell Scientific Publications, 1993.

Flenley DC. Interpretation of blood-gas and acid–base data. *Br J Hosp Med* 1978; **20**: 384–94.

Gibson GJ. *Clinical Tests of Respiratory Function*. Oxford: Oxford University Press, 2009.

Gibson GJ. Measurement of respiratory muscle strength. *Respir Med* 1995; **89**: 529–35.

Hanning CD, Alexander-Williams JM. Pulse oximetry: a practical review. *BMJ* 1995; **311**: 367–70.

Radiology of the chest

Chest X-ray

The chest X-ray has a key role in the investigation of respiratory disease. The standard view is the erect, **postero-anterior(PA) chest X-ray** taken at full inspiration with the X-ray beam passing from back to front. A **lateral X-ray** gives a better view of lesions lying behind the heart or diaphragm, which may not be visible on a PA X-ray, and allows abnormalities to be viewed in a further dimension. Supine and **antero-posterior (AP) views** are usually taken at the bedside using mobile equipment in patients who are too ill to be brought to the X-ray department. AP films are less satisfactory in defining many abnormalities, producing magnification of the cardiac outline, for example.

The main landmarks of the normal chest X-ray are shown in Figs 4.1 and 4.2. X-rays should be examined both close up and from a short distance on a viewing box or computer screen in an area with reduced background lighting. It is important to confirm the name and date on the X-ray and to check the technical quality of the film. Symmetry between the medial end of both clavicles and the thoracic spine confirms that the film has been taken without any rotation artefact. If the film has been taken in full inspiration the right hemidiaphragm is normally intersected by the anterior part of the sixth rib. The vertebral bodies are usually visible through the cardiac shadow if the X-ray exposure is satisfactory. It is helpful to examine the film systematically to avoid missing useful information. The shape and bony structures of the chest wall should be surveyed and the position of the hemidiaphragms and trachea noted. The shape and size of the heart and the appearances of the mediastinum and hilar shadows are examined. The size, shape and disposition of the vascular shadows are noted and the pattern of the lung markings in different zones are carefully compared. It is advisable to focus attention on areas of the chest X-ray where lesions are commonly missed such as the lung apices, hila and the area behind the heart. Any abnormality detected should be analysed in detail and interpreted in the context of all clinical information. It is often helpful to obtain previous X-rays or to monitor the evolution of abnormalities over time on follow-up X-rays. Some of the radiological features of the major lung diseases are shown in individual chapters. In some circumstances chest X-ray abnormalities follow a specific pattern that allows a differential diagnosis to be outlined.

Abnormal features

Collapse

Obstruction of a bronchus by a carcinoma, foreign body (e.g. inhaled peanut) or mucus plug causes loss of aeration with '**loss of volume**' and collapse of the lung distal to the obstruction. Collapse of each individual lobe of the lung produces its own

Respiratory Medicine Lecture Notes, Eighth Edition. Stephen J. Bourke and Graham P. Burns.
© 2011 John Wiley & Sons, Ltd. Published 2011 by John Wiley & Sons, Ltd.

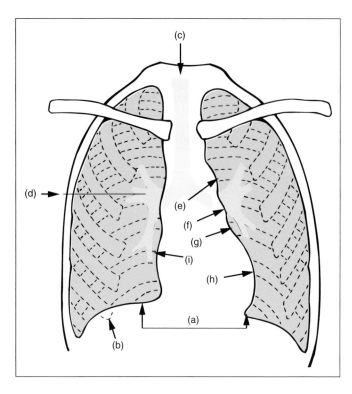

Figure 4.1 Diagram of chest X-ray (PA view). The right hemidiaphragm is 1–3 cm higher than the left (a) and on full inspiration it is intersected by the shadow of the anterior part of the sixth rib (b). The trachea (c) is vertical and central or very slightly to the right. The horizontal fissure (d) is found in the position shown and should be truly horizontal. It is a very valuable marker of change in volume of any part of the right lung. The left border of the cardiac shadow comprises: (e) aorta; (f) pulmonary artery; (g) concavity overlying the left atrial appendage; (h) left ventricle. The right border of the cardiac shadow normally overlies the right atrium (i) and above that of the superior vena cava.

particular appearance on chest X-ray (Figs 4.3 and 4.4) with **shift of landmarks** such as the mediastinum resulting from loss of volume. Obstruction of a main bronchus usually causes obvious asymmetry (Fig. 4.5). **Compensatory expansion** of other lobes may result in increased transradiency of adjacent areas of the lung. In right middle lobe collapse there may be little to see on a PA X-ray apart from lack of definition of the right heart border. This is a useful sign that helps to distinguish it from lower lobe collapse where the right border of the heart remains clearly defined. Left lower lobe collapse is manifest as a triangular area of increased density behind the heart shadow, often with a shift of the heart shadow to the left and increased transradiency of the left hemithorax because of compensatory expansion of the left upper lobe (Fig. 4.4). Collapse is a sinister sign often indicating an obstructing carcinoma that may be confirmed by bronchoscopy.

Consolidation

Air in the lungs appears black on X-ray. Consolidation appears as **areas of opacification** sometimes conforming to the outline of a lobe or segment of lung in which the air has been replaced by an inflammatory exudate (e.g. pneumonia), fluid (e.g. pulmonary oedema), blood (e.g. pulmonary haemorrhage) or tumour (e.g. alveolar cell carcinoma). Bronchi containing air passing through the consolidated lung are sometimes clearly visible as black tubes of air against the white background of the consolidated lung: **air bronchograms** (see Fig. 17.2). Structures such as the heart, mediastinum and diaphragm are usually clearly outlined as a silhouette on an X-ray because of the contrast between the blackness of aerated lung and the whiteness of these structures. When there is abnormal shadowing in the lung adjacent to these structures there is loss of the sharp outline, and this is often referred to as the **silhouette sign**.

Pulmonary masses (Table 4.1, Fig. 4.6)

Table 4.1, Fig. 4.6 Various descriptive terms such as 'rounded opacity', 'nodule' or 'coin lesion' are used to refer to pulmonary masses. Carcinoma of the lung is the most important cause of a mass on chest X-ray but several other diseases may cause a similar appearance. Features such as

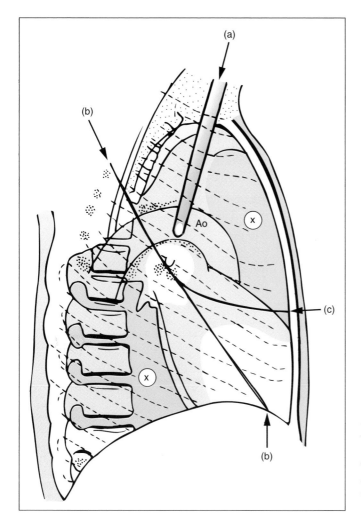

Figure 4.2 Diagram of chest X-ray (lateral view). (a) Trachea. (b) Oblique fissure. (c) Horizontal fissure. It is useful to note that in a normal lateral view the radiodensity of the lung field above and in front of the cardiac shadow is about the same as that below and behind (x). Ao, aorta.

cavitation, **calcification, rate of growth**, the presence of **associated abnormalities** (e.g. lymph node enlargement) and whether the lesion is **solitary** or whether **multiple** lesions are present, may provide clues to diagnosis. However, these features are often not reliable indicators of aetiology, and the X-ray appearances must be interpreted in the context of all the clinical information. Further investigations such as computed tomography (CT) and biopsy (bronchoscopic, percutaneous, surgical) are often necessary.

Cavitation

Cavitation is the presence of an area of radiolucency within a mass lesion. It is a feature of **bronchial carcinoma** (particularly squamous

carcinoma) (Fig. 4.7), **tuberculosis, lung abscess, pulmonary infarcts, Wegener's granulomatosis** and some **pneumonias** (e.g. *Staphylococcus aureus, Klebsiella pneumoniae*).

Fibrosis

Localised fibrosis produces **streaky shadows** with evidence of **traction** upon neighbouring structures. Upper lobe fibrosis causes traction upon the trachea and elevation of the hilar vascular shadows. Generalised interstitial fibrosis produces a hazy shadowing with a **fine reticular (net-like)** or **nodular pattern** (see Chapter 13). Advanced interstitial fibrosis results in a honeycomb pattern with diffuse opacification containing multiple circular translucencies a few millimetres in diameter.

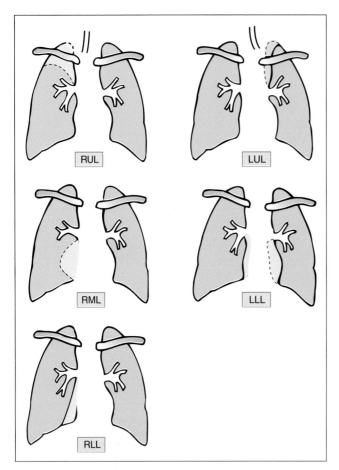

Figure 4.3 **Radiographic patterns of lobar collapse**. Collapsed lobes occupy a surprisingly small volume and are commonly overlooked on the chest X-ray. Helpful information may be provided by the position of the trachea, the hilar vascular shadows and the horizontal fissure. LLL, left lower lobe; LUL, left upper lobe; RLL, right lower lobe; RML, right middle lobe; RUL, right upper lobe.

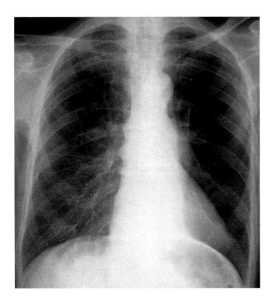

Figure 4.4 **Left lower lobe collapse**. The left lower lobe has collapsed medially and posteriorly and appears as a dense white triangular area behind the heart close to the mediastinum. The remainder of the left lung appears hyperlucent because of compensatory expansion. Bronchoscopy showed an adenocarcinoma occluding the left lower lobe bronchus.

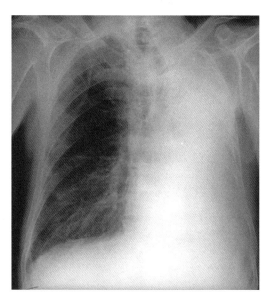

Figure 4.5 **Left lung collapse**. There is complete opacification of the left hemithorax with shift of the mediastinum to the left. Bronchoscopy showed a small-cell carcinoma occluding the left main bronchus.

Mediastinal masses

Metastatic tumour or lymphomatous involvement of the mediastinal lymph nodes are the most common causes of mediastinal masses but there are a number of other diseases that may cause mediastinal masses (Fig. 4.8). Thymic tumours, thyroid

Table 4.1 Causes of pulmonary masses

Neoplastic
- Primary bronchial carcinoma
- Metastatic carcinoma
- Benign tumours (hamartoma)

Non-neoplastic
- Tuberculoma
- Lung abscess
- Hydatid cyst
- Pulmonary infarct
- Arteriovenous malformation
- Encysted interlobar effusion ('pseudotumour')
- Rheumatoid nodule

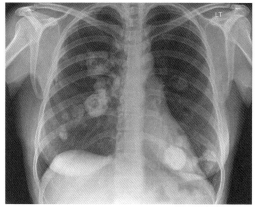

Figure 4.6 Chest X-ray showing multiple partially calcified rounded masses in both lungs due to benign chondromas.

masses and dermoid cysts are most commonly situated in the anterior mediastinum whereas neural lesions (e.g. neurofibroma) and oesophageal cysts are often situated posteriorly. Aneurysmal enlargement of the aorta or ventricle may produce masses in the middle compartment of the mediastinum. CT scans are helpful in delineating the

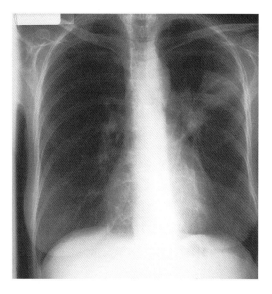

Figure 4.7 A cavitating lesion in the left upper lobe. A cavity appears as an area of radiolucency (black) within an opacity (white). Sputum cytology showed cells from a squamous carcinoma. Computed tomography showed left hilar and subcarinal lymphadenopathy.

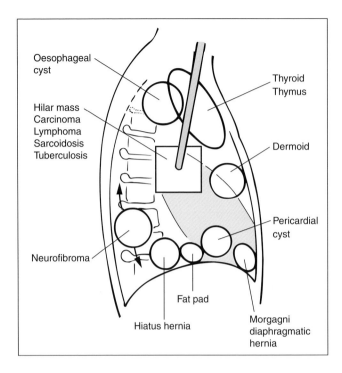

Oesophageal cyst

Hilar mass
Carcinoma
Lymphoma
Sarcoidosis
Tuberculosis

Neurofibroma

Thyroid
Thymus

Dermoid

Pericardial cyst

Fat pad

Hiatus hernia

Morgagni diaphragmatic hernia

Figure 4.8 Mediastinal masses. Diagram of lateral view of the chest, indicating the sites favoured by some of the more common mediastinal masses.

anatomy of mediastinal lesions. Thoracotomy with surgical excision is often necessary.

Ultrasonography of the chest

Normal air-filled lung does not transmit high-frequency sound waves so that ultrasonography is not useful in assessing disease of lung parenchyma. It is helpful in assessing lesions of the pleura and is particularly useful for localising loculated pleural effusions and guiding chest tube insertion (see Chapter 16).

Computed tomography

CT scanning uses a technique of multiple projection with reconstruction of the image from X-ray detectors by a computer so that structures can be displayed in cross-section. A number of different techniques can be used depending on the area of interest. CT scanning is particularly useful in

providing a detailed cross-sectional image of mediastinal disease, which is often difficult to assess on plain chest X-ray. Figure 4.9 shows the principal mediastinal structures with horizontal lines indicating the levels of the CT sections illustrated diagrammatically in Fig. 4.10. CT scanning is a key investigation in the staging of lung cancer (see Chapter 12), and has replaced bronchography (instillation of radiocontrast dye into the bronchial tree) in detecting and determining the extent of bronchiectasis (see Chapter 8). High-resolution CT scans are much more sensitive than plain X-ray in assessing the lung parenchyma and can provide a detailed image of emphysema (see Chapter 11) and interstitial lung disease. A 'ground glass' appearance on a high-resolution CT scan of a patient with interstitial lung disease, for example, often corresponds to alveolar inflammation whereas a 'reticular honeycomb pattern' indicates advanced fibrosis with less active inflammation and less response to steroids (see Chapter 13). Modern CT scanners have the capacity to perform very rapid spiral images and this imaging technique combined with injection of radiocontrast material into a peripheral vein can be used to identify emboli in central pulmonary arteries in thromboembolic disease (see Chapter 15).

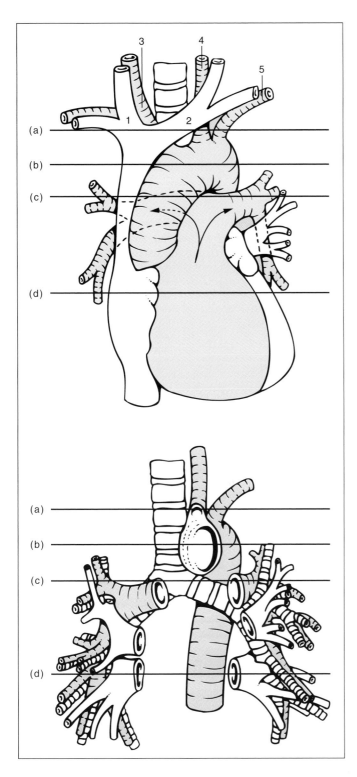

Figure 4.9 **Mediastinal structures**. Principal blood vessels and airways. *Top:* Heart and major blood vessels showing the aorta curling over the bifurcation of the pulmonary trunk into left and right pulmonary arteries (arrows). The horizontal lines (a)–(d) indicate the levels of the computed tomography sections illustrated in Fig. 4.10. 1, right brachiocephalic vein; 2, left brachiocephalic vein; 3, innominate or brachiocephalic artery; 4, left common carotid artery; 5, left subclavian artery.
Bottom: Structures with the heart removed. The aorta curls over the left main bronchus, which lies behind the left pulmonary artery. Pulmonary arteries are shown shaded, pulmonary veins unshaded and bronchi are shown striped. In general the arteries loop downwards, like a handlebar moustache; veins radiate towards a lower common destination – the left atrium. The veins are applied to the front of the arteries and bronchi and take a slightly different path to the respective lung segments. On the right, the order of structures from front to back is vein–artery–bronchus; on the left, the pulmonary artery loops over the left upper lobe bronchus and descends behind so that the order is vein– bronchus–artery.

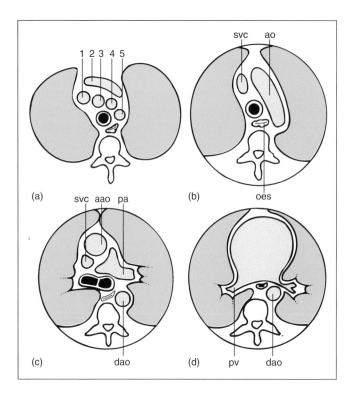

Figure 4.10 Principal mediastinal structures on computed tomography. The sections (a)–(d) are at levels (a)–(d) in Fig. 4.9. The sections should be regarded as being viewed from below **(i.e. the left of the thorax is on the right of the figure)**. (a) *Section above the aortic arch.* Many large vessels and an anterior sausage shape are seen; the trachea has not bifurcated (black circle). Numerals refer to Fig. 4.9 and its legend. (b) *Section at the level of aortic arch.* A large oblique sausage shape representing the aortic arch is seen (ao); oes, oesophagus which is visible in all of the sections; svc, superior vena cava.(c) *Section below the aortic arch.* Both ascending (aao) and descending (dao) aortas are visible, the trachea is bifurcating and the pulmonary arteries are seen; pa, left pulmonary artery. (d) *Section at the level of pulmonary veins (pv).* Lower lobe intrapulmonary arteries and bronchi are not shown in the diagram.

Positron emission tomography

Positron emission tomography (PET) scanning is being increasingly used in the diagnosis and staging of lung cancer. It is based on the concept that neoplastic cells have greater metabolic activity and a higher uptake of glucose than normal cells. ^{18}F-fluoro-2-deoxy-glucose (FDG) is a glucose analogue that is preferentially taken up by neoplastic cells after intravenous injection and which then emits positrons. PET scanning is particularly helpful in the **staging of lung cancer** to detect metastases and to determine involvement of lymph nodes in patients being considered for radical treatment such as surgical resection or high-dose radiotherapy (see chapter 12). PET scanning is also particularly useful in the differential diagnosis of an indeterminate **solitary pulmonary nodule**. Often such a nodule is small and not amenable to biopsy. Calcification or lack of growth of the lesion over time suggest that the nodule is benign (e.g. hamartoma, healed tuberculous granuloma). If the patient is a smoker at high risk

of cancer and otherwise fit it may be advisable to proceed directly to surgical resection of such a lesion without preoperative histological confirmation. Active accumulation of FDG in the lesion on PET scanning suggests malignancy. False-negative findings can occur in tumours <1 cm and false-positive uptake can occur in inflammatory conditions such as tuberculosis, sarcoidosis, histoplasmosis and coccidioidomycosis.

 KEY POINTS

- The chest X-ray has a key role in the investigation of lung disease. It should be studied in a systematic way and interpreted in the context of all clinical information.
- CT is more sensitive than the chest X-ray and is crucial in the staging of lung cancer, in assessing interstitial lung disease and in diagnosing pulmonary emboli.
- Ultrasonography is useful in assessing pleural effusions and is used to guide placement of a chest tube when draining a pleural effusion.
- PET is helpful in diagnosing and staging lung cancer.

📖 FURTHER READING

Hansell DM. Thoracic imaging. In: Gibson GJ, Geddes DM, Costabel U, Sterk PJ, Corrin B, eds., *Respiratory Medicine*. London: WB Saunders Co, 2003: 316–51.

Lynch DA, Godwin JD, Safrin S, et al. High-resolution computed tomography in idiopathic pulmonary fibrosis. *Am J Respir Crit Care Med* 2005; **172**: 488–93.

MacMahon H, Austin JHM, Gamsu G, et al. Guidelines for the management of small pulmonary nodules on CT scans: a statement from the Fleischner Society. *Radiology* 2005; **237**: 395–400.

Remy-Jardin M, Ghaye B, Remy J. Spiral computed tomography angiography of pulmonary embolism. *Eur Respir Monograph* 2004; **27**: 124–43.

Vansteenkiste JF. Imaging in lung cancer: position emission tomography scan. *Eur Respir J* 2002; **19** (suppl 35): 49–60.

Verschakelen JA, DeWever W, Bogaert J, Stroobants S. Imaging: staging of lung cancer. *Eur Respir Monograph* 2004; **30**: 214–44.

5

Upper respiratory tract infections and influenza

Introduction

Acute upper respiratory tract infections (URTIs) are a very common cause of morbidity, visits to doctors and absence from school or work. They are the most common respiratory complaint accounting for about **9% of all consultations in general practice**. A child suffers about eight, and an adult about four respiratory infections each year. Although unpleasant, most URTIs are mild and self-limiting, but a small number give rise to serious problems, most notably acute epiglottitis in children and influenza A in elderly patients debilitated by chronic underlying disease. Difficulties arise in distinguishing URTIs from more serious lower respiratory tract infections such as pneumonia (Fig. 5.1), and alertness combined with careful assessment and clinical judgement are required. Most URTIs are of viral origin but a variety of viruses and bacteria may produce the same clinical pattern of illness (e.g. pharyngitis, sinusitis).

Common cold

The common cold (coryza) is an acute illness characterised by rhinorrhoea, sneezing, nasal obstruction and sore throat (pharyngitis) with minimal fever or systemic symptoms. It may be caused by about 200 different strains of viruses including **rhinoviruses**, **coronaviruses**, **respiratory syncytial**, **parainfluenza** and **influenza viruses**. Infection is transmitted by droplet spread, and attack rates are highest in young children attending school who then transmit infection to their parents and siblings at home. The multiplicity of viral strains prevents the development of immunity. The bacterial flora of the nasopharynx remains unchanged for the first few days of the illness but then may show an increase in the number of *Haemophilus influenzae* and *Streptococcus pneumoniae* organisms, and there is the potential for secondary bacterial infection to occur with extension of infection beyond the nasopharynx, giving rise to sinusitis, otitis media, bronchitis or pneumonia. Most people with the common cold do not need to see their general practitioner and can be encouraged to manage the condition themselves or to seek advice from a pharmacist. No specific treatment is possible for the common cold but symptoms are often alleviated by use of paracetamol or aspirin.

Pharyngitis

Pharyngitis may occur as part of the common cold or as a separate illness. Most cases are caused by

Respiratory Medicine Lecture Notes, Eighth Edition. Stephen J. Bourke and Graham P. Burns.
© 2011 John Wiley & Sons, Ltd. Published 2011 by John Wiley & Sons, Ltd.

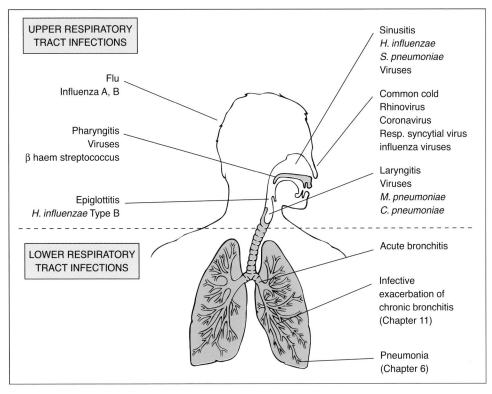

UPPER RESPIRATORY
TRACT INFECTIONS

Sinusitis
H. influenzae
S. pneumoniae
Viruses

Flu
Influenza A, B

Common cold
Rhinovirus
Coronavirus
Resp. syncytial virus
influenza viruses

Pharyngitis
Viruses
β haem streptococcus

Laryngitis
Viruses
M. pneumoniae
C. pneumoniae

Epiglottitis
H. influenzae Type B

LOWER RESPIRATORY
TRACT INFECTIONS

Acute bronchitis

Infective
exacerbation of
chronic bronchitis
(Chapter 11)

Pneumonia
(Chapter 6)

Figure 5.1 Acute respiratory infections.

viruses (Table 5.1) but pharyngitis may also be caused by group A **β-haemolytic streptococci**, *Mycoplasma pneumoniae* or *Chlamydophila pneumoniae*, for example. The patient complains of a sore throat and there is erythema of the pharynx often with enlargement of the tonsils. **Infectious mononucleosis** (glandular fever) often involves pharyngitis but is also associated with lymphadenopathy and splenomegaly, and is caused by the Epstein–Barr (EB) virus. A blood film may show atypical mononuclear cells and the Monospot or heterophile antibody test is positive. Characteristically, patients with infectious mono-nucleosis develop a rash if given amoxicillin as treatment of pharyngitis. It is not possible to dis-tinguish between viral and bacterial pharyngitis on clinical grounds. β-haemolytic streptococci may be found on microbiology of a throat swab but this does not differentiate between active infection and a carriage state. Even when pharyngitis is caused by bacterial infection antibiotics are not usually necessary, as the illness tends to be self-limiting.

Local extension of infection may result in otitis media, tonsillitis or quinsy (peritonsillar abscess). Streptococcal infection may be complicated by glomerulonephritis or rheumatic fever but these are rare nowadays. Antibiotic treatment of pharyngitis is usually only given to severe or complicated cases. Streptococci are sensitive to phenoxymethylpenicillin or amoxicillin. *Myco-plasma pneumoniae* or *Chlamydophila pneumo-niae* require a tetracycline or macrolide antibiotic (e.g. clarithromycin).

Sinusitis

Infection of the maxillary sinuses causes facial pain, nasal obstruction and discharge, often accompanied by fever and malaise. A variety of organisms may cause sinusitis including respira-tory **viruses**, *Haemophilus influenzae*, *Strepto-coccus pneumoniae*, *Staphylococcus aureus* and

Table 5.1 Principal respiratory viruses

Virus	Disease	Notes
Rhinovirus	Common cold, pharyngitis, chronic bronchitic exacerbations	More than 100 serotypes; identification and study difficult
Coronavirus	Common cold	Numerous serotypes; identification difficult
	Severe Acute Respiratory Syndrome (SARS)	SARS coronavirus (see Chapter 6)
Adenovirus	Pharyngitis, conjunctivitis, severe bronchitis in childhood, rarely severe pneumonia	About 30 serotypes
Respiratory syncytial virus	Bronchiolitis in infants, common cold in adults	One serotype, winter epidemics
Influenza A	Influenza – may be severe	Epidemics, continuous antigenic variation
Influenza B	Influenza	Milder illness, minor epidemics
Parainfluenza	Croup, other upper respiratory tract infections, some bronchiolitis	Serotypes 1–4, A and B
Measles	Measles, severe illness with pneumonia in immunocompromised	Vaccination effective
Cytomegalovirus	Silent infection or minor respiratory illness, pneumonia in immunosuppressed	One serotype
Herpes simplex	Stomatitis, rarely pharyngitis, pneumonia in immunosuppressed	One serotype, severe infection treatable with aciclovir or vidarabine
Herpes zoster	Pneumonia in adult infection	Severe infection treatable with aciclovir, leaves scattered calcific lesions
Coxsackie, enteroviruses and ECHO viruses	Minor part in respiratory infection, Coxsackie A may cause herpangina; B causes 'pleurodynia' and pericarditis/myocarditis	Local epidemics
Epstein–Barr virus	Pharyngitis, lymphadenitis, infectious mononucleosis	Heterophile antibody test, typical blood picture

ECHO, enteric cytopathic human organ.

anaerobic bacteria. In chronic sinusitis X-rays may show mucosal thickening, opacification or the presence of a fluid level in the sinus. Recurrent sinusitis may be accompanied by more widespread respiratory tract infection in patients with bronchiectasis caused by cystic fibrosis, hypogammaglobulinaemia or ciliary dyskinesia. Post-nasal drip from sinusitis is irritating to the larynx and may cause a persistent cough. Sinusitis is usually treated with antibiotics (e.g. amoxicillin, trimethoprim), nasal decongestants (e.g. ephedrine) and analgesia (e.g. paracetamol). Surgical drainage may be necessary for relief of chronic sinusitis.

Acute laryngitis

This term is used when temporary hoarseness or loss of voice occurs with pharyngitis or the common cold, and is caused by oedema of the vocal cords. No treatment is necessary.

Croup

Croup (acute laryngotracheobronchitis) is usually caused by **viruses** such as parainfluenza virus, respiratory syncytial virus, influenza A and B, rhinoviruses, adenovirus and measles. Characteristically, the child develops a harsh barking cough with an upper respiratory infection and this may progress to stridor. Often no treatment is required but some children develop more severe lower respiratory infections and progressive respiratory distress requiring intubation and ventilation. Oral prednisolone is sometimes beneficial in severe croup and nebulised high-dose budesonide may be associated with more rapid recovery in less severely affected patients.

Acute epiglottitis

Epiglottitis is a very serious disease that is usually caused by virulent strains of *Haemophilus influenzae* **type B**, and there is often an accompanying septicaemia. Death may result from occlusion of the airway by the inflamed oedematous epiglottis. It is most common in children of about 2–3 years of age, but cases have also occurred in adults. The patient is ill with pyrexia, sore throat, laryngitis and painful dysphagia. Symptoms of upper airway obstruction may develop rapidly with stridor and respiratory distress. A lateral neck X-ray may show epiglottic swelling. Blood cultures often isolate *Haemophilus influenzae* type B. Patients with suspected epiglottitis should be admitted to hospital and attempts at examining the upper airway should only be performed when facilities are available for tracheal intubation and ventilation. Because of possible amoxicillin resistance chloramphenicol or cefuroxime are appropriate antibiotics. The widespread use of vaccination against *Haemophilus influenzae* in childhood is making epiglottitis increasingly rare.

Influenza

Seasonal influenza

Influenza is an acute illness characterised by pyrexia, malaise, myalgia, headache and prostration as well as upper respiratory symptoms. Lethargy and depression may persist for several days afterwards. Although the term 'flu' is used very loosely by the public, it is the systemic features that characterise true infection with the influenza viruses. Influenza virus type A undergoes frequent spontaneous changes in its haemagglutinin and neuraminidase surface antigens. Minor changes, referred to as '**antigenic drift**', result in outbreaks of seasonal influenza in the winter months each year. Major changes, referred to as '**antigenic shift**', result in epidemics and **pandemics** of infection reflecting the lack of immunity in the population to the new strain. Type B is more antigenically stable and produces less severe disease. Type C causes only mild sporadic cases of upper respiratory infection.

Influenza is highly infectious so that all members of a household often become ill together. Outbreaks of influenza cause considerable morbidity even in healthy adults. It is usually a self-limiting illness but can be complicated by bronchitis, otitis media and secondary bacterial pneumonia (e.g. *Staphylococcus aureus*, *Streptococcus pneumoniae* or *Haemophilus influenzae*). The greatest morbidity and mortality occur in patients who are elderly with underlying cardiac or respiratory disease and seasonal influenza outbreaks cause an average annual excess mortality of about 12 000 deaths in the UK.

The diagnosis of influenza can be confirmed by immunofluorescent microscopy of nasal secretions or by serology. **Oseltamivir** and **zanamivir** are drugs that reduce the replication of influenza viruses by inhibiting viral neuraminidase. Oseltamivir is given orally whereas zanamivir is only available by inhalation. These drugs have to be given within 48 hours of the onset of symptoms to be effective. They reduce the duration of illness by about 1 day and they may reduce complications in at-risk patients with severe influenza. They can also be given for post-exposure prophylaxis in at-risk adults not protected by vaccination. Vaccination remains the most effective way of preventing illness from seasonal influenza. However, if new pandemic strains of influenza emerge it will take time to develop vaccines. **Amantadine** is an older antiviral agent that blocks the ion channel function of a protein in the influenza virus, but some strains are resistant to this drug and it is not currently recommended for the treatment of influenza in the UK. Use of aspirin or paracetamol relieves symptoms. Antibiotics are used when there are features of secondary bacterial infection (e.g. otitis media, sinusitis). Pneumonia associated with influenza may be severe and requires treatment with broad-spectrum antibiotics including antibiotics against *Staphylococcus aureus* (e.g. co-amoxiclav, cefuroxime, flucloxacillin).

Influenza vaccination

The influenza vaccine is prepared each year using the virus strains most likely to be prevalent that year. The vaccine contains inactivated virus and is about 70–80% effective in protecting against infection. Where infection occurs despite vaccination it is usually less severe and associated with less morbidity and mortality than the disease seen in unvaccinated patients. Selective immunisation is recommended to protect those most at risk of serious illness or death from influenza. Annual vaccination is recommended for those over the age of 65 years and those with chronic respiratory disease (e.g. chronic obstructive pulmonary disease, asthma, bronchiectasis, etc.), chronic heart disease, renal failure, diabetes mellitus, immunosuppression and for patients living in nursing homes.

Adverse reactions to influenza vaccine are usually mild, consisting of fever and malaise in some patients and local reactions at the site of injection. The vaccine is contraindicated in patients with egg allergy. Patients should be advised that the vaccine will not protect them from all respiratory viruses.

Pandemic influenza

Influenza pandemics have occurred sporadically and unpredictably over the last century. They arise when there are major changes in the haemagglutinin and neuraminidase surface antigens of the influenza A virus. In 1918 a pandemic of influenza caused by the H1N1 strain (Spanish flu) killed about 30 million people worldwide. In this pandemic the mortality was particularly high in those aged 20–40 years. There were further pandemics in 1957, caused by the H2N2 strain (Asian flu), and in 1968, caused by the H3N2 strain (Hong Kong flu), each killing about 1 million people worldwide. In recent years there is concern about the transmission of an avian strain of influenza (H5N1) from birds such as ducks and poultry to humans. This has occurred mainly in South East Asia and has produced severe influenza pneumonia in humans, with a high death rate. Spread of infection was contained by slaughtering large numbers of birds in affected areas. In 2009/2010 a further pandemic, caused by H1N1 ('swine flu') occurred. It first appeared in Mexico but then spread globally. This virus was not particularly pathogenic and therefore the number of deaths was relatively low. There is the potential for influenza viral strains to undergo mutations that might increase their virulence and the capacity for transmission from human to human. During pandemics the number of patients with influenza can overwhelm the normal health-care systems and contingency plans have been developed for such circumstances.

 KEY POINTS

- Most upper respiratory infections are self-limiting, caused by viruses, and antibiotics are not usually indicated.
- Seasonal influenza A causes an acute systemic illness with substantial morbidity and mortality, particularly in elderly at-risk patients.
- Influenza A vaccine is prepared each year for the prevalent strains and gives effective protection against seasonal influenza.
- Pandemic influenza occurs when there are major mutations in the virus that result in increased virulence and a lack of immunity in the population.

 FURTHER READING

British Infection Society, British Thoracic Society, Health Protection Agency in collaboration with the Department of Health. Pandemic flu: clinical management of patients with an influenza-like illness during an influenza pandemic. *Thorax* 2007; **62** (suppl 1): 1–46.

Husby S, Agertoft L, Mortensen S, Pedersen S. Treatment of croup with nebulised steroid (budesonide): a double-blind placebo controlled study. *Arch Dis Child* 1993; **68**: 352–6.

Lagace-Wiens PR, Rubinstein E, Gurnel A. Influenza epidemiology – past, present and future. *Crit Care Med* 2010; **38** (suppl): e1–e9.

Little PS, Williamson I, Shvartzman P. Are antibiotics appropriate for sore throats? *BMJ* 1994; **309**: 1010–12.

Mansel JK, Rosenow EC, Smith TF, Martin JW. *Mycoplasma pneumoniae*. *Chest* 1989; **95**: 639–46.

Nguyen-Van-Tam JS, Openshaw PJ, Hashim A, et al. Risk factors for hospitalization and poor outcome with pandemic A/H1N1 influenza. *Thorax* 2010; **65**: 645–51.

Vernon DD, Sarnaik AP. Acute epiglottitis in children: a conservative approach to diagnosis and management. *Crit Care Med* 1986; **14**: 23–5.

Wilson R. Influenza vaccination. *Thorax* 1994; **49**: 1079–80.

Wong SSY, Yuen KY. Avian influenza virus infections in humans. *Chest* 2006; **129**: 156–68.

6

Pneumonia

Lower respiratory tract infections

The lower respiratory tract, below the larynx, is normally sterile. Infections can reach the lungs by a number of routes: **inhalation**, **aspiration**, **direct inoculation** (e.g. stab wound to chest) and **blood borne** (e.g. from intravenous drug misuse). In some situations lower respiratory tract infection may be regarded as a **primary exogenous event** in which inhalation of a large dose of a virulent pathogen produces a severe infection in a previously healthy person. Thus, *Legionella pneumophila* may be inhaled from a contaminated water system, or *Chlamydophila psittaci* from an infected bird resulting in a severe pneumonia. In other circumstances infection is a **secondary endogenous event**. Thus, a patient who is debilitated by major trauma and requiring endotracheal ventilation in an intensive therapy unit (ITU) may develop pneumonia. Typically in these circumstances the patient's oropharynx becomes colonised by Gram-negative enteric bacteria that are usually acquired from endogenous sources within the patient such as the upper gastrointestinal tract, subgingival dental plaque and periodontal crevices. These bacteria may then reach the lower airway by microaspiration.

Pneumonia

Pneumonia is a general term denoting inflammation of the gas exchange region of the lung. Usually it implies **parenchymal lung inflammation caused by infection**, and the term 'pneumonitis' is sometimes used to denote inflammation caused by physical, chemical or allergic processes. Pneumonia is an important cause of morbidity and mortality in all age groups. Globally it is estimated that 5 million children under the age of 5 years die from pneumonia each year (95% in the developing countries). In the UK about 1 in 1000 of the population are admitted to hospital with pneumonia each year and the mortality in these patients is about 10%. There are about 3000 deaths from pneumonia each year in the age group 15–55 years. About 25% of all deaths in elderly people are related to pneumonia, although this is often the terminal illness in a patient with serious concomitant disease.

Classification in relation to clinical context (Fig. 6.1)

A microbiological approach to pneumonia focuses primarily on identification of the pathogen and its susceptibility to antibiotics. However, many of the major respiratory pathogens may be present

Respiratory Medicine Lecture Notes, Eighth Edition. Stephen J. Bourke and Graham P. Burns.
© 2011 John Wiley & Sons, Ltd. Published 2011 by John Wiley & Sons, Ltd.

Previously well infant
1 RSV
2 Adenovirus and other viruses
3 Bacterial

Previously ill infant
1 Staphylococcus
2 *E. coli* and Gram-negative bacteria
3 Viruses and opportunistic organisms

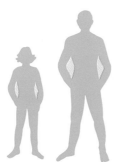

Children
1 Viruses
2 Pneumococcus
3 Mycoplasma
4 Others

Previously fit adults
1 Pneumococcus
2 Mycoplasma
3 *H. influenzae*
4 Viruses
5 Staphylococcus
6 *Legionella*
7 Others

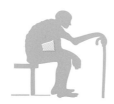

Previous respiratory illness;
elderly and debilitated
1 Pneumococcus
2 *H. influenzae*
3 Staphylococcus
4 *Klebsiella* and
   Gram-negative organisms

If no response think of:
TB, *Mycoplasma, Legionella,*
carcinoma

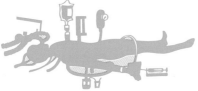

Severely immunocompromised
and AIDS
1 Pneumocystis pneumonia
2 Cytomegalovirus
3 Adenovirus
4 Herpes simplex
5 Bacteria (*Legionella,*
   Staphylococcus, Pneumococcus)
6 Opportunistic mycobacteria;
   tuberculosis

Hospital-acquired pneumonia
1 Gram-negative bacteria
   (*Pseudomonas, Klebsiella,*
   Proteus)
2 Staphylococcus
3 Pneumococcus
4 Anaerobic bacteria, fungi
5 NB aspiration pneumonia
6 Others

Figure 6.1 Likely causes of pneumonia in different clinical circumstances. Age and previous health are important factors.

in the oropharynx in a normal person so that identification of an organism in respiratory tract secretions may not be sufficient to implicate it as the cause of the illness. Conversely the same pathogen can cause various illnesses at different levels in the respiratory tract such as sinusitis, bronchitis or pneumonia, and different bacteria may cause an identical clinical syndrome such as pneumonia. A clinical approach to pneumonia focuses on the clinical context of the illness, the patient's previous health status and on the circumstances of the illness. Pneumonia is the result of a complex interaction between the **patient**, the **environment** and the **infecting organism**, and the pattern of the disease depends on the **virulence** of the pathogen and the **vulnerability** of the patient. The circumstances of the illness include the following:

- site of infection in the respiratory tract;
- age of the patient;
- community- or hospital-acquired infection;
- concurrent disease;
- environmental and geographical factors;
- severity of the illness; and
- microbiology of the pneumonia.

Site of infection

The term 'chest infection' is an imprecise term often used by lay people to refer to non-specific respiratory symptoms. In assessing and treating respiratory tract infections it is important to define the site of infection as clearly as possible. **Upper respiratory tract infections** (above the larynx) are often viral in origin and self-limiting, not requiring treatment (see Chapter 5). **Lower respiratory tract infections** may affect the bronchial tree such as **bronchitis**, or the lung parenchyma such as **pneumonia**. Infective exacerbations of chronic bronchitis (see Chapter 11) are often caused by organisms of low virulence (e.g. non-typeable *Haemophilus influenzae*) when the patient's defences against infection are compromised by smoking-induced damage to the bronchial mucosa. Penetration of antibiotics into the scarred mucosa and viscid secretions may be difficult. Extension of bronchial infection into the surrounding lung parenchyma is often referred to as **bronchopneumonia**. Infection of the lung parenchyma with extensive consolidation of a lobe of a lung – **lobar pneumonia** – is usually caused by organisms of greater virulence (e.g. *Streptococcus pneumoniae*). Infection may spread to the pleura resulting in **empyema** or to the bloodstream causing **septicaemia**.

Age of the patient

In **children** under the age of 2 years pneumonia is commonly caused by viruses such as respiratory syncytial virus (RSV), adenovirus, influenza and parainfluenza viruses. *Chlamydia trachomatis* infection may be transmitted to the infant from the mother's genital tract during birth resulting in pneumonia. In older children and **adults** of all ages *Streptococcus pneumoniae* is the most common cause of primary pneumonia. *Mycoplasma*

pneumoniae infection is rare in elderly people and particularly affects young adults. The incidence of pneumonia increases greatly in **elderly people** and the high frequency of underlying chronic diseases (e.g. chronic obstructive pulmonary disease (COPD), heart failure) in this group is associated with a high mortality.

Community- or hospital-acquired pneumonia

The characteristics of the patients and the spectrum of pathogens differ greatly depending on whether pneumonia is contracted in the community or in hospital. When pneumonia is acquired in the community it may be a primary infection in a previously healthy individual or it may occur in association with concomitant disease (e.g. COPD), but a few pathogens (notably *Streptococcus pneumoniae*) account for the majority of cases and Gram-negative organisms are rare. Most patients are treated at home with only about 25% needing hospital admission. The most important organisms identified as causing **community-acquired pneumonia** are as follows:

- *Streptococcus pneumoniae*   50–60%
- *Mycoplasma pneumoniae*   10%
- *Chlamydophila pneumoniae*   10%
- Viruses (e.g. influenza)   10%
- *Haemophilus influenzae*   5%
- *Staphylococcus aureus*   3%
- *Legionella pneumophila*   2%
- Others   2%

  Hospital-acquired (nosocomial pneumonia) is defined as pneumonia developing 2 or more days after admission to hospital for some other reason. It is therefore a secondary infection in patients with other illnesses. In those with milder pneumonia on general wards the causative organisms may be similar to those found in the community. However, pneumonia in the context of endotracheal ventilation on ITU or in those who have already received antibiotics is different. In these circumstances Gram-negative organisms (e.g. *Pseudomonas aeruginosa*, *Escherichia coli*) are the most important pathogens, and meticillin-resistant *staphylococcus aureus* (MRSA) is an increasing problem. A variety of factors, including use of broad-spectrum antibiotics and impaired host defences, promote the colonisation of the nasopharynx of hospitalised patients with Gram-negative organisms. Aspiration of infected nasopharyngeal secretions into the lower respiratory tract is facilitated by factors that compromise the defence mechanisms of the lung (e.g. endotracheal intubation in ITU) impaired cough associated with anaesthesia, surgery or cerebrovascular disease. The spectrum of causative organisms varies depending on the exact circumstances but the most common pathogens in hospital-acquired pneumonia are as follows:

- Gram-negative bacteria   50%
- *Staphylococcus aureus*   20%
- *Streptococcus pneumoniae*   15%
- Anaerobes and fungi   10%
- Others (e.g. *Legionella pneumophila*)   5%

Concurrent disease

Alcohol misuse, **malnutrition**, **diabetes** and underlying **cardiorespiratory disease** predispose to pneumonia and are associated with a greatly increased mortality. Patients with **COPD** have impaired mucociliary clearance and organisms of quite low virulence (e.g. *Haemophilus influenzae*) may spread from the bronchi into the peribronchial lung parenchyma causing bronchopneumonia. Mortality from **influenza infection**, either as a cause of primary pneumonia or associated with secondary bacterial pneumonia, is highest in **elderly** people. **Aspiration pneumonia** is likely to occur in patients with impaired swallowing as a result of oesophageal or neuromuscular disease, or in patients with impaired consciousness (e.g. epileptic fits, anaesthesia). Patients who have undergone **splenectomy** are particularly vulnerable to pneumococcal pneumonia and septicaemia and are usually given pneumococcal vaccination and maintained on life-long penicillin prophylaxis.

Environmental and geographical factors

Although in some cases pneumonia arises by aspiration of endogenous infective organisms from the oropharynx, in other cases the patient's environment is the source of infection with the inhalation of infected droplets from **other patients** (e.g. influenza, tuberculosis), from an **animal source** (e.g. *Chlamydophila psittaci* from birds, *Coxiella burnetti* from farm animals) or from other **environmental sources** (e.g. *Legionella pneumophila* from contaminated water systems).

Some infections have a particular **geographical distribution** (e.g. histoplasmosis in North America, *Burkholderia pseudomallei* in East Asia, typhoid in tropical countries) and need to be considered in patients who live in, or have recently visited, these areas. A knowledge of the **local pattern of prevalent infections** and **antibiotic resistance** in a community is important. For example, *Mycoplasma pneumoniae* infection particularly occurs in outbreaks about every 4 years and requires treatment with tetracycline or a macrolide (e.g. clarithromycin) antibiotic. Although *Streptococcus pneumoniae* in the UK is usually sensitive to penicillin, about 30% of strains isolated in Spain are resistant and this should be borne in mind when choosing initial antibiotic therapy.

Severity of pneumonia (Fig. 6.2)

Community-acquired pneumonia has a wide spectrum of severity from a mild self-limiting illness to a fatal disease. It is therefore vital to assess accurately the severity of the pneumonia, as this is an important factor in determining the choice of antibiotics, the extent of investigations and in deciding whether a patient should be treated **in hospital** rather than **at home** or in an **ITU** rather than on a general ward. Severe pneumonia can rapidly develop into multiorgan failure with respiratory, circulatory and renal failure. Patients who have certain core adverse prognostic features have a greatly increased risk of death: acute **confusion**, elevated **urea** (>7 mmol/L), increased **respiratory rate** (≥30/min) and low **blood pressure** (systolic <90 mmHg, diastolic <60 mmHg), age over 65 years. A **CURB-65 score** (confusion, elevated urea, respiratory rate, blood pressure, age >65 years) is useful in assessing the severity of pneumonia (Fig 6.2). Patients with severe pneumonia are likely to benefit from more intensive monitoring (arterial catheter, central venous catheter, urinary catheter) and treatment (rapid correction of hypovolaemia, inotropic support, ventilatory support) in an ITU.

Clinical features

Patients with pneumonia typically present with **cough**, **purulent sputum** and **fever**, often accompanied by **pleuritic pain** and **breathlessness**. There may be a history of a recent upper respiratory tract infection. Diagnosing the site and severity of respiratory tract infection is notoriously

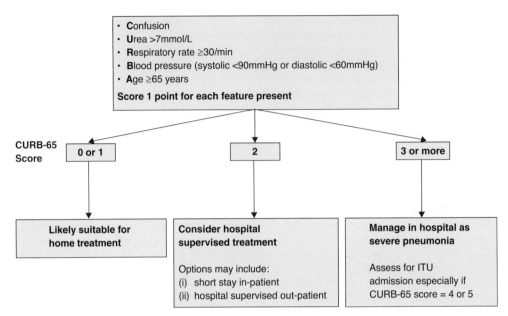

Figure 6.2 CURB-65 Severity Score. The severity of pneumonia can be assessed using a scoring system based on the key parameters of new onset confusion, an elevated urea, respiratory rate, blood pressure and age >65 years, giving a CURB-65 score. Patients with a score of >3 are at high risk of death and may need to be treated in an intensive therapy unit (ITU). Patients with a score < 1 may be suitable for treatment at home. Clinical judgement, social circumstances and the stability of comorbid illness are also important in assessing disease severity.

difficult and careful assessment combined with good clinical judgement is important. Early review of the situation is crucial in the event of deterioration because the severity of the illness is often underestimated by the patient and doctor alike. **Localised chest signs** such as crackles, dullness or bronchial breathing indicate pneumonia rather than bronchitis, for example, but may not always be present. Cyanosis and tachypnoea are features of respiratory failure. Rigors, high fever or prostration suggest septicaemia. Elderly patients, in particular, may present with non-respiratory symptoms such as confusion.

The initial clinical approach focuses on an **assessment of the circumstances and severity** of the illness because these guide decisions as to how and where the patient should be treated. Rather than diagnosing a patient as having a 'chest infection' an effort should be made to use an appropriate descriptive phrase such as: 'a previously fit adult with severe community-acquired pneumonia and suspected septicaemia (rigors, prostration)' or 'probable bronchopneumonia (crackles) and respiratory failure (cyanosis) in a patient with COPD'.

Investigation

Patients with mild pneumonia that responds rapidly to antibiotics are usually treated at home and in this situation investigations do not usually influence management or outcome. Nonetheless, microbiology laboratories will often request that general practitioners send sputum and serology samples from some patients treated in the community so as to be able to alert clinicians to outbreaks of influenza or *Mycoplasma pneumoniae* for example, and to provide information on local patterns of bacterial resistance to antibiotics. More extensive investigations are indicated for patients requiring admission to hospital.

General investigations

- **Chest X-ray** (Fig. 6.3) confirms the diagnosis of pneumonia by demonstrating consolidation, detects complications such as lung abscess or empyema, and helps to exclude any underlying disease (e.g. bronchial carcinoma).
- **Haematology and biochemistry tests** are useful in assessing the severity of the disease.

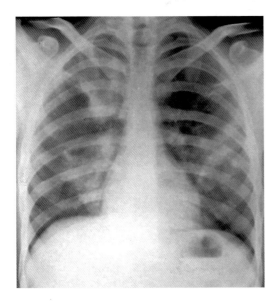

Figure 6.3 This 60-year-old man was admitted to hospital with a 2-week history of myalgia, headache, dyspnoea and cough without sputum. He was severely ill, cyanosed and confused with a fever of 39 °C, tachycardia of 110/min, respiratory rate 40/min and blood pressure of 110/60 mmHg. Po_2 was 5.7 kPa (43 mmHg), Pco_2 4.9 kPa (37 mmHg), white cell count 4.6×10^9/L and urea 31 mmol/L. He had received amoxicillin for 6 days before admission without improvement. Chest X-ray shows extensive bilateral multilobar consolidation. He kept birds as a hobby and one of his budgerigars had died recently. The clinical diagnosis of psittacosis was subsequently confirmed by serology tests. He was treated with intravenous fluids, oxygen and tetracycline and recovered fully.

- **Oxygenation** is assessed by pulse **oximetry** and those with O_2sat $< 94\%$ should have **arterial blood gas** measurements.

Further investigations may be indicated if alternative diagnoses are being considered (e.g. computed tomographic angiography for pulmonary embolism). Where there is a suspicion of aspiration pneumonia a radiocontrast oesophagogram (e.g. 'Gastrografin swallow') is useful in assessing swallowing problems. Recurrent pneumonia may be an indication of an immunodeficiency state and tests such as measurement of immunoglobulin levels or human immunodeficiency virus (HIV) testing should be performed as appropriate. Measurement of C-reactive protein may help in differentiating pneumonia from non-infective diseases and in monitoring response to treatment.

Specific investigations

These are aimed at detecting the pathogen causing the pneumonia.

- **Sputum Gram stain** may give a valuable and rapid clue to the responsible organism in an ill patient.
- **Sputum culture** is the main test used to detect bacterial causes of pneumonia but contamination of the sample by oropharyngeal organisms, prior use of antibiotics and inability to produce sputum limit the sensitivity and specificity of the test.
- **Blood cultures** should be performed on all patients admitted to hospital with moderate or severe pneumonia but are positive in only about 15% of cases.
- **Pleural fluid** should be aspirated in all patients with pleural effusions and may yield a causative organism or reveal empyema (see Chapter 16).
- **Antigen detection tests** are available for some pathogens. Pneumococcal antigen may be identified in sputum, urine, pleural fluid or blood and may be positive in cases where prior antibiotics limit the sensitivity of cultures. Direct fluorescent antibody staining may detect *Legionella pneumophila* in bronchoalveolar lavage fluid, and tests for *Legionella* antigen in urine are available. Pneumococcal and Legionella urine antigen tests should be performed in those with severe pneumonia.
- **Serological tests** allow a retrospective diagnosis of the infecting organism if a rising titre is found between acute and convalescent samples. This is most useful for some viruses and pneumonia caused by atypical organisms such as *Mycoplasma pneumoniae* or *Chlamydophila pneumoniae*.

Invasive investigations such as bronchoscopy with bronchoalveolar lavage may be indicated in severe pneumonia and in immunocompromised patients.

Treatment

General

Mild pneumonia in a fit patient can be treated **at home**. Admission to **hospital** is necessary for patients who demonstrate features of severe pneumonia, who have concomitant disease or who do not have adequate family help at home. The severity of the pneumonia should be formally assessed at the time of admission to hospital and elective transfer to an **ITU** should be considered for patients with severe disease.

Sufficient **oxygen** should be given to maintain arterial Po_2 >8 kPa (60 mmHg) and an oxygen saturation of 94–98%. Adequate non-sedative **analgesia** (e.g. paracetamol or non-steroidal anti-inflammatory drugs) should be given to control pleuritic pain. **Fluid balance** should be optimised, using intravenous rehydration as required for dehydrated patients. Chest physiotherapy may be beneficial to patients with COPD and copious secretions but is not helpful in patients without underlying lung disease. Nutritional support (e.g. oral dietary supplements, nasogastric feeding) should be given in prolonged illnesses. The patient's general condition, pulse, blood pressure, temperature, respiratory rate and oxygen saturation should be monitored frequently and any deterioration should prompt reassessment of the need for transfer to ITU. Prophylaxis of venous thromboembolism with low molecular weight heparin should be given to patients who are not fully mobile.

Antibiotic treatment

The initial choice of antibiotics is based upon an assessment of the circumstances and severity of the pneumonia. Treatment is then adjusted in accordance with the patient's response and the results of microbiology investigations. Careful patient selection for treatment and appropriate antibiotic choice are important in reducing the risks of antibiotic resistance, MRSA and *Clostridium difficile* infection. Hospitals often have their own antibiotic policies based on their particular circumstances, and specialist advice should be sought for complex problems. For **community-acquired pneumonia**, *Streptococcus pneumoniae* is the most likely pathogen and **amoxicillin** 500 mg t.d.s. orally is an appropriate antibiotic. **Doxycycline** or clarithromycin are alternatives for those allergic to penicillins. Where there is a suspicion of an 'atypical pathogen' (e.g. *Mycoplasma pneumoniae*, *Chlamydophila psittaci*) addition of a macrolide antibiotic, such as **clarithromycin** 500 mg b.d. is required. In **severe pneumonia** the initial antibiotic regimen must cover all likely pathogens and allow for potential antibiotic

resistance, and intravenous **co-amoxiclav** 1.2g t.d.s. **and clarithromycin** 500 mg b.d. are appropriate. **Cefuroxime** is an alternative for those with allergy to penicillin. In severe **hospital-acquired pneumonia**, Gram-negative bacteria are common pathogens, and a combination of an **aminoglycoside** (e.g. tobramycin) and a **third-generation cephalosporin** (e.g. ceftazidime) or an **anti-pseudomonal penicillin** (e.g. piperacillin with tazobactam) is commonly used.

Patients should be reviewed frequently and switched from intravenous to oral antibiotics when improving. Failure to respond or failure of the C-reactive protein level to fall by 50% within 4 days suggests the occurrence of a complication (e.g. empyema), infection with an unusual pathogen (e.g. *Legionella pneumophila*), the presence of antibiotic resistance or incorrect diagnosis (e.g. pulmonary embolism).

Specific pathogens

Pneumococcal pneumonia (Fig. 6.4)

Streptococcus pneumoniae is the causative organism in about **60% of community-acquired pneumonias** and in about 15% of hospital-acquired pneumonias. Research studies using tests for pneumococcal antigen suggest that it may account for many cases where no organism is identified. It is a Gram-positive coccus, which can cause infections at all levels in the respiratory tract including sinusitis, otitis media, bronchitis and pneumonia. Up to 60% of people carry *Streptococcus pneumoniae* as a **commensal in the nasopharynx** and infection is transmitted in airborne droplets. Nasopharyngeal carriage may progress to infection where there is a breach in the respiratory tract defences, and smoking and viral infections are important factors disrupting surface defence mechanisms. There are many **different serotypes that vary in their virulence**, but virulent strains can render a previously fit and healthy person critically ill within a few hours.

Pneumococcal infection in asplenic patients (e.g. post-splenectomy) is severe with a high mortality, such that these patients are usually given pneumococcal vaccination and long-term prophylactic phenoxymethylpenicillin 500 mg b.d. *Streptococcus pneumoniae* is usually **sensitive to penicillin antibiotics** (e.g. amoxicillin or

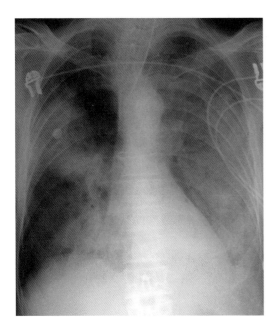

Figure 6.4 Pneumococcal pneumonia. This 70-year-old man was admitted to hospital with severe community-acquired pneumonia. He was confused with a fever of 39 °C, respiratory rate 32/min, blood pressure 90/50 mmHg and a urea of 22 mmol/L. His CURB-65 score was 5, indicating severe pneumonia. He was admitted to the ITU but died despite treatment with antibiotics, mechanical ventilation and full supportive care. Blood cultures isolated Streptococcus pneumonia. In the UK about 1 in 1000 of the population are admitted to hospital each year with community-acquired pneumonia and about 10% of these patients die.

benzylpenicillin) but antibiotic **resistance is an emerging problem** particularly in certain countries such as Spain, where about 30% of isolates are resistant, so that it is necessary to give broad antibiotic cover to a patient who has acquired pneumonia in a country with a high prevalence of antibiotic-resistant pneumococcus. **Pneumococcal vaccine** is recommended for those above 65 years of age and for patients with chronic lung disease, diabetes, renal and cardiac disease and for patients who are asplenic or immunodeficient (e.g. hypogammaglobulinaemia, HIV).

Haemophilus influenzae pneumonia

Haemophilus influenzae is a **Gram-negative bacillus**. Virulent strains are encapsulated and divided into six serological types. *Haemophilus influenzae* **type B (Hib)** is a virulent encapsulated form that causes **epiglottitis, bacteraemia, meningitis** and **pneumonia**. Hib vaccine is given to children to reduce the risk of meningitis and this vaccine also provides protection against epiglottitis. However, it is the less virulent form of the organism – **non-typeable unencapsulated *Haemophilus influenzae*** – that is a common cause of respiratory tract infection, predominantly where there has been damage to the bronchial mucosa by smoking or viral infection. *Haemophilus influenzae* often forms part of the normal pharyngeal flora. Deficient mucociliary clearance in patients with smoking-induced chronic bronchitis facilitates spread of the organism to the lower respiratory tract, where it gives rise to **exacerbations of COPD**. Spread of infection into the lung parenchyma causes **bronchopneumonia**. It is usually treated with **amoxicillin** but about 10% of strains are resistant and alternative antibiotics include co-amoxiclav (amoxicillin with clavulanic acid), trimethoprim and moxifloxacin.

Staphylococcal pneumonia

Staphylococcus aureus is a **Gram-positive coccus** that forms clusters resembling a bunch of grapes. Although it is a relatively uncommon cause of either community- or hospital-acquired pneumonia it may produce a very **severe illness with a high mortality**. It particularly occurs as a **sequel to influenza** so that anti-staphylococcal antibiotics should be given to patients who develop pneumonia after influenza. Infection may also reach the lungs via the bloodstream when staphylococcal bacteraemia arises from intravenous cannulae in hospitalised patients or from intravenous drug misuse, for example. The production of toxins (e.g. Panton-Valentine leukocidin) may cause tissue necrosis with cavitation, pneumatocele formation and pneumothoraces. It is usually sensitive to flucloxacillin, co-amoxiclav or cefuroxime. MRSA is an increasing problem. Most isolates are susceptible to vancomycin and linezolid.

Klebsiella pneumonia

Klebsiella pneumoniae is a **Gram-negative organism** that generally causes pneumonia only in **patients who have impaired resistance** to infection (e.g. **alcohol misuse, malnutrition, diabetes**) or **underlying lung disease** (e.g. bronchiectasis). It often produces severe infection with destruction of lung tissue, **cavitation** and **abscess formation**. Treatment requires attention to the underlying disease state and prolonged antibiotic therapy, guided by the results of microbiology culture and sensitivity. Often a **third-generation cephalosporin** (e.g. ceftazidime) or piperacillin with tazobactam is appropriate.

Pseudomonas aeruginosa pneumonia

Pseudomonas aeruginosa is a **Gram-negative bacillus** that is a common cause of **pneumonia in hospitalised patients**, particularly those with neutropenia and those receiving endotracheal ventilation in ITU. It is usually treated with a combination of an aminoglycoside (e.g. tobramycin) and a third-generation cephalosporin (e.g. ceftazidime) or **anti-pseudomonal penicillin** (e.g. meropenem or piperacillin with tazobactam).

Pneumonia caused by 'atypical pathogens'

'Atypical pathogens' is an imprecise term that is sometimes used in clinical practice to refer to certain pathogens that cause pneumonia such as *Mycoplasma pneumoniae*, chlamydial organisms and *Legionella pneumophila*. Characteristically, these organisms are **not sensitive to penicillins** and require treatment with **tetracycline or macrolide (e.g. clarithromycin)** antibiotics. These organisms are **difficult to culture** in the laboratory and the diagnosis is often made retrospectively by demonstrating a rising antibody titre on serological tests.

Mycoplasma pneumonia

Mycoplasma pneumoniae is a small free-living organism, which does not have a rigid cell wall and which is therefore not susceptible to antibiotics such as penicillin that act on bacterial cell walls. Infection is transmitted from person to person by infected respiratory droplets. It **particularly affects children and young adults** although any age group may be affected. Infection typically occurs in **outbreaks every 4 years** and spreads throughout families, schools and colleges. *Mycoplasma pneumoniae* typically causes an initial upper respiratory tract infection with pharyngitis, sinusitis and otitis, followed by pneumonia in about 30% of cases. A variety of **extrapulmonary syndromes** may occur and may be related to immune responses to infection. These include lymphocytic meningoencephalitis, cerebellar ataxia, peripheral neuropathy, rashes, arthralgia, splenomegaly and hepatitis. **Cold agglutinins** to type O red cells are often present and haemolytic anaemia may occur. *Mycoplasma pneumoniae* causes significant protracted morbidity but is rarely life threatening.

Chlamydial respiratory infections

There are three chlamydial species that cause respiratory disease.

- *Chlamydophila psittaci* is primarily an infection of **birds** that is transmitted to humans as a **zoonosis** (a disease contracted from animals) by inhalation of contaminated droplets. Psittacosis or ornithosis is the name given to the resultant illness which is often severe and characterised by high fever, headache, delirium, a macular rash and severe pneumonia.
- *Chlamydophila pneumoniae* was identified as a respiratory pathogen in 1986. Infection is confined to **humans** and there is no avian or animal reservoir of infection. Infection with this organism is extremely common in all age groups and spreads directly from **person to person**, with **outbreaks occurring in families, schools and colleges**. It typically produces upper respiratory disease including pharyngitis, otitis and sinusitis but may also cause pneumonia that is usually mild. Other bacterial pathogens (e.g. *S. pneumoniae*) are often identified at the same time so that the direct pathogenic role of *C. pneumoniae* is uncertain.
- *Chlamydia trachomatis* is a common cause of sexually transmitted genital tract infection and **infants** may acquire respiratory tract infection with this organism from their mother's genital tract during birth.

Legionella pneumonia

Legionella pneumophila is a **Gram-negative bacillus** that is widely distributed in nature in **water**. The organism was first identified in 1976 when an outbreak of severe pneumonia affected delegates at a convention of the American Legion, who contracted infection from a contaminated humidifier system (**Legionnaires' disease**). In sporadic cases there is often no apparent source for the infection.

Sometimes infection can be traced back to a **contaminated water system** such as a shower in a hotel room. Epidemics of infection may occur from a common source such as a contaminated humidification plant, water storage tanks or heating circuits. Infection does not spread from patient to patient. *Legionella pneumophila* typically causes a **severe pneumonia** with prostration, confusion, diarrhoea, abdominal pain and respiratory failure, with an associated high mortality. Direct fluorescent antibody staining may detect the organism in bronchoalveolar lavage fluid, and tests to detect *Legionella* antigen in urine are available, and allow rapid diagnosis. A combination of clarithromycin or a fluoroquinolone (e.g. levofloxacin, moxifloxacin, ciprofloxacin) and rifampicin is often used to treat severe *Legionella* pneumonia.

Severe acute respiratory syndrome

In 2003 there was a global epidemic of a severe acute respiratory syndrome (SARS) characterised by a severe pneumonia with a high mortality. The causative organism was identified as a new coronavirus that was named **SARS coronavirus**, and it is likely to have evolved from coronaviruses which infect civet cats and bats. The epidemic seems to have emerged from the Guandong province of China and then spread explosively with outbreaks in Hong Kong, Beijing, Taiwan, Singapore, Hanoi and Toronto. A particular feature of the epidemic was the very rapid global spread of infection by **airplane travel**. For example, an infected person travelled by plane from Hong Kong to Toronto resulting in spread of infection to a new continent. Passengers on the plane and taxi drivers in contact with the index case developed infection. The SARS coronavirus is very virulent and highly infectious spreading from person to person by direct aerosol transmission or by indirect aerosolisation from contaminated surfaces. Secondary spread of infection from patients to **healthcare workers** and medical students was a major feature of the epidemic. Tertiary cases then occurred in the families of healthcare workers. Aerosolising procedures (e.g. nebulisation, suctioning of secretions, tracheal intubation) are particularly hazardous for transmission of infection from patients to healthcare workers. Many of the patients also had diarrhoea and in some outbreaks transmission may also have occurred by aerosolisation from sewage drainage systems. In total during 2003 approximately 8500 cases of SARS occurred in 29 countries with 916 deaths, giving a global case fatality of 11%. Patients presented with fevers, rigors, myalgia, cough, vomiting and diarrhoea and typically had peripheral consolidation on chest X-ray. Treatment mainly consisted of supportive care and 20% of patients required care on an ITU. Broad-spectrum antibiotics were given for potential secondary bacterial infections and some patients seemed to benefit from corticosteroids. Currently available antiviral drugs do not seem to be effective against the SARS coronavirus. The global epidemic was brought to an end by late 2003 using **public health measures** including rapid case detection, case isolation, contact tracing and strict **infection control procedures** such as isolation of patients in negative pressure cubicles, use of respiratory protective masks, gowns, goggles and gloves. Vigilance is needed as there is the potential for the SARS coronavirus to re-emerge, and contingency plans emphasise the importance of infection control procedures in limiting spread of infection.

Immunocompromised patients

There is an increasing number of patients who are severely immunocompromised by a variety of diseases and by use of immunosuppressive drugs. Patients with neutropenia are particularly vulnerable to **bacterial infections** (e.g. *Streptococcus pneumoniae*, Gram-negative bacteria) and invasive **fungal infections** (e.g. *Aspergillus fumigatus*, *Candida albicans*), and patients with depressed T-lymphocyte function are vulnerable to **Pneumocystis pneumonia(PCP)**, **tuberculosis** and **cytomegalovirus** (**CMV**) **infection**, for example.

There are three particular situations where profound immunosuppression commonly arises:

1 Patients with cancer receiving **anti-neoplastic chemotherapy**.
2 Patients with inflammatory diseases (e.g. connective tissue diseases, Wegener's granulomatosis, inflammatory bowel disease, etc.) receiving **immunosuppressive drugs** (e.g. corticosteroids, cyclophosphamide, methotrexate, infliximab).
3 **Patients post-organ transplantation** (bone marrow, renal, lung, etc.) receiving immunosuppressive drugs (e.g. ciclosporin, azathioprine).

The problem is often that of a patient with one of these conditions presenting with pulmonary infiltrates on chest X-ray accompanied by breathlessness and sometimes fever. The infiltrates in these circumstances may be caused by pulmonary involvement by the underlying disease process, a reaction to drug treatment, infection resulting from immunosuppression or to other coincidental disease processes. Treatment is crucially dependent upon accurate diagnosis.

Assessment involves a careful clinical history and examination focusing on the clinical context and clues to aetiology (Table 6.1). Microbiology of sputum, urine and blood may identify specific pathogens. Induced sputum is particularly useful in diagnosing PCP. If these initial tests are not diagnostic it is often advisable to proceed directly to bronchoscopy with bronchoalveolar lavage for detailed microbiology. Transbronchial lung biopsy is useful in obtaining tissue for histological diagnosis but carries the risk of pneumothorax or haemorrhage. Occasionally, surgical lung biopsy is warranted.

Pulmonary complications of HIV infection (Table 6.2)

The human immunodeficiency virus (HIV) is a retrovirus that binds to the CD4 molecule of T-lymphocytes resulting in a progressive fall in the number and function of CD4 lymphocytes. The occurrence of various infections reflects the CD4 T-lymphocyte count and depends on the patient's previous and current exposure to pathogens (e.g. reactivation of previous tuberculosis or re-infection with tuberculosis in areas with a high prevalence, e.g. Africa). As the CD4 T-lymphocyte count falls there is initially an increase in the frequency of infection with common **standard pathogens** (e.g. *Streptococcus pneumoniae, Mycobacterium tuberculosis*). Then, as the CD4 count falls below about $200/mm^3$, infections with **opportunistic pathogens** (e.g. *Pneumocystis jirovecii*) develop. These are infections that do not usually cause disease in immunocompetent people. In the later stages of

---

Table 6.1 Differential diagnosis of pulmonary infiltrates in immunocompromised patients

Chest X-ray infiltrates
- Is it the underlying disease?
- Is it a reaction to drugs?
- Is it infection?
- Is it some other disease process?

Disease	Cancer	Inflammatory disease	Organ transplant
	(e.g. lymphoma, carcinoma)	(e.g. rheumatoid disease)	(e.g. bone marrow, renal)
	Lymphangitis	Interstitial lung disease	Graft versus host disease
	Lung metastases		
Drugs	Lung fibrosis or pneumonitis (e.g. bleomycin, busulfan, cyclophosphamide, methotrexate, gold, penicillamine)		
Infection	Bacterial or opportunistic infections (PCP, CMV)		
Other process	Pulmonary oedema, haemorrhage, embolism, etc.		

Pulmonary infiltrates

Clinical assessment
Microbiology of sputum, urine, blood (e.g. TB, bacteria)
Induced sputum (e.g. PCP)
Bronchoscopy and bronchoalveolar lavage (CMV, PCP, TB)
Transbronchial lung biopsy
Surgical lung biopsy (histology)

Diagnosis ⟶ **Specific treatments**

CMV, cytomegalovirus; PCP, pneumocystis pneumonia; TB, tuberculosis.

Table 6.2 Pulmonary complications of HIV infection

Infectious diseases

Bacterial infections

    Streptococcus pneumoniae

    Haemophilus influenzae

Pseudomonas aeruginosa

Tuberculosis

Opportunistic infections

    Fungal

        Pneumocystis jirovecii

        Aspergillus fumigatus

        Candida albicans

    Viral

        Cytomegalovirus

        Herpes simplex

    Mycobacterial

        Mycobacterium avium–intracellulare

Immune reconstitution syndromes

Sarcoid-like syndrome

Paradoxical deterioration of pneumonia

Non-infectious diseases

Neoplastic

    Kaposi's sarcoma

    B-cell lymphoma

    Primary effusion cell lymphoma

Inflammatory

    Lymphocytic alveolitis ($\downarrow T_L$co)

    Non-specific interstitial pneumonitis

    Lymphocytic interstitial pneumonitis

    Airways disease and emphysema

    Primary pulmonary hypertension

AIDS **neoplastic diseases** (e.g. Kaposi's sarcoma, B-cell lymphomas) occur. There is an increased incidence of **airways** disease and **emphysema** in HIV patients due to pathogenic synergy between HIV and smoking.

Bacterial respiratory infections

Patients with HIV have an increased incidence of respiratory tract infections with **sinusitis**, **bronchitis**, **bronchiectasis** and **pneumonia** occurring as a result of standard bacterial pathogens. Infection with *Streptococcus pneumoniae*, *Haemophilus influenzae* and *Staphylococcus aureus* are common, and may precede the diagnosis of HIV infection or the onset of opportunistic infections. Infection with Gram-negative organisms (e.g. *Pseudomonas aeruginosa*) occurs in more advanced disease. The clinical features may be unusual with a higher frequency of complications such as bacteraemia, abscess formation, cavitation and empyema. Pneumococcal and influenza vaccination may be helpful and sometimes long-term prophylactic antibiotics are used. With the advent of highly active anti-retroviral treatment (HAART) HIV is now a treatable condition with a good prognosis, but it is estimated that in the UK one-third of people do not know that they are infected such that they do not get the benefits of HAART. Late diagnosis is a major factor in HIV-related morbidity and mortality. Patients with a wide range of conditions (e.g. pneumonia, bronchiectasis, tuberculosis) should now be offered HIV testing.

Pneumocystis pneumonia

Pneumocystis jirovecii (formerly known as *carinii*) is a fungus that only causes disease in immuno-compromised individuals, and in HIV infection it typically occurs at the stage when the CD4 T-lymphocyte count has fallen to below 200/mm^3. PCP typically presents as a subacute illness over a few weeks with cough, dyspnoea, fever, hypoxaemia, reduced transfer factor for carbon monoxide and bilateral perihilar interstitial infiltrates on chest X-ray (Fig. 6.5). These clinical features are not specific to PCP and can be caused by a variety of other infections, and more than one pathogen may be present. The chest X-ray may be normal in early PCP and high-resolution computed tomography is more sensitive. Sometimes the radiological features are unusual showing unilateral consolidation, nodules or upper lobe consolidation, for example. Cavitating lesions may occur and pneumothorax is a recognised complication.

The **diagnosis** is usually confirmed by detecting *Pneumocystis jirovecii* using a monoclonal antibody immunofluorescent technique on specimens obtained by **sputum induction** or by bronchoscopy and **bronchoalveolar lavage**. To induce sputum the patient is given 3% hypertonic saline by nebulisation followed by chest physiotherapy. If this test is negative it is usual to proceed to bronchoalveolar lavage whereby a bronchoscope is advanced into a subsegmental bronchus and

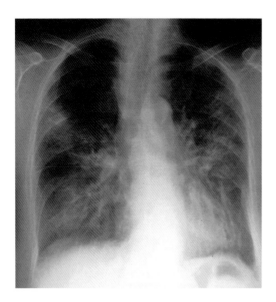

Figure 6.5 Pneumocystis pneumonia. This 28-year-old woman, who was an intravenous drug misuser, presented with fever, dyspnoea and hypoxaemia (Po_2 8.2 kPa (62 mmHg)). Chest X-ray shows diffuse bilateral perihilar and lower zone shadowing. HIV antibody test was positive and CD4 T-lymphocyte count was 100/mm^3 (normal 600–1600/mm^3). Induced sputum was positive for *Pneumocystis jirovecii* on immunofluorescent monoclonal antibody testing. The patient responded fully to high-dose intravenous co-trimoxazole, prednisolone and oxygen, and she was then commenced on long-term secondary prophylaxis with oral co-trimoxazole 3 days/week. When her pneumocystis pneumonia had been fully treated highly active anti-retroviral therapy was started.

60 mL aliquots of warmed sterile saline are instilled and aspirated. More invasive procedures, such as **transbronchial** or **surgical lung biopsy**, are usually only performed in complex cases where the aetiology of lung infiltrates cannot be determined by other tests and where a histological diagnosis is considered essential for guiding treatment decisions.

Treatment of PCP consists of high-dose intravenous **co-trimoxazole** (trimethoprim 15 mg/kg/day and sulfamethoxazole 75 mg/kg/day in four divided doses) subsequently converted to oral therapy, usually continued for 3 weeks. Side-effects (e.g. allergic rashes, nausea, marrow suppression) are common and intravenous **pentamidine or clindamycin with primaquine** are alternatives.

Patients with moderate or severe PCP (e.g. Po_2 < 9.5 kPa (70 mmHg)) benefit from the addition of **corticosteroids** (e.g. prednisolone 40 mg/day) to reduce the pulmonary inflammatory response. High-flow **oxygen** is often required and use of **continuous positive airway pressure (CPAP)** may reduce the need for **ventilation** in severe cases.

Primary prophylaxis is given to HIV-infected patients whose CD4 T-cell count is < 200/mm^3, to prevent first infection. **Secondary prophylaxis** is given to prevent recurrence in patients who have already suffered an episode of PCP. Co-trimoxazole (trimethoprim and sulfamethoxazole) 960 mg given on 3 days/week is the regimen of choice. Nebulised pentamidine given once monthly, atovaquone or a combination of oral pyrimethamine and dapsone are alternatives for patients who cannot tolerate co-trimoxazole. PCP prophylaxis may be stopped in patients who have responded well to HAART with control of viral replication and recovery of CD4 cell counts.

Mycobacterial infection

Mycobacterium tuberculosis (see also Chapter 7)

Patients with HIV infection and impaired CD4 lymphocyte function are highly susceptible to developing **reactivation** of previously acquired latent tuberculosis and to **contracting the disease from an exogenous source**, with rapid **progression to active disease**. Early in HIV disease, tuberculosis resembles the typical disease seen in non-HIV patients, with upper lobe consolidation and cavitation. In severely immunocompromised patients the clinical features may be very non-specific with fever, weight loss, malaise, diffuse shadowing on chest X-ray and a high incidence of extrapulmonary disseminated disease. Standard anti-tuberculosis treatment is given using isoniazid, rifampicin, pyrazinamide and ethambutol (see Chapter 7). Bacillus Calmette– Guérin (BCG) vaccination is contraindicated in HIV infection because of the risk of active infection developing with the live attenuated vaccine bacillus in severely immunocompromised patients. Because of their impaired cellular immunity, patients with HIV are very susceptible to contracting and transmitting tuberculosis so that strict isolation precautions are warranted, particularly for patients with multidrug-resistant tuberculosis.

Mycobacterium avium–intracellulare complex

This is an opportunistic mycobacterium that does not usually cause disease in normal subjects but which commonly infects patients with advanced AIDS, particularly when the CD4 count is $< 100/$ mm^3. Extrapulmonary disease is more common than pulmonary disease and the diagnosis of disseminated *Mycobacterium avium–intracellulare* complex (MAIC) is usually made when the organism is cultured from blood, bone marrow, lymph node or liver biopsy. The organism is not usually responsive to standard anti-tuberculosis drugs and it is treated with a combination of rifabutin, ethambutol, ciprofloxacin and clarithromycin or azithromycin.

Viral infections

Cytomegalovirus (CMV) infection is common in AIDS, usually causing systemic infection with hepatitis, retinitis, encephalitis and colitis, rather than overt pulmonary infection. CMV is often isolated from the lungs of AIDS patients but it is not always pathogenic, sometimes being present as a commensal. It is treated with ganciclovir. **Epstein–Barr virus**, **adenovirus**, **influenza** and **herpes simplex virus** may cause pneumonia in AIDS patients. Herpes simplex virus is frequently present in the mouth of HIV-infected patients so that its isolation from the respiratory tract often indicates colonisation rather than infection.

Fungal pulmonary infections

Invasive pulmonary infections with *Aspergillus fumigatus* or *Candida albicans* are unusual but may occur late in the course of AIDS. **Cryptococcal** pneumonia may occur as part of a disseminated infection but usually meningoencephalitis dominates the clinical picture. Treatment is with fluconazole, flucytosine and amphotericin. Pulmonary **histoplasmosis** and **coccidioidomycosis** may occur in areas where these fungi are endemic (e.g. USA).

HIV-related neoplasms

Kaposi's sarcoma

This is the most common malignancy in HIV-infected patients. Characteristically, it occurs in HIV-infected homosexual men and it is thought that this may relate to **co-infection with human herpes virus 8**. Pulmonary Kaposi's sarcoma is nearly always accompanied by lesions in the skin or buccal mucosa. Chest X-ray appearances are variable as the tumour may affect the bronchi, lung parenchyma, pleura or mediastinal lymph nodes. At bronchoscopy Kaposi's sarcoma appears as red or purple lesions. The diagnosis is usually made on the basis of the visual appearances in the context of mucocutaneous Kaposi's sarcoma as biopsy of the bronchial lesions is often non-diagnostic and may cause haemorrhage. Anti-retroviral therapy (HAART) may lead to regression of Kaposi's sarcoma but anti-neoplastic chemotherapy (e.g. doxorubicin, paclitaxel) is often needed.

Lymphoma

Late in the course of AIDS, high-grade **B-cell lymphomas** arise. The lungs are often involved as part of multiorgan involvement. **Primary effusion lymphoma** can occur and may present with pleural, pericardial or peritoneal effusions. The response to chemotherapy is often poor.

Interstitial pneumonitis

Patients with HIV infection may develop **nonspecific interstitial pneumonitis (NSIP)**. This presents as episodes of dyspnoea with pulmonary infiltrates, reduced gas diffusion and hypoxaemia. Bronchoalveolar lavage is negative for infection and lung biopsy shows evidence of lymphocytic inflammation. It may be a manifestation of direct HIV infection of the lung. It is often self-limiting but prednisolone may be beneficial.

Lymphoid interstitial pneumonitis is usually seen only in children with HIV infection, and the pneumonitis may be part of more widespread lymphocytic infiltration of liver, bone marrow and parotid glands with hypergammaglobulinaemia. Its aetiology is uncertain but it may be related to Epstein–Barr virus co-infection.

Primary pulmonary hypertension (see Chapter 15)

This is a rare complication of HIV infection and may result from the effect of inflammatory mediators and cytokines, produced by infection of the lung with the HIV virus, on the pulmonary circulation.

Immune reconstitution syndromes

When anti-retroviral therapy (HAART) inhibits viral replication there is a corresponding increase in the population of T-cells, enhancement of lympho-proliferative responses and increased 1L-2 receptor expression. These proinflammatory effects may give rise to certain syndromes associated with immune reconstitution. Some patients develop a **sarcoid-like granulomatous disorder** with diffuse opacities on chest X-ray, lymphadenopathy, salivary gland enlargement and elevated serum angiotensin-converting enzyme levels. **Pulmonary hypersensitivity** reactions to anti-retroviral drugs have also been described. **Paradoxical deterioration** of opportunistic pneumonia (e.g. PCP, tuberculosis), despite antibiotic therapy, may occur as the patient mounts an inflammatory response. This may be severe enough to cause acute respiratory failure and requires corticosteroid therapy. In patients presenting with HIV infection and low CD4 counts, opportunistic infections should be sought and treated before starting HAART.

 Respiratory emergencies Pneumonia

- Urgent chest X-ray is key in confirming the diagnosis.
- Enquire about travel, recent influenza, contact with animals, allergy to antibiotics.
- Full blood count, urea/electrolytes, C-reactive protein.
- Assess severity: CURB-65 score – **C**onfusion, **U**rea, **R**espiratory rate, **B**lood pressure, age.
- Assess oxygenation (O$_2$sat/blood gases), social circumstances, comorbid illness.
- In severe pneumonia send blood and sputum for microbiology cultures, and urine for pneumococcal and legionella antigen.
- Give antibiotics urgently: mild – amoxicillin 500 mg t.d.s. orally, moderate/severe – IV co-amoxiclav 1.2 g t.d.s. + clarithromycin 500 mg b.d.;
- Consider prophylaxis for venous thrombosis e.g. tinzaparin 3500 units subcutaneously daily;
- Monitor respiratory rate, O$_2$sat, pulse, blood pressure, temperature;
- Review frequently. Switch from intravenous to oral antibiotics when improving. If not improving consider other diagnoses (e.g. pulmonary embolism) or complications (e.g. empyema);
- Arrange clinical review and chest X-ray 6 weeks after discharge from hospital.

 KEY POINTS

- Pneumonia is an important cause of morbidity and mortality in all age groups.
- About 1 in 1000 of the UK population are admitted to hospital each year with pneumonia and the mortality is 10%.
- *Streptococcus pneumoniae* is the most common cause of community-acquired pneumonia, but atypical pathogens (e.g. *Mycoplasma pneumoniae*) are also important such that treatment is often with a combination of amoxicillin and a macrolide antibiotic (e.g. clarithromycin).
- Gram-negative organisms (e.g. *Pseudomonas aeruginosa*) are the main cause of hospital-acquired pneumonia such that treatment is often with antibiotics such as ceftazidime, meropenem or piperacillin with tazobactam.
- The severity of community-acquired pneumonia should be assessed using the CURB-65 score (confusion, elevated urea, respiratory rate, blood pressure, age >65 years)
- Patients with HIV are initially vulnerable to lung infections with bacteria (e.g. *Streptococcus pneumoniae, Mycobacterium tuberculosis*). When the CD4 count falls below 200/mm^3 opportunistic infections (e.g. PCP) develop.

 FURTHER READING

American Thoracic Society. Guidelines for the management of adults with hospital-acquired, ventilation-associated and healthcare-associated pneumonia. *Am J Respir Crit Care Med* 2005; **171**: 388–416.

Barlow G, Nathwani D, Davey P. The CURB65 pneumonia severity score outperforms generic sepsis and early warning scores in predicting mortality in community- acquired pneumonia. *Thorax* 2007; **62**: 253–9.

British Society for Antimicrobial Chemotherapy. Report of the working party on hospital-acquired pneumonia of the British Society for Antimicrobial Chemotherapy. *JAC* 2008; **62**: 5–34.

British Thoracic Society Community Acquired Pneumonia in Adults Guideline Group. Guidelines for the management of community acquired pneumonia in adults: update 2009. *Thorax* 2009; **64** (Suppl III): 1–61.

Hoare Z, Lim WS. Pneumonia: update on diagnosis and management. *BMJ* 2006; **332**: 1077–9.

Hull MW, Phillips P, Montaner JSG. Changing global epidemiology of pulmonary manifestations of HIV/AIDS. *Chest* 2008; **134**: 1287–98.

Ong ELC. Common AIDS-associated opportunistic infections. *Clin Med* 2008; **8**: 539–43.

Woodhead M, Blasi F, Ewig S, et al. European Society Task Force. Guidelines for the management of adult lower respiratory tract infections. *Eur Respir J* 2005; **26**: 1138–80.

World Health Organization. Consensus document on the epidemiology of severe acute respiratory syndrome (SARS). WHO, 2003 (http://www.who.int/csr/sars/en/WHOconsensus.pdf)

7

Tuberculosis

Tuberculosis is an infection caused by *Mycobacterium tuberculosis* that may affect any part of the body but most commonly affects the lungs. It is spread by a person inhaling the bacterium in droplets coughed or exhaled by someone with infectious tuberculosis.

Epidemiology

The World Health Organization estimates that **2 billion people (one-third of the world's population) have latent infection with *Mycobacterium tuberculosis*, 15–20 million people have active disease and 1.8 million deaths occur each year** from tuberculosis (95% in the developing world). One hundred years ago in the UK more than 30000 people died from tuberculosis each year (about the same as for lung cancer at present). Mortality and notification rates declined steadily from 1900 onwards because of improvement in nutritional and social factors, with a sharper decline occurring from the late 1940s onwards after the introduction of effective treatment (Fig. 7.1). Notification rates in England and Wales reached a low point of about 5000 a year in 1987 but have increased again to about 8500 a year recently. This increased incidence of tuberculosis is mainly seen in those born abroad and in ethnic minority groups. The notification rates for tuberculosis are highest in the Black African (211 per 100 000 population), Pakistani (145 per 100 000) and Indian (104 per 100 000)

ethnic groups and lowest in the White ethnic group (4 per 100 000). The recent increase in notification rates is partly the result of patterns of immigration and increasing international travel. Other groups of people with a high incidence of tuberculosis are the homeless, those misusing drugs and alcohol and people co-infected with the human immunodeficiency virus (HIV). In younger age groups tuberculosis is often newly acquired infection whereas in the older age groups it is often reactivation of latent infection acquired many years previously. Factors that reduce resistance and precipitate reactivation include ageing, alcohol misuse, poor nutrition, debility from other diseases, use of immunosuppressive drug therapy and co-infection with HIV. In the UK, overlap between the population with HIV infection (mainly young White men) and the population with tuberculosis (mainly older White people and younger immigrants from the Indian subcontinent) is limited so that only 5% of patients with acquired immune deficiency syndrome (AIDS) have tuberculosis and about 6% of patients with tuberculosis are identified as having HIV infection. However, **4.5 million people worldwide are estimated to be co-infected with HIV and tuberculosis** (98% in developing countries).

Clinical course (Fig. 7.2)

The clinical course of tuberculosis often evolves over many years and represents a complex

Respiratory Medicine Lecture Notes, Eighth Edition. Stephen J. Bourke and Graham P. Burns.
© 2011 John Wiley & Sons, Ltd. Published 2011 by John Wiley & Sons, Ltd.

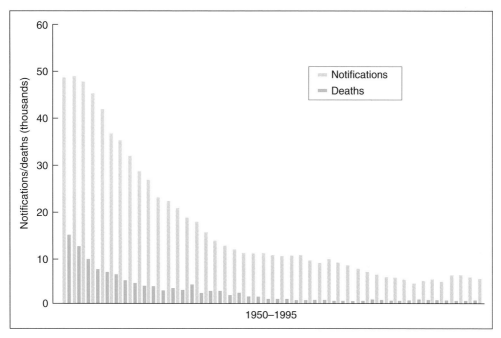

Figure 7.1 Notifications of tuberculosis and deaths in England and Wales, 1950–1995. Notifications of tuberculosis have declined from about 50 000 in 1950 to 5000 in 1987, since when notifications have increased to about 6500 per year. The recent increase is related to factors such as immigration, international travel and co-infection with HIV. (Reproduced with permission from *The Prevention and Control of Tuberculosis in the United Kingdom*, Department of Health, 1996.)

interaction between the infecting organism (*Mycobacterium tuberculosis*) and the person's specific immune response and non-specific resistance to infection. Traditional descriptions of tuberculosis divide the disease into two main patterns, **primary** and **post-primary** tuberculosis, although these are mainly based upon the characteristic evolution of the disease in the days before effective chemotherapy.

Primary tuberculosis

Primary tuberculosis is the pattern of disease seen with **first infection** in a person (often a child) **without specific immunity** to tuberculosis. Infection is acquired by inhalation of organisms from an infected individual, and the initial lesion typically develops in the peripheral subpleural region of the lung followed by a reaction in the hilar lymph nodes. The **primary complex** appears on chest X-ray as a peripheral area of consolidation (Gohn focus) with hilar adenopathy. Occasionally, erythema nodosum develops at this stage. An

immune response develops, the tuberculin test becomes positive and **healing** often takes place. This stage of the disease is often asymptomatic but may leave calcified nodules on chest X-rays representing the healed primary focus. Active **progression** of first infection may occur. Bronchial spread of infection may cause progressive consolidation and cavitation of the lung parenchyma, and pleural effusions may develop. Lymphatic spread of infection may cause progressive lymph node enlargement, which in children may compress bronchi with obstruction, distal consolidation and the development of collapse and bronchiectasis. Bronchiectasis of the middle lobe is a very typical outcome of hilar node involvement by tuberculosis in childhood. Haematogenous spread of infection results in early generalisation of disease that may cause miliary tuberculosis, and the lethal complication of tuberculous meningitis (particularly in young children). Infection spread during this initial illness may lie **dormant** in any organ of the body (e.g. bone, kidneys) for many years only to **reactivate** many years later.

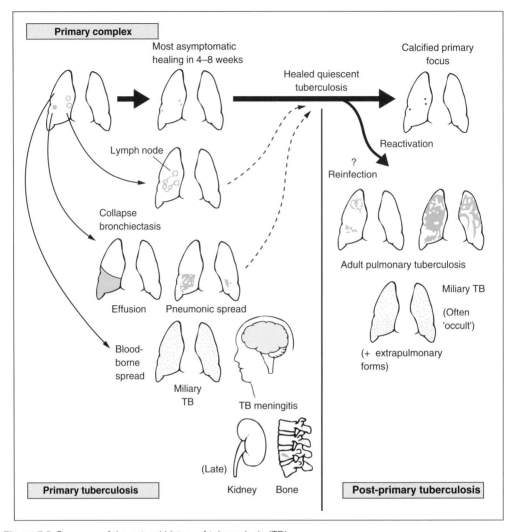

Figure 7.2 Summary of the natural history of tuberculosis (TB).

Post-primary tuberculosis

Post-primary tuberculosis is the **pattern of disease seen after the development of specific immunity**. It may occur following direct progression of the initial infection or result from endogenous **reactivation** of infection or from exogenous **re-infection** (inhalation of *Mycobacterium tuberculosis* from another infected individual) in a patient who has had previous contact with the organism and has developed a degree of specific immunity. Reactivation particularly occurs in old age and in circumstances where immunocompetence is impaired (e.g. illness, alcohol misuse, immunosuppressive drug treatment). The lungs are the most usual site of post-primary disease and the apices of the lungs are the most common pulmonary site.

Diagnosis

Clinical features

Definitive diagnosis requires identification of *Mycobacterium tuberculosis* because the clinical features of the disease are non-specific. The most typical **chest symptoms** are persistent cough, sputum production and haemoptysis. **Systemic symptoms** include fever, night sweats, anorexia and

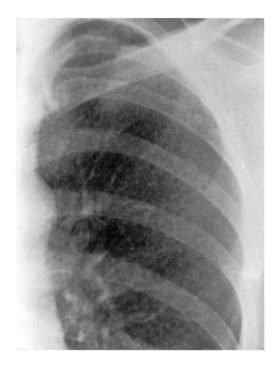

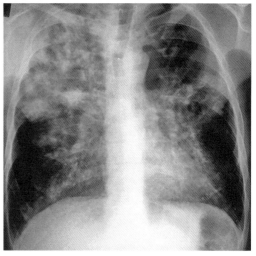

Figure 7.3 This 24-year-old man presented with malaise, fever and weight loss without any respiratory symptoms. Six months previously he had immigrated to the UK from Pakistan. X-ray shows multiple 1–2 mm nodules throughout both lungs characteristic of miliary tuberculosis. Sputum and bronchoalveolar lavage did not show acid- and alcohol-fast bacilli (AAFB). Transbronchial biopsies, however, showed caseating granulomas characteristic of tuberculosis. His symptoms resolved and the chest X-ray appearances returned to normal after 6 months of anti-tuberculosis chemotherapy.

Figure 7.4 This 68-year-old man was persuaded to consult a doctor because of a 6-month history of cough, haemoptysis, night sweats and weight loss. He suffered from alcoholism and lived in a hostel for homeless men. His chest X-ray shows cavitating consolidation throughout the right upper lobe with further areas of consolidation in the left upper and right lower lobes. Sputum acid- and alcohol-fast bacilli (AAFB) stains were positive and cultures yielded *Mycobacterium tuberculosis* sensitive to standard drugs. He was treated with directly observed anti-tuberculosis therapy. Six of 38 residents of the hostel were found to have active tuberculosis. DNA fingerprinting techniques showed that this cluster of six cases was caused by three different strains of *Mycobacterium tuberculosis* arising as a result of both reactivation of latent tuberculosis in debilitated elderly men and spread of infection within the hostel.

weight loss. A range of **chest X-ray** abnormalities occur (Figs 7.3 and 7.4). Cavitating apical lesions are characteristic of tuberculosis but such lesions may also be caused by lung cancer. Irregular mottled shadowing (particularly of the lung apices), streaky fibrosis, calcified granuloma, miliary mottling, pleural effusions and hilar gland enlargement may all be features of tuberculosis.

Diagnosis depends on the doctor having a high level of awareness of the many presentations of tuberculosis and undertaking appropriate investigations (e.g. sputum **acid- and alcohol-fast bacilli** (AAFB) staining and culture for tuberculosis) in patients with persistent chest symptoms or abnormal X-rays. A high index of suspicion is required in assessing patients who have recently immigrated from a high-prevalence area (e.g. Africa, Indian subcontinent), and in patients at risk for reactivation of infection because of factors that lower their resistance (age, alcohol misuse, debilitating disease, use of immunosuppressive drugs).

Although tuberculosis most commonly affects the lungs, **any organ in the body may be involved** and the diagnosis needs to be considered in patients with a **pyrexia of unknown origin** and in patients with a variety of indolent chronic lesions (e.g. in bone, kidney or lymph nodes). The term **miliary tuberculosis** refers to a situation where there has been widespread haematogenous dissemination of tuberculosis, usually with multiple 'millet-seed' size nodules evident on chest X-ray. Chest symptoms are often minimal and typically the patient is ill and pyrexial with anaemia and weight loss.

Laboratory diagnosis

Identification of *Mycobacterium tuberculosis* by laboratory tests may take some time and anti-tuberculosis treatment may have to be commenced based on clinical and radiological features while awaiting the results of laboratory tests. Once the diagnosis is suspected, repeated **sputum** samples should be examined by the **Ziehl–Neelsen** (ZN) method looking for AAFB that appear as red rods on a blue background. **Sputum cultures** require special media (e.g. Löwenstein–Jensen medium) and the tubercle bacillus grows slowly taking 4–7 weeks to give a positive culture and a further 3 weeks for the *in vitro* testing of antibiotic sensitivity. **Biopsy** of an affected site (e.g. pleura, lymph node, liver, bone marrow) may show the characteristic features of **caseating granuloma** (central cheesy necrosis of a lesion formed by macrophages, lymphocytes and epithelial cells). Biopsy specimens should also be submitted for mycobacterial cultures. Newer techniques are being developed to improve the speed, sensitivity and specificity of the laboratory diagnosis of tuberculosis. The **Bactec radiometric system**, for example, uses a liquid medium containing a radioactively labelled ^{14}C-labelled substance that releases $^{14}CO_2$ when metabolised, and detection of this reflects the growth of *Mycobacterium tuberculosis*. DNA techniques using the **polymerase chain reaction** are being developed and may, for example, prove useful in detecting evidence of infection in cerebrospinal fluid in tuberculous meningitis. **DNA fingerprint techniques make it possible to distinguish different strains of *Mycobacterium tuberculosis*.** This can give useful insights into the likely sources and spread of infection and help assess the relative contribution of newly acquired and reactivated infection in different populations.

Treatment (Table 7.1)

Before effective antibiotics became available in the late 1940s, about 50% of patients with sputum-positive tuberculosis died of the disease. Patients were admitted to sanatoria for bed rest, 'sunshine and fresh air' therapy and nutritional support in an attempt to enhance their own resistance to the disease. When large tuberculous cavities developed in the lungs attempts were made to collapse the cavities by inducing an artificial pneumothorax, crushing the phrenic nerve, instilling various materials outside the pleura to compress the lung (plombage) or performing thoracoplasty, whereby the ribs were excised and the lung compressed

Table 7.1 Treatment of tuberculosis

Drug	Children	Adult	Duration	Adverse effects
		Dose		
Isoniazid	10 mg/kg	300 mg	6 months	Hepatitis, neuropathy
Rifampicin	10 mg/kg	< 50 kg 450 mg	6 months	Hepatitis, rashes
		> 50 kg 600 mg		Enzyme induction
Pyrazinamide	35 mg/kg	< 50 kg 1.5 g	Initial	Hepatitis, rashes
		> 50 kg 2.0 g	2 months	Elevated uric acid
Ethambutol	15 mg/kg	15 mg/kg	2 months	Optic neuritis

- 6 months of rifampicin and isoniazid, with pyrazinamide and ethambutol for first 2 months
- Monitor treatment meticulously (e.g. monthly review)
- Check compliance
- Use directly observed therapy if problems with compliance
- Notify the diagnosis to Public Health Authorities
- Contact tracing of close family contacts.

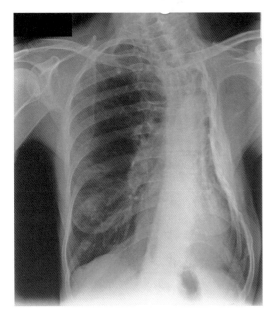

Figure 7.5 **Thoracoplasty**. Before effective antibiotics became available in the late 1940s about 50% of patients with sputum-positive tuberculosis died of the disease. At that time attempts were sometimes made to collapse large tuberculous cavities by performing a thoracoplasty, an operation in which the ribs were resected and the lung was compressed against the mediastinum

against the mediastinum (Fig. 7.5). In the late 1940s **streptomycin** and **para-amino salicylic acid** (PAS) were introduced into clinical practice and the outlook for patients with tuberculosis was revolutionised. It soon became apparent that treatment had to be **prolonged** and **combinations** of antibiotics had to be used because of the capacity of the tubercle bacillus to lie dormant in lesions for long periods and to develop resistance to antibiotics.

The current standard treatment of tuberculosis consists of **6 months** of **rifampicin** and **isoniazid**, supplemented by **pyrazinamide and ethambutol** for the first 2 months. All drugs are usually given in a single daily dose. Rifampicin and isoniazid are bactericidal drugs that kill extracellular bacilli which are actively metabolising. Both rifampicin and pyrazinamide are effective against intracellular bacilli within macrophages. Prolonged treatment is needed to eradicate bacilli lying dormant. The use of the combination of drugs also prevents the emergence of resistance from the small number of bacilli that are naturally resistant to any one of the antibiotics. Ethambutol is bacteriostatic and is included in the treatment regimen to prevent the emergence of resistance to other drug. Meticulous **supervision** of treatment is essential and patients should be seen at least monthly for prescription of medication, checking of **compliance** with treatment and monitoring for side-effects (e.g. liver function tests). Errors in the prescription of medication or failure of the patient to comply with treatment may have serious consequences with the emergence of resistant organisms. **Directly observed therapy** should be instituted for patients who have difficulty complying with treatment, whereby the patient is observed to ensure that he or she swallows the medication. Sometimes this can be achieved by giving high doses of the antituberculosis medication three times per week with the patient attending a hospital or general practice clinic to be given the medication under the supervision of a doctor or nurse. Flexible strategies are required to ensure compliance of patients with social (e.g. homelessness) or psychological (e.g. alcohol misuse, mental illness) problems and there is an important role for community health workers or trained laypersons in these circumstances.

At present, **drug-resistant tuberculosis** is rare in the initial treatment of patients from the White ethnic group in the UK, but is more common in patients who have had previous treatment or who come from Africa or the Indian subcontinent. Overall about 7.8% of isolates of *Mycobacterium tuberculosis* are resistant to isoniazid, 1.7% are resistant to rifampicin and 1.2% have multiple drug resistance. **Multidrug-resistant tuberculosis** results from inadequate previous treatment. The development of resistant organisms in a patient failing to comply with treatment may make the tuberculosis very difficult to treat, and such a patient poses a risk to public health because he or she may infect others with drug-resistant tuberculosis. Some outbreaks of multidrug-resistant tuberculosis have occurred in prisons and hospitals with high mortality rates.

The most dangerous of the **adverse reactions** to anti-tuberculosis treatment is **hepatotoxicity**, and patients should be advised to stop treatment and report for medical advice if they develop fever, vomiting, malaise or jaundice. Isoniazid, rifampicin and pyrazinamide may all cause hepatitis and allergic reactions such as **rashes**. Isoniazid may cause a **peripheral neuropathy** and this is preventable by pyridoxine 10 mg/day, which is given routinely to those at risk of neuropathy (e.g. patients with diabetes or alcohol misuse). Intermittent rifampicin may cause 'flu-like' symptoms, and the **induction of microsomal hepatic enzymes** reduces the serum half-life of drugs such as warfarin, steroids, phenytoin and oestrogen contraceptives so that patients may need adjustment in dosage of medications and may need to use alternative contraceptive measures. Rifampicin produces a reddish discoloration of urine (which may be used to monitor compliance) and may cause staining of soft contact lenses. Pyrazinamide sometimes causes initial facial flushing, and may cause an **elevation of uric acid levels** with arthralgia. Ethambutol causes a dose-related **optic neuritis**, which is rare at doses below 15 mg/kg/day. Patients should have their visual acuity checked before starting treatment and should stop the drug if visual symptoms occur, and the drug should be avoided if possible in patients with impaired renal function or pre-existing visual problems.

Latent tuberculosis

The term **'latent tuberculosis'** refers to the situation where a person has been infected with *Mycobacterium tuberculosis* at some time but does not currently have active disease. The immune response has controlled the primary infection but all viable organisms might not have been eliminated. It is estimated that there is a 5–10% risk of a person with latent tuberculosis developing active disease at some stage over the course of their life. The greatest risk of progression to disease is within 2 years of the initial infection and this is particularly relevant when undertaking contact tracing procedures of people who may have acquired infection recently from a patient with active tuberculosis. Factors that increase the risk of reactivation of latent infection include ageing, alcohol misuse, poor nutrition, co-infection with HIV and use of immunosuppressive drugs. Recently, for example, tumour necrosis factor alpha antagonists are being used in the treatment of Crohn's disease and rheumatoid arthritis, and these immunosuppressive treatments are associated with a significant risk of reactivation of latent tuberculous infection such that latent infection should be sought and treated before starting such treatments. People with latent tuberculosis are asymptomatic and usually have a normal chest X-ray. Detection of latent infection depends on demonstrating an immune response to *Mycobacterium tuberculosis* using a tuberculin test or an interferon-gamma-based blood test.

Tuberculin testing (Fig. 7.6)

Hypersensitivity to the tubercle bacillus can be detected by the intradermal injection of a purified protein derivative (PPD) of the organism. The response is of the type IV cell-mediated variety and results in a raised area of induration and reddening of the skin. In the **Mantoux test** 0.1 mL of tuberculin solution is injected intradermally (not subcutaneously) and the test is read at 48–72 hours. A positive result is indicated by redness and induration at least 10 mm in diameter. If active tuberculosis is suspected the lowest dilution may be used initially to prevent a severe reaction, and higher concentrations used if there is no reaction. The **Heaf test** is performed with a spring-loaded needled 'gun'. A drop of undiluted PPD (100 000 TU/mL) is placed on the volar surface of the forearm and the 'gun' is used to puncture through the PPD solution. The reaction is graded from I to IV according to the formation of papules and the extent of induration. A positive tuberculin test indicates the presence of hypersensitivity to tuberculin resulting from either previous infection with tubercle bacillus or from bacillus Calmette–Guérin (BCG) vaccination. A weak reaction may be non-specific and indicate contact with other non-tuberculous environmental mycobacteria. A strongly positive test in a child who has not received BCG vaccination is likely to indicate primary infection. If there is evidence of

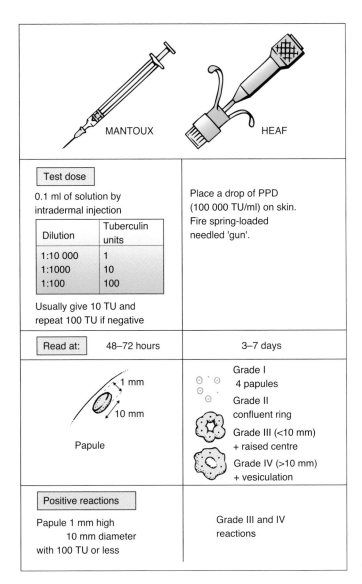

MANTOUX	HEAF
Test dose	
0.1 ml of solution by intradermal injection	Place a drop of PPD (100 000 TU/ml) on skin. Fire spring-loaded needled 'gun'.
Dilution / Tuberculin units: 1:10 000 → 1; 1:1000 → 10; 1:100 → 100	
Usually give 10 TU and repeat 100 TU if negative	
Read at: 48–72 hours	3–7 days
1 mm / 10 mm — Papule	Grade I — 4 papules; Grade II — confluent ring; Grade III (<10 mm) + raised centre; Grade IV (>10 mm) + vesiculation
Positive reactions Papule 1 mm high 10 mm diameter with 100 TU or less	Grade III and IV reactions

Figure 7.6 Tuberculin testing. In order to standardise procedures the Mantoux test is nowadays preferred to the previous Heaf test.

active disease, full anti-tuberculosis treatment is required; if there is no evidence of active disease chemoprophylaxis is advisable. A source among adult contacts of the child must be carefully sought. A negative tuberculin test makes active tuberculosis unlikely and indicates a lack of immunity so that BCG vaccination is recommended.

Interferon-gamma release assays

Tuberculin skin tests lack specificity in diagnosing *Mycobacterium tuberculosis* infection since a positive reaction may be the result of previous BCG vaccination or to exposure to non-tuberculous mycobacteria. In recent years laboratory assays have been developed that measure the release of interferon gamma from a patient's T-cells when exposed to specific antigens from *Mycobacterium tuberculosis*. There are currently two such assays available in the UK: the Quantiferon Gold assay (Cellestis Limited, Australia) and the T-spot TB assay (Oxford Immunotec, Oxford, UK). These tests require only a single blood test but it needs to be analysed in the laboratory within a few hours. These interferon-gamma blood tests are most useful in more specific diagnosis of latent *Mycobacterium tuberculosis* infection, but they should not be used as a routine diagnostic tool for active tuberculosis.

Control

Treating active disease

Prompt **identification** and **treatment** of patients with active tuberculosis limits the spread of infection. Sputum-positive patients (AAFB positive) should be considered as potentially infectious until they have completed 2 weeks of treatment. The patient's family will already have been exposed to the risk of infection so that segregation of the patient from contact with his or her family at the time of diagnosis is not useful, and most patients can be treated as outpatients. Where patients with suspected or confirmed tuberculosis are admitted to hospital they should be kept in a single room. Particular care is required if the patient has multidrug-resistant tuberculosis and these patients should be treated in a negative pressure ventilation room to prevent transmission of infection to other patients or healthcare workers.

Contact tracing

When a diagnosis of tuberculosis is made there is a statutory requirement in the UK for the doctor to **notify** the patient to the public health authorities who are then responsible for undertaking **screening of contacts**. The index patient may have acquired infection from, or transmitted infection to, someone in his or her close environment. It is usual to limit contact tracing to household contacts and to close friends sharing a similar level of contact with the index patient. If initial investigations reveal a large number of contacts with tuberculosis, consideration should be given to widening the circle of contacts who are offered screening. Typically about 1–3% of close contacts of smear-positive cases are found to have active disease, and many more have latent infection.

Screening of contacts consists of a combination of checking for symptoms of tuberculosis, **chest X-ray**, **tuberculin testing, interferon-gamma tests** and assessment of **BCG status**. Most cases of active tuberculosis are found at the first clinic visit in unvaccinated close contacts of smear-

positive disease. If the contact has not had **BCG vaccination** a tuberculin test is performed and if this is negative vaccination is recommended. For children a tuberculin test is the usual initial screening test. Children with a strongly positive tuberculin test should have a chest X-ray. A strongly positive tuberculin test with a normal chest X-ray suggests that the child has been infected with tubercle bacillus, has not developed active disease but remains at risk of doing so in the future. The risk of future activation of such latent infection is reduced by **chemoprophylaxis**; which consists of treatment for 6 months with isoniazid alone or for 3 months with isoniazid and rifampicin. In latent tuberculosis there are many thousand times fewer bacteria than in active tuberculosis and treatment with a single drug for 6 months or two drugs for 3 months is sufficient to kill dormant bacteria. Those with a negative tuberculin test should have it repeated 6 weeks later (to ensure they are not in the process of developing immunity to recently acquired infection), and if they remain tuberculin-negative BCG vaccination is advisable.

Screening of immigrants

Immigrants from areas with a high prevalence of tuberculosis (e.g. Africa, Indian subcontinent) should be screened for tuberculosis on arrival in a country of low prevalence such as the UK. Adults should have a chest X-ray and children should have a tuberculin test. Thereafter the procedure is as for close contacts, with treatment of active disease, chemoprophylaxis of latent infection or BCG vaccination as appropriate.

BCG vaccination

BCG is a live attenuated strain of tuberculosis that **provides about 75% protection against tuberculosis for about 15 years**. It is given by intradermal injection (not subcutaneous injection) and produces a local skin reaction. In the UK BCG vaccination used to be offered to children at the age of 13 years. In 2005 this policy was changed from routine to **targeted vaccination** whereby BCG vaccination is offered to infants in communities with a high incidence of tuberculosis (>40 per 100 000) and to unvaccinated individuals who come from, or whose parents come from, countries with a high prevalence of tuberculosis.

Non-tuberculous mycobacteria (atypical opportunist mycobacteria)

There are a number of other mycobacteria that can cause pulmonary disease and that do not belong to the *Mycobacterium tuberculosis* complex. These are called 'atypical' or 'opportunist' mycobacteria and the most common of these are ***Mycobacterium kansasii***, ***Mycobacterium avium-intracellulare*** complex, ***Mycobacterium malmoense***, ***Mycobacterium xenopi***, ***Mycobacterium abscessus*** and ***Mycobacterium chelonae***. They are widespread in nature and can be found in water and soil so that sometimes contamination of clinical specimens occurs from environmental sources. They act as low-grade pathogens that do not usually pose a risk to normal individuals. Infections occur mainly in patients with impaired immunity (e.g. AIDS, see Chapter 6) or in those with damaged lungs (e.g. advanced emphysema, cystic fibrosis, bronchiec-

tasis). They are often associated with chronic symptoms such as cough, sputum production, haemoptysis and weight loss. Diagnosis is made on the basis of their characteristics on laboratory culture tests. Treatment is often difficult requiring prolonged (e.g. 2 years) treatment with rifampicin and ethambutol because these organisms often show resistance to some standard anti-tuberculosis antibiotics. Some more recently developed antibiotics (e.g. clarithromycin or ciprofloxacin) may be useful in treatment. These organisms are low-grade pathogens and do not pose a threat to contacts of infected patients so that there is no need for contact tracing procedures.

 FURTHER READING

Ahmed AB, Abubakar I Delpech V, et al. The growing impact of HIV infection on the epidemiology of tuberculosis in England and Wales: 1999–2003. *Thorax* 2007; **62**: 672–6.

American Thoracic Society/Centers for Disease Control and Prevention/Infectious Diseases Society of America: Controlling tuberculosis in the United States. *Am J Respir Crit Care Med* 2005; **172**: 1169–227.

British Thoracic Society. Recommendations for assessing risk and for managing *Mycobacterium tuberculosis* infection and disease in patients due to start anti-TNF-α treatment. *Thorax* 2005; **60**: 800–5.

British Thoracic Society. Management of opportunist mycobacterial infections: Joint Tuberculosis Committee guidelines. *Thorax* 2000; **55**: 210–18.

British Thoracic Society. Chemotherapy and management of tuberculosis in the United Kingdom. *Thorax* 1998; **53**: 536–48.

Davies PDO, Drobniewski F. The use of interferon-gamma-based blood tests for the detection of latent tuberculosis infection. *Eur Respir J* 2006; **28**: 1–3.

Moore-Gillon J, Davies PD, Ormerod LP. Rethinking TB screening: politics, practicalities and the press. *Thorax* 2010; **65**: 663–5.

National Institute for Health and Clinical Excellence. *Clinical Guideline 33: Tuberculosis: Clinical Diagnosis and Management of Tuberculosis, and Measures for its Prevention and Control.* London: NICE, 2006. (http://www.nice.org.uk/CG33).

 KEY POINTS

- Worldwide, 2 billion people have latent infection with *Mycobacterium tuberculosis* and 15–20 million people have active tuberculosis.
- In the UK the incidence of tuberculosis is highest in the African, Pakistani and Indian ethnic groups, in homeless people and in people with reduced immunity because of ageing, alcohol misuse, poor nutrition, immunosuppressive drug treatments and co-infection with HIV.
- Diagnosis depends on having a high level of awareness of the presentations of tuberculosis and undertaking appropriate investigations (e.g. sputum AAFB staining) to identify *Mycobacterium tuberculosis*.
- Treatment consists of 6 months of rifampicin and isoniazid with pyrazinamide and ethambutol for the first 2 months.
- Control of tuberculosis involves detection and meticulous treatment of cases of active tuberculosis, notification of the diagnosis to the public health authorities, contact tracing to detect active or latent infection in contacts of the index case, and targeted vaccination of groups with a high incidence of tuberculosis.

8

Bronchiectasis and lung abscess

Bronchiectasis

Bronchiectasis is a chronic disease characterised by irreversible **dilatation of bronchi** caused by bronchial wall damage resulting from infection and inflammation. These morphological changes are usually accompanied by chronic **suppurative lung disease** with cough productive of purulent sputum.

Pathogenesis

Bronchiectasis represents a particular type of bronchial injury that may result from a number of different underlying disease processes. Damage to the bronchial wall causes disruption of the mucociliary escalator and allows bacteria to adhere to the respiratory epithelium and colonise the lung. **Adherence of bacteria** to the respiratory epithelium often involves specific interactions between adhesive structures on the bacterial membrane and receptors on the mucosal surface. After injury the airway epithelium undergoes a process of repair that involves the spreading, migration and proliferation of epithelial cells. During this process epithelial cells synthesise fibronectin, which is

required for cell migration, and integrin, that is important for cell-to-cell adhesion. These fibronectin and integrin epithelial receptors are used by the outer membrane protein of bacteria such as *Pseudomonas aeruginosa* as sites of bacterial adherence. Thus, key elements in the repair process of epithelium are also major receptors for bacterial adherence. The presence of bacteria at a normally sterile site stimulates an inflammatory response as part of the body's attempt to eradicate infection. However, in bronchiectasis this inflammatory response is ineffective in eradicating infection and a persistent cycle of chronic infection and inflammation ensues resulting in further tissue damage.

Bronchiectasis may be confined to one area of the lung if there is a **local** cause (e.g. bronchial obstruction by a foreign body) or may be **diffuse** if there is a generalised cause (e.g. immunoglobulin deficiency). The walls of the bronchi are infiltrated by inflammatory cells, and are scarred and dilated with reduced elastin content. The exact mechanisms giving rise to bronchiectasis are not fully understood but the disease may become self-perpetuating through a vicious circle of steps that may be initiated in a variety of ways (Fig. 8.1).

- **Impaired mucociliary clearance** leads to accumulation of secretions.
- Accumulated secretions predispose to bacterial **infection.**

Respiratory Medicine Lecture Notes, Eighth Edition. Stephen J. Bourke and Graham P. Burns.
© 2011 John Wiley & Sons, Ltd. Published 2011 by John Wiley & Sons, Ltd.

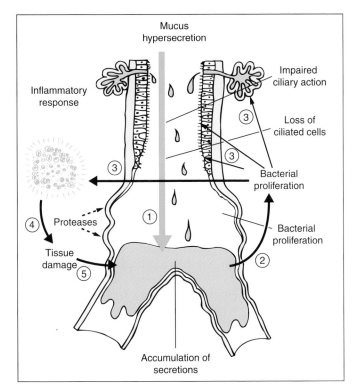

Figure 8.1 Bronchiectasis is often a progressive disease because bronchial damage results in impaired ciliary function with the accumulation of secretions, secondary bacterial infection, a destructive inflammatory response and further bronchial damage in a vicious self-perpetuating circle.

- Infection provokes an **inflammatory response**, increased mucus production and impaired ciliary function.
- Excessive inflammation causes **tissue damage.**
- Damage to the bronchial wall produces **dilatation of bronchi** and disruption of mucociliary clearance, and the vicious circle of injury progresses.

Aetiology (Table 8.1)

Infections

Severe infections are one of the most common causes of bronchial wall damage and bronchiectasis. In childhood, **pertussis (whooping cough)** or **measles** are important causes that are declining in frequency as a result of childhood vaccination programmes. In adults, bronchiectasis may complicate **pneumonia** resulting from virulent organisms such as *Streptococcus pneumoniae, Staphylococcus aureus* or *Klebsiella pneumoniae*. Better use of antibiotics has resulted in an overall decline in postinfective bronchiectasis. **Tuberculosis** is still a common cause of bronchiectasis in developing countries. Recurrent aspiration pneumonia may also lead to bronchiectasis. Many adults with **idiopathic** lower lobe bronchiectasis attribute their disease to childhood lung infections.

Bronchial obstruction

Bronchiectasis may develop in an area of lung obstructed by a bronchial **carcinoma**. In children, inhalation of a **foreign body** (e.g. peanut) may give rise to bronchial obstruction and distal bronchiectasis. **Lymph node enlargement** as part of tuberculosis may compress a bronchus and give rise to bronchiectasis. This particularly occurs in the middle lobe.

Immunodeficiency states

Patients with congenital **hypogammaglobulinaemia** or **selective immunoglobulin deficiencies** usually present with recurrent respiratory tract infections in childhood. Sometimes the diagnosis is not established until adulthood when bronchiectasis may have developed. All patients with bronchiectasis should have measurement of immunoglobulins IgG, IgA and IgM with serum electrophoresis. Patients with immunoglobulin deficiencies require specialist immunology assessment

Table 8.1 **Aetiology of bronchiectasis**

Severe infection
   Childhood pertussis
   Bacterial pneumonia
   Recurrent aspiration pneumonia
   Tuberculosis

Bronchial obstruction
   Foreign body (e.g. peanut)
   Bronchial carcinoma
   Lymph node enlargement

Immunodeficient states
   Hypogammaglobulinaemia
   Immunodeficiency as a result of lymphoma
   HIV infection

Allergic bronchopulmonary aspergillosis
   Cystic fibrosis (see Chapter 9)
   Ciliary dysfunction
   Primary ciliary dyskinesia
   Kartagener's syndrome

Associated diseases
   Ulcerative colitis
   Rheumatoid arthritis
   Idiopathic bronchiectasis

with regard to intravenous immunoglobulin replacement therapy. Baseline specific antibody levels to tetanus toxoid and the capsular polysaccharides of *Streptococcus pneumoniae* and *Haemophilus influenzae* type b should be measured. If baseline levels are low the adequacy of the humoral response should be assessed by immunisation with appropriate vaccines and re-measurement of antibody levels after 21 days. Immunoglobulin deficiencies may also arise secondary to malignancies such as **lymphoma** or **myeloma**. Patients with **human immunodeficiency virus(HIV) infection** are also susceptible to recurrent bacterial infections and bronchiectasis, and HIV testing should be offered when appropriate (see Chapter 6).

Allergic bronchopulmonary aspergillosis (Fig. 8.2)

Aspergillus fumigatus is a ubiquitous fungus that may **colonise** the respiratory tract as an incidental finding without giving rise to symptoms. Patients with lung cavities (e.g. post-tuberculosis or sarcoidosis) may develop an **aspergilloma**, which is a ball of fungal hyphae that appears on X-ray as a mass in the centre of a cavity surrounded by a halo of radiolucency (Fig. 8.3). This is often asymptomatic, but associated inflammation may cause bronchial artery hypertrophy and haemoptysis requiring surgical resection or therapeutic bronchial artery embolisation. **Invasive aspergillosis** (e.g. necrotising pneumonia or fungaemia) occurs in immunocompromised patients.

Patients with **asthma** may develop an allergic reaction to *Aspergillus* and demonstrate **precipitating antibodies** to *Aspergillus* in their serum and positive responses to **skin prick tests**. Some of these patients develop **allergic bronchopulmonary aspergillosis** in which there is intense bronchial inflammation with **eosinophilia** and **high IgE** levels in the blood. Eosinophilic infiltrates in the lung give rise to **fleeting X-ray shadows**. Thick **mucus plugs** cause obstruction of small bronchi and give rise to **bronchiectasis** that is usually proximal in location. All patients with bronchiectasis should have measurement of serum IgE, skin prick testing or specific serum IgE to *Aspergillus fumigatus* and aspergillus precipitins. Treatment requires suppression of the inflammatory immune response by oral prednisolone and high-dose inhaled corticosteroids.

Ciliary dyskinesia

The epithelial cells of the bronchi possess cilia that beat in an organised way so as to move particles in the layer of mucus on their surface upwards and out of the lung. This **mucociliary escalator** is an essential clearance mechanism. Ciliary function is impaired by cigarette smoke and bacterial toxins. Viral infections may cause widespread shedding of ciliated respiratory cells. Bronchial damage of whatever cause often disrupts the mucociliary clearance mechanism impairing the lung defence mechanisms and perpetuating the vicious circle of bronchiectasis.

Primary ciliary dyskinesia is an autosomal recessive condition in which there is an abnormality of the ultrastructure of cilia throughout the body such that they do not beat in a coordinated fashion. Failure of ciliary function in the respiratory tract gives rise to otitis, sinusitis and bronchiectasis. The tail of sperm is also a ciliary structure and males with primary ciliary dyskinesia are subfertile. It is thought that cilia are also responsible for the

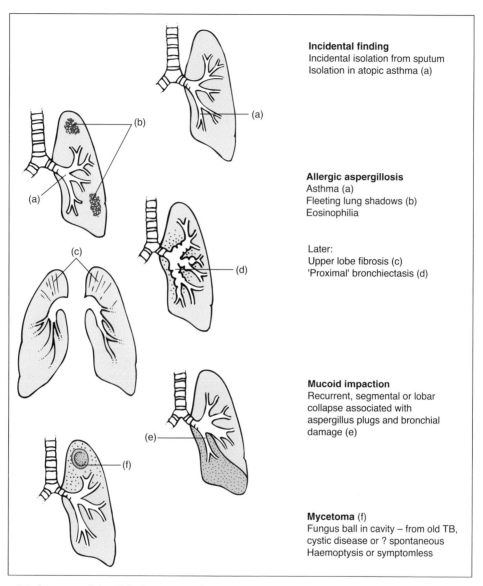

Incidental finding
Incidental isolation from sputum
Isolation in atopic asthma (a)

Allergic aspergillosis
Asthma (a)
Fleeting lung shadows (b)
Eosinophilia

Later:
Upper lobe fibrosis (c)
'Proximal' bronchiectasis (d)

Mucoid impaction
Recurrent, segmental or lobar
collapse associated with
aspergillus plugs and bronchial
damage (e)

Mycetoma (f)
Fungus ball in cavity – from old TB,
cystic disease or ? spontaneous
Haemoptysis or symptomless

Figure 8.2 Summary of the clinical spectrum of *Aspergillus* lung disease. TB, tuberculosis.

normal rotation of internal structures in embryonic life so that failure of ciliary function results in random rotation with about 50% of patients having dextrocardia and situs inversus (e.g. appendix in left iliac fossa). Ciliary dyskinesia with situs inversus is known as **Kartagener's syndrome** (Fig. 8.4).

An estimate of ciliary function can be obtained by timing the nasal clearance of saccharin. In this test a 1-mm cube of saccharin is placed on the inferior turbinate of the nose. The time from placing the particle to the patient tasting the saccharin is usually less than 30 minutes, and is a measure of nasal ciliary clearance. However, this test is difficult to perform and a simple cold can disrupt mucociliary clearance for up to 6 weeks. Patients with primary ciliary dyskinesia characteristically have low exhaled nasal nitric oxide levels. In men, sperm motility may be assessed by microscopy of seminal fluid. However, definitive testing for primary ciliary dyskinesia requires referral to a designated specialist centre where a brush biopsy of nasal mucosa is performed. The ultrastructure

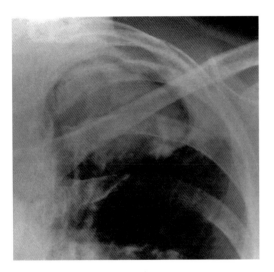

Figure 8.3 This 70-year-old woman had suffered from tuberculosis in the 1950s that had resulted in bilateral apical lung fibrosis and severely impaired lung function (forced expiratory volume in 1 second, 0.5 L; forced vital capacity, 1.1 L). She presented with recurrent major haemoptysis, and chest X-ray showed features characteristic of an aspergilloma with an opacity in the left apex surrounded by a halo of radiolucency. *Aspergillus* hyphae were seen on sputum microscopy and *Aspergillus* precipitins were present in her blood. Tests for carcinoma and tuberculosis were negative. Bronchial arteriography showed marked hypertrophy of the bronchial artery to the left upper lobe and therapeutic embolisation was performed resulting in resolution of the haemoptysis.

of cilia can then be assessed by electron microscopy and ciliary function can be assessed by microscope photometry that assesses the ciliary beat frequency and pattern.

Cystic fibrosis

Cystic fibrosis usually presents in early childhood with recurrent respiratory infections and failure to thrive due to pancreatic insufficiency (see chapter 9). Nowadays it is usually detected by newborn screening. However more than 1700 mutations of the cystic fibrosis gene have been described and the clinical spectrum of the disease has been extended to include patients with less severe lung disease and normal pancreatic function. Some of these patients present with bronchiectasis in adulthood. As such it is recommended that all children and adults up to the age of 40 years should have **sweat**

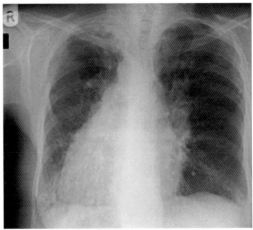

Figure 8.4 This 60-year-old woman has primary ciliary dyskinesia, which is an autosomal recessive disorder in which abnormalities of ciliary structure and function give rise to chronic upper and lower respiratory tract infections such as otitis, sinusitis and bronchiectasis. Cilia are also involved in the normal rotation of internal structures in embryonic life and failure of ciliary function results in random rotation such that 50% of these patients have dextrocardia and situs inversus (e.g. heart on the right side and appendix in the left iliac fossa).

tests and gene analysis for cystic fibrosis. The diagnosis of cystic fibrosis should also be considered in older patients with persistent isolation of *Staphylococcus aureus*, progressive bronchiectasis or associated features such as malabsorption, pancreatitis, nasal polyposis or male infertility.

Associated diseases

Patients with certain diseases seem to have an increased incidence of bronchiectasis. These diseases include rheumatoid arthritis, ulcerative colitis, Crohn's disease and coeliac disease but the mechanism by which bronchiectasis arises in these diseases is unclear.

Clinical features

The cardinal feature of bronchiectasis is **chronic cough** productive of copious **purulent sputum**. There is considerable variation in the severity of the disease and mild cases are often misdiagnosed as chronic bronchitis. **Haemoptysis** is common and may occasionally be severe, requiring therapeutic embolisation of hypertrophied bronchial arteries to control the bleeding source. Infective exacerbations may be associated with **fever** and **pleuritic pain**. Chronic severe bronchiectasis may cause **malaise**, **weight loss** and **halitosis** (foul breath). Coarse **crackles** may be audible over affected areas and **clubbing** is sometimes present. Systemic spread of infection (e.g. cerebral abscess) and secondary amyloidosis are now very rare because of control of infection by antibiotics.

Investigations (Fig. 8.5)

A **chest X-ray** may show features of bronchiectasis such as peribronchial thickening, which is evident as parallel tramline shadowing, or cystic dilated bronchi. However, the chest X-ray is often normal in less severe cases and high-resolution **computed tomography(CT)** is the key investigation in confirming the diagnosis and in determining the location and extent of the disease. The CT features of bronchiectasis are bronchial dilatation (internal bronchial lumen diameter greater than the accompanying pulmonary artery) and lack of the normal tapering of the bronchi peripherally. Diffuse bronchiectasis is seen in immune deficiency, ciliary dyskinesia and cystic fibrosis. Localised bronchiectasis may follow an episode of pneumonia.

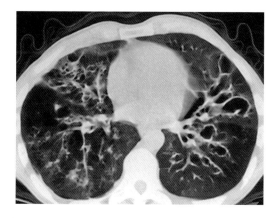

Figure 8.5 This 50-year-old man had suffered pertussis pneumonia at the age of 18 months. He had chronic cough productive of copious purulent sputum isolating *Pseudomonas aeruginosa* on culture. CT showed extensive bilateral bronchiectasis with dilatation of bronchi, cyst formation and patchy peribronchial consolidation. He was treated with postural drainage physiotherapy, salbutamol, long-term nebulised antibiotics (colistin) and intermittent courses of oral ciprofloxacin or intravenous ceftazidime.

Having confirmed the presence of bronchiectasis, an attempt should be made to diagnose the underlying cause of the bronchiectasis, and further specific tests performed as indicated, for example *Aspergillus* **precipitins** and skin prick tests (allergic bronchopulmonary aspergillosis), **immunoglobulin level** (hypogammaglobulinaemia), **ciliary function tests** (ciliary dyskinesia), and **sweat tests** with genetic analysis for cystic fibrosis. **Bronchoscopy** is useful in detecting any endobronchial obstruction in cases of localised bronchiectasis. **Sputum microbiology** should be performed to define what infective organisms are present as a guide to antibiotic treatment. Mycobacterial cultures should also be performed as non-tuberculous mycobacteria (e.g. Mycobacterium avium complex) are sometimes associated with bronchiectasis (see chapter 7). **Lung function tests** define the level of any deficit and help determine whether bronchodilator drugs may be helpful.

Treatment

- **Specific treatment** of the underlying cause is rarely possible but relief of endobronchial obstruction (e.g. foreign body) is the key treatment for some patients, intravenous immunoglobulin replacement therapy is essential for patients with hypogammaglobulinaemia, and suppression of the inflammatory response by oral or inhaled corticosteroids is important in allergic aspergillosis.
- **Chest physiotherapy** is an effective treatment in clearing secretions. Patients should receive instruction from a physiotherapist in airway clearance techniques such as the active cycle of breathing technique, oscillating positive expiratory pressure devices (e.g. flutter, Acapella devices), autogenic drainage and postural drainage using gravity-assisted positions based on the location of the bronchiectasis on CT scans. Nebulised 7% **hypertonic saline** may be useful in improving sputum clearance. It sometimes provokes bronchoconstriction such that pre-treatment with a bronchodilator (e.g. salbutamol, terbutaline) is needed. Oral carbocisteine is sometimes used as a **mucolytic agent** but nebulised DNase, used in cystic fibrosis, is not effective in other forms of bronchiectasis.
- **Antibiotics** are used to suppress chronic infection and to treat exacerbations. High doses are sometimes required to penetrate the scarred bronchial mucosa and purulent secretions and

it is often recommended that treatment should be prolonged for 14 days. The choice of antibiotics is guided by the results of sputum microbiology. *Haemophilus influenzae* and *Streptococcus pneumoniae* are common and are usually sensitive to amoxicillin. Long-term oral antibiotics (e.g. amoxicillin, doxycycline) are sometimes used in severe disease but there is a risk of promoting antibiotic resistance. *Moraxella catarrhalis* is usually associated with the production of beta-lactamase so that co-amoxiclav or ciprofloxacin may be useful. *Pseudomonas aeruginosa* is common in severe disease and may be treated by oral ciprofloxacin or intravenous anti-pseudomonal antibiotics (e.g. meropenem, ceftazidime, tobramycin). Chronic pseudomonas infection is an adverse feature associated with more severe bronchiectasis. When this organism is first identified an attempt should be made to eradicate it using oral ciprofloxacin 750 mg b.d. for 14 days. If this is not successful options include a 4-week course of ciprofloxacin with nebulised colistin, or a course of intravenous anti-pseudomonas antibiotics. If pseudomonas is isolated persistently long-term nebulised antibiotics (e.g. colistin, tobramycin) may be used to suppress the infection and associated inflammation.. Long-term treatment with a macrolide antibiotic (e.g. azithromycin) may reduce the frequency of exacerbations of bronchiectasis, possibly by an anti-inflammatory rather than an anti-microbial effect. Pneumococcal and influenza vaccinations are recommended for patients with bronchiectasis.

- **Bronchodilator drugs** (e.g. salbutamol, terbutaline) and an **inhaled steroid** (e.g. beclometasone, budesonide, fluticasone) are indicated only where there is associated reversible airways obstruction.
- **Surgical excision** is a potential treatment for the few patients who have localised disease and troublesome symptoms. **Lung transplantation** is an option for some patients whose disease has progressed to respiratory failure.

Lung abscess (Fig. 8.6)

A lung abscess is a **localised collection of pus within a cavitated necrotic lesion in the lung parenchyma**. The chest X-ray characteristically shows a cavitating lesion containing a fluid level. The patient typically complains of cough with expectoration of large amounts of foul material often accompanied by haemoptysis, fever, weight loss and malaise. It is important to distinguish between a lung abscess and other causes of cavitating lung lesions, such as a squamous cell carcinoma, and bronchoscopy or percutaneous fine-needle aspiration of the lesion may be required.

The infection giving rise to a lung abscess may arise via a number of routes. Oropharyngeal

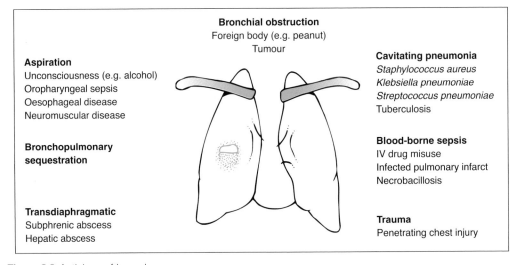

Bronchial obstruction
Foreign body (e.g. peanut)
Tumour

Aspiration
Unconsciousness (e.g. alcohol)
Oropharyngeal sepsis
Oesophageal disease
Neuromuscular disease

Bronchopulmonary sequestration

Transdiaphragmatic
Subphrenic abscess
Hepatic abscess

Cavitating pneumonia
Staphylococcus aureus
Klebsiella pneumoniae
Streptococcus pneumoniae
Tuberculosis

Blood-borne sepsis
IV drug misuse
Infected pulmonary infarct
Necrobacillosis

Trauma
Penetrating chest injury

Figure 8.6 Aetiology of lung abscess.

aspiration is the most common cause and occurs in states of unconsciousness (e.g. alcohol excess, epilepsy, anaesthesia), and where there is dysphagia as a result of oesophageal or neuromuscular disease. Infection of the upper airways (e.g. sinusitis, dental abscess) may be an important source of bacteria, and anaerobic organisms (e.g. *Fusobacteria, Prevotella*) are common. Infection may arise distal to **bronchial obstruction** caused by a tumour or foreign body (e.g. inhaled peanut). The centre of an area of destructive **pneumonia** may break down to form a lung abscess particularly when the pneumonia results from *Staphylococcus aureus* or *Klebsiella pneumoniae*. Tuberculosis may present as a lung abscess. **Blood-borne** infection may occur by intravenous injection of infected material by drug addicts. Pulmonary emboli may cause pulmonary infarction, with secondary infection giving rise to an abscess. Penetrating **chest trauma** is an unusual cause of lung abscess. **Transdiaphragmatic** spread of infection may occur from a subphrenic abscess (e.g. post-cholecystectomy) or a hepatic abscess (e.g. amoebic abscess).

Drainage of pus from the abscess cavity is a key aspect of treatment. This can often be achieved by bronchial drainage using postural drainage physiotherapy. Sometimes percutaneous drainage is achieved by positioning a catheter drainage tube under radiological guidance. Prolonged **antibiotic** therapy is given in accordance with the likely organism and the results of microbiology tests (e.g. metronidazole for anaerobic infections). **Surgical excision** of the abscess cavity is sometimes required where medical treatment fails.

Necrobacillosis

Necrobacillosis (Lemière's disease) is an unusual cause of lung abscess that is associated with a very characteristic clinical picture first described by Lemière. Typically, a young adult develops a **severe sore throat** with **cervical adenopathy** because of infection with the anaerobe, *Fusobacterium necrophorum*. This is associated with a local venulitis followed by a **septicaemic illness** with haematogenous spread of infection. The lungs are frequently involved with multiple **abscesses** forming, often with a **pleural empyema** and evidence of infection elsewhere (e.g. **septic arthritis**, **osteomyelitis**). Prolonged anaerobic blood culture is

required to identify the organism, which is sensitive to metronidazole.

Bronchopulmonary sequestration

Bronchopulmonary sequestration is a congenital anomaly in which an **area of lung is not connected to the bronchial tree** (i.e. 'sequestered') and has an **anomalous blood supply** usually from the aorta. If infection develops in the sequestration it often progresses to an abscess because of lack of drainage to the bronchial tree. Surgical resection is required but pre-operative bronchial arteriography is necessary to identify the anomalous blood supply.

 KEY POINTS

- Bronchiectasis is characterised by permanent dilatation of bronchi due to bronchial damage caused by infection and inflammation.
- High-resolution CT is the key investigation in confirming the diagnosis.
- Investigations for specific causes of bronchiectasis include sweat tests (cystic fibrosis), immunoglobulin levels (hypogammaglobulinaemia), *Aspergillus* preciptins (allergic aspergillosis) and ciliary tests (primary ciliary dyskinesia).
- Treatment involves chest physiotherapy, antibiotics, inhaled bronchodilators, and specific treatment of any underlying cause.
- A lung abscess is a localised collection of pus within a cavitated necrotic lesion in the lung parenchyma.

 FURTHER READING

Barbato A, Frischer T, Kuehni CE, et al. Primary ciliary dyskinesia: a consensus statement on diagnostic and treatment approaches in children. *Eur Respir J* 2009; **34**: 1264–76.

Davies G, Wilson R. Prophylactic antibiotic treatment of bronchiectasis with azithromycin. *Thorax* 2004; **59**: 540–1.

DeBoeck K, Wilschanski M, Castellani C, et al. Cystic fibrosis: terminology and diagnostic algorithms. *Thorax* 2006; **61**: 627–35.

Ooi GC, Khong PL, Chan-Yeung M, et al. High-resolution CT quantification of bronchiectasis: clinical and functional correlation. *Radiology* 2002; **225**: 663–72.

Pasteur MC, Bilton D, Hill AT on behalf of the British Thoracic Society Guideline for (non-CF) Bronchiectasis Group. British Thoracic Society guideline for non-CF bronchiectasis. *Thorax* 2010; **65**: Suppl 1: 1–64.

Shoemark A, Ozerovitch L, Wilson R, et al. Aetiology in adult patients with bronchiectasis. *Respir Med* 2007; **101**: 1163–70.

Ten Hacken NH, Van der Molen T. Bronchiectasis. *BMJ* 2010; **341**: 146–7.

The primary ciliary dyskinesia family support group (www.pcdsupport.org.uk/).

Cystic fibrosis

Introduction

Cystic fibrosis is the most common life-limiting inherited disease of Caucasians. **It affects about 1 in 2500 live births** in the UK and is inherited in an autosomal recessive manner. About **1 in 25 of the population is a carrier** of the disease.

The basic defect

Cystic fibrosis is caused by mutations of a large gene on the long arm of chromosome 7 that codes for a 1480-amino-acid protein, named **cystic fibrosis transmembrane conductance regulator (CFTR)**. The most common mutation is traditionally designated ΔF508 (F508del), in which deletion of three base pairs of the gene results in the loss of phenylalanine ('delta F') at position 508 of the protein. This causes misfolding of the mutant CFTR that is then degraded in the endoplasmic reticulum such that no CFTR protein reaches the cell membrane. CFTR functions as a cyclic AMP-dependent **chloride channel** in the apical membrane of epithelial cells and the primary physiological defect in cystic fibrosis is reduced chloride conductance at epithelial membranes, most notably in the respiratory, gastrointestinal, pancreatic, hepato-biliary and reproductive tracts. Other ion channels such as the epithelial sodium channel (ENaC) and calcium activated chloride channels (CaCC) also play an important role in membrane physiology (Figure 9.1). Although CFTR's main function is as a chloride channel it has other regulatory roles including inhibition of sodium transport through ENaC, inhibition of CaCC, regulation of intracellular vesicle transport and regulation of bicarbonate– chloride exchange. In sweat ducts, failure of reabsorption of chloride ions results in elevated concentrations of chloride and sodium in the sweat, a characteristic feature of the disease and the basis for the sweat test used in diagnosis.

More than 1800 mutations of the CFTR gene have now been identified and these are divided into five major classes according to their effect on CFTR function:

- class I: defective protein synthesis (e.g. G542X);
- class II: defective protein processing (e.g. ΔF508);
- class III: defective protein activation (e.g. G551D);
- class IV: impaired chloride conductance (e.g. R117H);
- class IV: reduced amount of functioning CFTR (e.g. A455E).

Generally mutations in classes I–III result in no CFTR function at the cell membrane. This is typically associated with more severe clinical disease. In class IV and V mutations the mutant CFTR may have some degree of function and this may be associated with less severe clinical disease. However, many other factors influence the clinical phenotype.

Respiratory Medicine Lecture Notes, Eighth Edition. Stephen J. Bourke and Graham P. Burns.
© 2011 John Wiley & Sons, Ltd. Published 2011 by John Wiley & Sons, Ltd.

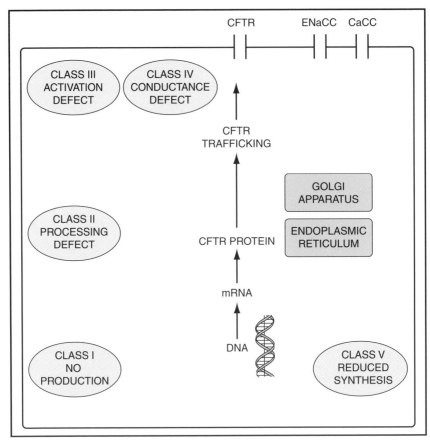

Figure 9.1 The cystic fibrosis gene codes for a 1480-amino-acid protein named cystic fibrosis transmembrane conductance regulator (CFTR) that is trafficked through the cell via the endoplasmic reticulum and Golgi apparatus and inserted into the apical membrane where it functions as a cAMP-dependent chloride channel. Class I mutations disrupt synthesis of CFTR and include nonsense and frameshift mutations leading to premature termination codons (PTC) and lack of protein production. Class II mutations result in misfolded CFTR that is then degraded in the endoplasmic reticulum. In class III mutations CFTR reaches the apical membrane but is not activated. Class IV mutations result in reduced CFTR conductance. In Class V mutations there is reduced synthesis of normal CFTR and therefore reduced CFTR function at the cell membrane. CFTR has additional regulatory effects on epithelial sodium channels (ENaC) and on calcium activated chloride channels (CaCC).

Lungs

In the bronchial mucosa reduced chloride secretion and increased sodium reabsorption results in **secretions of abnormal viscosity** with reduced water content of the airway surface liquid and reduced depth of the periciliary fluid, which disrupts mucociliary clearance. The **high salt content** of the airway surface fluid **inactivates defensins** that are naturally occurring antimicrobial peptides on the epithelial surface. There is some evidence that the CFTR also has a role in the normal uptake and processing of *Pseudomonas aeruginosa* from the respiratory tract. Patients with cystic fibrosis also have abnormal mucus glycoproteins that act as binding sites such that **bacteria adhere to the mucosa** and proliferate. Thus, the gene defect results in dysfunction of CFTR and predisposes to severe chronic lung infection by a variety of mechanism at the cellular level. The inflammatory response is unable to clear the infection and a vicious cycle of **infection** and **inflammation** develops, progressing to lung damage, **bronchiectasis**, **respiratory failure** and **death**.

Gastrointestinal tract

In the **pancreas** the abnormal ion transport results in the plugging and obstruction of ductules with progressive destruction of the gland. The pancreatic enzymes (e.g. lipase) fail to reach the small intestine and this results in **malabsorption** of fats with steatorrhoea and failure to gain weight. Progressive destruction of the endocrine pancreas may cause **diabetes**. Abnormalities of bile secretion and absorption cause an increased incidence of **gallstones** and **biliary cirrhosis**. Sludging and desiccation of intestinal contents probably accounts for the occurrence of **meconium ileus** (neonatal intestinal obstruction) in about 10% of babies with cystic fibrosis, and for the development of **distal intestinal obstruction syndrome** (meconium ileus equivalent) in older children and adults.

Clinical features (Fig. 9.2)

Infants and young children

About 10% of children with cystic fibrosis present at birth with **meconium ileus**, a form of intestinal obstruction caused by inspissated viscid faecal material resulting from lack of pancreatic enzymes and from reduced intestinal water secretion. More than half of children affected by cystic fibrosis have obvious malabsorption by the age of 6 months with **failure to thrive** associated with abdominal distension and copious offensive stools from **steatorrhoea** as a result of malabsorbed fat. **Rectal prolapse** occasionally occurs. Recurrent **respiratory infections** rapidly become a prominent feature with cough, sputum production and wheeze. Newborn screening programmes are being introduced that allow the early diagnosis of cystic fibrosis, before the onset of symptoms and complications.

Older children and adults

Respiratory disease (Fig. 9.3)

Persistent cough and purulent sputum characterise the development of **bronchiectasis**. Progressive lung damage is associated with the development of digital clubbing and progressive **airways obstruction**, sometimes associated with wheeze. Serial measurements of forced expiratory volume in 1 second (FEV_1) give an indication of the severity and progression of the disease. Some patients show a significant asthmatic component with reversible airways obstruction and some develop colonisation of the bronchi by *Aspergillus fumigatus* and may show features of allergic bronchopulmonary

aspergillosis (see Chapter 8). Initially, the typical organisms isolated in sputum cultures are ***Staphylococcus aureus***, *Haemophilus influenzae* and *Streptococcus pneumoniae*. By the teenage years many have become infected with mucoid strains of ***Pseudomonas aeruginosa***. ***Burkholderia cepacia complex*** is a group of Gram-negative plant pathogens that cause onion rot. It was initially thought that these organisms were not pathogenic to humans but in the 1980s it became apparent that patients with cystic fibrosis were vulnerable to these bacteria and that infection could spread from patient to patient in an epidemic way, particularly among children with cystic fibrosis in close social contact in holiday camps, for example. The clinical course of patients with *Burkholderia cepacia* complex infection is very variable but some show an accelerated rate of decline in lung function and some develop a fulminant necrotising pneumonia, the so-called **'cepacia syndrome'** (Fig. 9.4). It is now recognised that there are many different strains of this bacterium but *Burkholderia cenocepacia* genomovar III is associated with the worst prognosis. Because of the potential for transmission of infection between patients with cystic fibrosis it is now standard practice to segregate patients with different infections such that they attend different clinics and wards, and social contact between patients with cystic fibrosis is discouraged. Non-tuberculous mycobacteria (e.g. *Mycobacterium abscessus*) can also colonise and infect the lungs in cystic fibrosis.

As the cycle of infection and inflammation progresses, lung damage worsens with deteriorating airways obstruction, destruction of lung parenchyma, impairment of gas exchange and the development of **hypoxaemia**, **hypercapnia** and **cor pulmonale**. The persistent pulmonary inflammation provokes hypertrophy of the bronchial arteries, and **haemoptysis** becomes common. Occasionally, when severe bleeding occurs, therapeutic embolisation of the bronchial arteries may be required. **Pneumothorax** occurs in about 5–10% of patients with advanced disease and may require prompt tube drainage. Pleurodesis may be required for recurrent pneumothoraces but this should be performed with care so as not to compromise future potential lung transplantation.

Gastrointestinal disease

About 85% of patients with cystic fibrosis have **pancreatic insufficiency** with **malabsorption of**

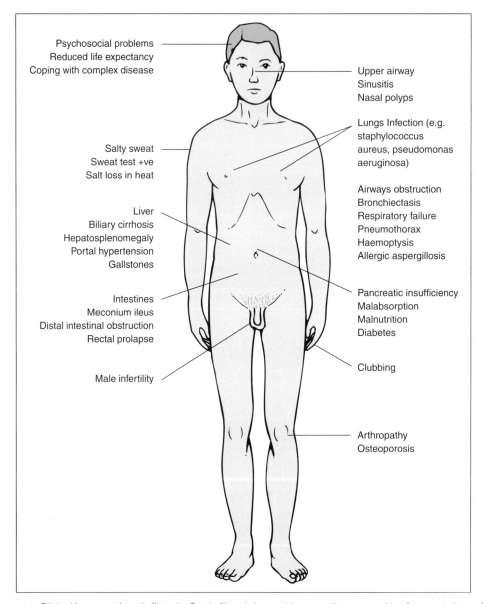

Figure 9.2 Clinical features of cystic fibrosis. Cystic fibrosis is a multisystem disease resulting from mutations of the gene that codes for a protein, cystic fibrosis transmembrane conductance regulator (CFTR), that functions as a chloride channel on epithelial membranes. Failure of chloride conductance results in abnormal secretions and organ damage in the respiratory, pancreatic, hepatobiliary, gastrointestinal and reproductive tracts.

fat because of lack of lipase. Unless these patients receive adequate pancreatic enzyme supplements they develop steatorrhoea with frequent bulky offensive stools and failure to gain weight. Progressive destruction of the endocrine pancreas is manifest by an increasing incidence of **diabetes** as these patients get older. A variety of **hepatobiliary** **abnormalities** occur including fatty liver, gallstones and focal biliary fibrosis, and about 5% of patients develop multinodular cirrhosis with hepatosplenomegaly, portal hypertension, oesophageal varices and liver failure. **Distal intestinal obstruction syndrome** (meconium ileus equivalent) (Fig. 9.5) results from inspissated fatty semi-solid

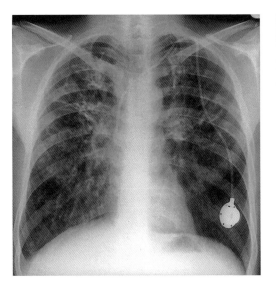

Figure 9.3 Chest X-ray of this 37-year-old man with cystic fibrosis shows hyperinflation, peribronchial thickening, cystic bronchiectasis and perihilar fibrosis. A Portacath central venous system is in place with the access port situated subcutaneously in the left lower chest. He has chronic *Pseudomonas aeruginosa* infection and receives about three courses of intravenous ceftazidime and tobramycin at home each year. His FEV$_1$ is 1.5 L (42% of predicted) and his general condition and lung function have remained stable over the last 5 years on treatment including long-term nebulised colistin, nebulised deoxyribonuclease, physiotherapy and nutritional supplements.

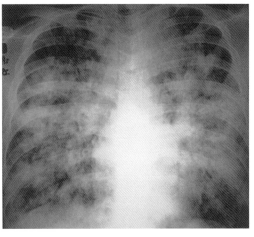

Figure 9.4 'Cepacia syndrome': chest X-ray of this 23-year-old man with cystic fibrosis shows the typical appearance of 'cepacia syndrome' with fulminant bilateral necrotising pneumonia. He had acquired *Burkholderia cenocepacia* genomovar III infection 7 years previously during an outbreak of infection among patients with cystic fibrosis attending a holiday camp. His lung function showed an accelerated rate of decline in the years after infection and he then developed a severe exacerbation that failed to respond to treatment and progressed to a fatal fulminant pneumonia over a 2-week period.

faecal material obstructing the terminal ileum. A number of factors contribute to the development of this complication including malabsorption of fat, disordered intestinal motility and dehydrated intestinal contents resulting from defective intestinal chloride transport. The clinical features vary depending on the severity of the obstruction. Typically, the patient suffers recurrent episodes of colicky abdominal pain and constipation, and there is often a palpable mass in the right iliac fossa. In severe cases complete intestinal obstruction may develop with abdominal distension, vomiting and multiple fluid levels in distended small bowel on an erect X-ray of abdomen. It is treated by a balanced intestinal lavage solution (e.g. Klean-Prep®) that is taken orally or by nasogastric tube. The radiocontrast Gastrografin® (sodium diatrizoate) may also be used as this agent has detergent properties that allow it to penetrate the inspissated fatty material and its hypertonicity then draws fluid into the faecal bolus. Other measures include rehydration, stool softeners (e.g. lactulose) and *N*-acetylcysteine; which probably acts by cleaving disulphide bonds in the mucoprotein faecal bolus. Prevention of recurrence requires adequate pancreatic enzyme supplements, avoidance of dehydration and sometimes use of laxatives.

Other complications

Nearly all **male patients are infertile** because of congenital bilateral absence of the vas deferens. The exact mechanism by which this complication occurs is not known but it has been suggested that it may result from resorption of the vas deferens after it has become plugged with viscid secretions in foetal life. Techniques such as microsurgical sperm aspiration from the epididymis or testes, with in vitro fertilisation by intracytoplasmic sperm injection can facilitate parenthood for men. Females have near normal fertility although some abnormalities of cervical mucus are present. **Pregnancy** places additional burdens on the mother's

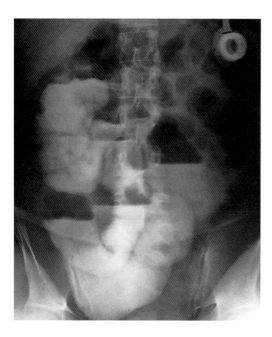

Figure 9.5 Meconium ileus equivalent. This 31-year-old woman with cystic fibrosis was admitted to hospital complaining of abdominal distension, colicky pain and constipation. A mass of inspissated faecal material was palpable in the right iliac fossa. Erect abdominal X-ray (after taking Gastrografin) shows distended loops of small bowel containing multiple fluid levels. A diagnosis of meconium ileus equivalent (distal intestinal obstruction syndrome) was made and she was treated with Gastrografin (orally and by enema), N-acetylcysteine orally, intravenous fluids, followed by flushing of the bowel using balanced intestinal lavage solution.

health and is sometimes associated with deterioration in the disease because of increased nutritional stress and impaired bronchial clearance. However, the main risk is of the mother failing to maintain all aspects of her own treatment as she focuses on the care of the baby.

Upper airway involvement causes troublesome **sinusitis** and **nasal polyps**. Cystic fibrosis **arthropathy** probably results from the deposition in joints of antigen–antibody complexes produced by the immune response to bacterial lung infections. Vasculitic **rashes** may also occur. In hot weather, patients with cystic fibrosis are at risk of developing **heat prostration** as a result of excess loss of salt in sweat. As these patients are living longer, a number of other complications are being described such as **osteoporosis** and **amyloidosis**.

Patients with cystic fibrosis face major **social and emotional stresses** relating to their reduced life expectancy, outlook for employment, ability to form relationships and undertake marriage and their general capacity to cope with a complex disease and its treatment.

Diagnosis

The diagnosis of cystic fibrosis is based upon the demonstration of **elevated sweat chloride** concentrations on a sweat test, in association with **characteristic clinical features** such as recurrent respiratory infections or evidence of pancreatic insufficiency. Nowadays the diagnosis is usually confirmed by the demonstration of **two known cystic fibrosis mutations** (e.g. ΔF508/G542X) on DNA analysis. It is possible to detect abnormal chloride conductance directly by measuring the potential difference of the nasal mucosa although this is a specialist research technique.

Sweat testing

In cystic fibrosis the ion-transport defect results in a failure to reabsorb chloride ions from the sweat, so that elevated sweat chloride and sodium concentrations are a characteristic feature of the disease. Sweating is induced by **pilocarpine iontophoresis**, the sweat is collected on filter paper and then analysed for sodium and chloride. Pilocarpine is placed on the skin of the forearm and a small electrical current is passed across it to enhance its penetration of the skin and stimulation of the sweat ducts. Meticulous technique is required to avoid evaporation of secretions or contamination. A sweat flow rate of at least $100\,\mu L/min$ is required for accurate analysis and sweat chloride levels above $60\,mmol/L$ on repeated tests are highly suggestive of cystic fibrosis. Sweat chloride values of $30\text{--}59\,mmol/L$ are considered intermediate and may be associated with atypical cystic fibrosis.

DNA analysis

The discovery of the cystic fibrosis gene in 1989 led to the development of **genotyping as an aid to diagnosis**. Genotyping can also be used to detect **carrier status**, and can be applied to chorionic villus biopsy material for **antenatal diagnosis**. However, there are more than 1800 mutations of the cystic fibrosis gene currently identified and routine analysis assesses only the most common mutations so that it can be difficult to exclude cystic fibrosis resulting from rare mutations. DNA analysis has established the diagnosis in some individuals with only mild clinical features, and this has extended our knowledge of the clinical spectrum of the disease to include some very rare older, less severely affected patients. Affected individuals have two gene mutations, one inherited from each of their parents. Carriers of the disease have only one abnormal gene, and do not show any evidence of the disease.

Atypical cystic fibrosis

As an increasing number of mutations of the CFTR gene are identified the clinical spectrum of the disease has been extended to include **atypical** or **non-classic** cystic fibrosis. The vast majority of patients with two mutations of the CFTR gene develop **classic cystic fibrosis**, characterised by the development of pancreatic malabsorption and recurrent respiratory infections in early childhood, with progressive severe lung disease over the years. About 5–10% of patients have a **late-diagnosis** of cystic fibrosis in later childhood or adulthood, having been misdiagnosed as having other diseases such as asthma, bronchitis or bronchiectasis. Sometimes these patients have had less severe lung disease and may also have had normal pancreatic function. It is recommended that all children and adults up to the age of 40 years presenting with bronchiectasis should have sweat tests and CFTR gene analysis. The diagnosis of cystic fibrosis should also be considered in older patients with bronchiectasis who have persistent *Pseudomonas aeruginosa* or *Staphylococcal aureus* infections, progressive disease or additional features such as malabsorption, pancreatitis, nasal polyps or male infertility. Although diagnosed late these patients have classic cystic fibrosis and have often already developed severe lung disease by the time of diagnosis with the risk of progressive disease over time. In contrast a small number of patients are now being identified who have truly atypical or non-classic disease associated with CFTR gene dysfunction. Sometimes these patients present with isolated manifestations such as **male infertility** due to congenital bilateral absence of the vas deferens, **nasal polyps**, recurrent **pancreatitis**, **sclerosing cholangitis**, neonatal hypertrypsinogenaemia or excessive **skin wrinkling** in water.

These patients often have intermediate sweat chloride levels of 30–59 mmol/L and rare, class IV or V mutations with some residual CFTR function that may protect them from more severe lung disease. These patients need careful assessment and follow-up in specialist cystic fibrosis centres.

Newborn screening

Early diagnosis of cystic fibrosis allows specific treatment to be commenced rapidly, and this is associated with an improved prognosis. Infants with cystic fibrosis have elevated serum **immunoreactive trypsin activity**. This can be measured on a single dried blood spot obtained on a Guthrie card as part of the newborn screening programme for diseases such as phenylketonuria and hypothyroidism.

Treatment

Cystic fibrosis is a complex multisystem disease, and skills from several disciplines are needed in treating these patients. The optimal use of currently available treatments and the introduction of new treatments is best achieved by concentrating the care of these patients in regional **specialist centres,** with a comprehensive multidisciplinary team. The basic elements of treatment comprise clearance of bronchial secretions by **physiotherapy**, treatment of pulmonary infection by **antibiotics** and correction of nutritional deficits by use of **pancreatic enzyme supplements** and **dietary support**. Patients and their families require continuous encouragement and support in coping with this complex disease. The Cystic Fibrosis Trust acts as a focus of **information and support**, and coordinates fund raising for research.

Chest physiotherapy

The viscid purulent sputum results in airways obstruction, and clearance of airway secretions by chest physiotherapy is important at all stages of the disease. A variety of techniques can be used including **postural drainage** (using gravity-assisted positions to aid drainage), chest **percussion** and **positive expiratory pressure devices** to aid dislodgement and expectoration of sputum from the peripheral airways. As patients mature it is important that they learn to perform bronchial clearance themselves. The 'active cycle of breathing technique' is often effective and popular with adult patients. This involves a **cycle of breathing control**, thoracic expansion exercises and the **forced expiratory technique** ('huffing') which releases secretions from peripheral bronchi. Some patients benefit from using oscillating positive expiratory pressure devices (e.g. flutter, Acapella devices). Exercise is an excellent adjunct to physiotherapy but should not replace it.

Antibiotics

Children with cystic fibrosis should be **immunised** against pertussis and measles as part of the childhood vaccination programme, and should receive annual influenza vaccination thereafter. They should avoid contact with people with respiratory infections and avoid inhalation of cigarette smoke. A variety of antibiotic strategies are used. *Staphylococcus aureus* is a major pathogen in the disease from early childhood and long-term continuous **flucloxacillin** is often used to suppress this infection. Further oral antibiotics are given during exacerbations in accordance with sputum cultures and sensitivity testing. Common pathogens include *Haemophilus influenzae* and *Streptococcus pneumoniae* which are usually sensitive to **amoxicillin**.

Infection with *Pseudomonas aeruginosa* becomes an increasing problem as children get older, and an important strategy in antibiotic therapy is to postpone for as long as possible the colonisation of the airways by this organism. Frequent sputum cultures are performed and intensive anti-pseudomonal antibiotic therapy is given when the organism is first isolated. This often comprises an **initial prolonged course of oral ciprofloxacin** and **nebulised colistin or tobramycin**. If this does not eradicate infection then **intravenous anti-pseudomonal antibiotics** are recommended. Eventually, chronic infection with *Pseudomonas aeruginosa* becomes established. Attempts at suppressing the effects of this infection involve long-term use of **nebulised antibiotics** such as colistin or tobramycin with additional courses of intravenous anti-pseudomonal antibiotics during infective exacerbations or when there is a decline in lung function. Usually an aminoglycoside (e.g. gentamicin, tobramycin) is given in combination with a third-generation cephalosporin (e.g. ceftazidime) or a modified penicillin (e.g. piperacillin). Treatment is usually given for 14 days and high doses are required to achieve adequate penetration of antibiotics into scarred bronchial mucosa because patients with cystic fibrosis have increased renal clearance of antibiotics.

Intravenous antibiotic treatment is often given **at home** by the patient after training. Where venous access is difficult a totally implanted central venous device can be inserted (e.g. Portacath). This comprises a central venous cannula connected to a subcutaneous port that is accessed by inserting a special non-cutting needle through the skin and the diaphragm of the subcutaneous chamber.

Burkholderia cepacia complex organisms are usually resistant to many of the commonly used anti-pseudomonal antibiotics such as colistin, ciprofloxacin and aminoglycosides, but are often sensitive to ceftazidime or meropenem.

Bronchodilator medication

Some patients with cystic fibrosis have a reversible component to their airways obstruction, and benefit from bronchodilator drugs (e.g. salbutamol, terbutaline) and inhaled steroids (e.g. beclometasone, budesonide, fluticasone).

Mucolytic medication

The sputum of patients with cystic fibrosis contains high levels of DNA, which is derived from the nuclei of decaying neutrophils. This makes the sputum very viscid and difficult to expectorate. Recombinant human **deoxyribonuclease (Dnase**/dornase alfa) is a genetically engineered enzyme that cleaves DNA. This treatment is administered by nebulisation and improves the lung function and reduces the number of exacerbations in some patients. Nebulised **7% hypertonic saline** improves mucociliary clearance by drawing water into the dehydrated periciliary layer. It sometimes provokes bronchoconstriction such that pre-treatment with a bronchodilator (e.g. salbutamol, terbutaline) is needed. **Mannitol**, administered via a dry powder inhaler, is an osmotic agent that also increases the water content of the airway surface liquid with improved mucociliary clearance.

Anti-inflammatory

The inflammatory response is unable to eradicate infection and contributes to the progressive lung damage. Corticosteroid drugs (e.g. **prednisolone**) may have a beneficial effect but their use is limited by adverse effects. High-dose **ibuprofen** may also be useful in reducing lung injury by inhibiting the migration and activation of neutrophils. **Macrolide antibiotics** (e.g. azithromycin) have been shown to improve lung function in patients with cystic fibrosis. This seems to be due to an anti-inflammatory effect by suppression of inflammatory cytokines, reducing neutrophil function and impairing biofilm formation around *Pseudomonas aeruginosa*.

Nutrition

Pancreatic enzyme supplements (e.g. Creon®, Pancrease®, Nutrizym®) are taken with each meal and with snacks containing fat. Enteric-coated preparations protect the lipase from inactivation by gastric acid, and use of antacid medication (e.g. omeprazole, lansoprazole) may improve effectiveness. The dose of enzyme is adjusted according to the dietary intake to optimise weight gain and growth and to control steatorrhoea. Use of high doses of pancreatic enzymes has been associated with the development of strictures of the ascending colon – so-called 'fibrosing colonopathy' – in a small number of children so that it is recommended that the dose of lipase should not exceed 10000 U/kg/day. Supplements of **fat-soluble vitamins** (A, D, E) are routinely given.

Patients with cystic fibrosis suffer from nutritional deficiencies as a result of malabsorption and the increased energy requirements resulting from increased energy expenditure because of chronic lung infection. Most patients with cystic fibrosis require 120–150% of the recommended daily calorie intake for individuals without cystic fibrosis, so that healthy eating for a patient with cystic fibrosis includes **high-energy foods** and frequent snacks between main meals. **Dietary supplements** (e.g. Fortisip®, Scandishake®) are useful when factors such as anorexia limit intake. In advanced disease **nocturnal enteral feeding** of high-energy formulas, through a nasogastric tube or gastrostomy, may be required.

Advanced disease

The clinical course of cystic fibrosis is very variable but an FEV$_1$ of less then 30% of the predicted value, for example, is associated with a 50% 2-year mortality rate. An awareness of the stage of the disease and the likely prognosis assists in planned management. Oxygen saturation should be measured by oximetry at each clinic visit in patients with advanced disease and when hypoxaemia develops domiciliary **oxygen** may alleviate the complications of respiratory failure. **Lung transplantation** is the main option to be considered for patients with advanced disease but the lack of donor organs severely limits the use of this treatment (see Chapter 19). Some patients will opt for a **palliative care** approach avoiding unpleasant interventions and focusing on measures that alleviate symptoms. Death is usually peaceful after a short coma due to ventilatory failure.

Prognosis

The prognosis of patients with cystic fibrosis has improved dramatically over the years. In the 1950s, survival beyond 10 years was unusual. Now the median survival is about 38 years and it is predicted to be at least 50 years for children now being born with the disease. There are now about 9000 patients with cystic fibrosis in the UK, and more than 50% are adults (aged 16 or over). Patients entering adulthood with cystic fibrosis face a number of problems, particularly relating to their chronic lung disease and reduced life expectancy (e.g. life insurance, choice of career, relationships, marriage, pregnancy, fertility). The improved survival of patients with cystic fibrosis has been attributed to a combination of factors including improved management of meconium ileus in neonates, earlier diagnosis, better dietary management and pancreatic enzyme supplementation and meticulous attention to physiotherapy and antibiotic treatments in specialist centres. Although cystic fibrosis typically produces severe progressive lung disease there is a wide **clinical spectrum of severity**. Some 'milder mutations' are associated with residual chloride conductance and less severe clinical disease but there is generally a poor correlation between specific gene mutations and clinical manifestations. Environmental factors, therapeutic regimens and additional 'modifier genes' that influence cytokine responses, for example, are important. Some patients are well and leading relatively normal lives, well into adulthood, and there is a need to adapt treatment to the stage and severity of the disease. With improved survival treatments need to be planned with care over decades to avoid adverse effects (e.g. aminoglycoside nephrotoxicity, antibiotic allergy and resistance) and to prevent long-term complications of the disease (e.g. osteoporosis, diabetic complications)

Prospective treatments

Ongoing refinements of conventional care in specialist centres continue to improve survival rates. New formulations of inhaled antibiotics (e.g. inhaled ciprofloxacin, nebulised aztreonam) may help control of airway infection. The identification of the cystic fibrosis gene in 1989 has revolutionised our understanding of the detailed molecular biology of this disease and offers the prospect of developing treatments directed against the basic underlying defects. Perhaps the most exciting approach is the direct replacement of the defective gene by **gene therapy**. The cystic fibrosis gene has been cloned and given to patients in experimental trials using liposomes or inactivated viruses as gene transfer agents to introduce the gene into epithelial cells. Expression of the gene can be detected by measuring transepithelial potential differences. Gene transfer and expression have been achieved and clinical trials are now underway to establish the clinical effectiveness and role of gene therapy. Substantial progress is being made in **pharmacological treatments** that address the molecular biology processes of CFTR transcription from DNA, trafficking through the cell, and activation and regulation at the apical membrane. Thus, **PTC124** is a **small molecule** that induces ribosomes to read through premature termination codons (PTC) during mRNA translation. It **corrects** the electrophysiological defect in patients with some class I mutations (e.g. G542X, W1282X). Vx770 (Vertex pharmaceuticals) is a CFTR **potentiator** that improves CFTR function in patients with the class III mutation, G551D. Some agents (e.g. phenylbutyrate, milrinone) regulate the expression of **molecular chaperons** (e.g. heat shock proteins) that improve the trafficking of CFTR through the cell, rescuing the mutant CFTR from degradation by the endoplasmic reticulum (e.g. ΔF508, class II mutation). Sometimes the term 'protein repair therapy' is used for mutant-specific therapies using a combination of correctors, chaperons and potentiators to improve CFTR function. A further approach is to attempt to correct the ion channel defect by stimulating **alternative chloride channels** (e.g. CaCC) or **inhibiting sodium channels** (e.g. ENaC). Amiloride and benzamil inhibit ENaC but have not yet shown clinical benefit. **Denufosol** is a purinergic receptor agonist that stimulates chloride and fluid transport via a non-CFTR mechanism, and initial trials show promising clinical results. Attempts at modifying the inflammatory response involve the assessment of the role of some currently available (e.g. ibuprofen, azithromycin) and some novel **anti-inflammatory agents** (e.g. glutathione, anti-elastases, lipoxins). Improvements in the field of **lung transplantation** (e.g. extending the donor pool by use of reconditioned lungs) offer the best hope for patients in the advanced stages of the disease. Advances in many different areas of scientific research are being brought into clinical practice in order to improve the outlook for patients with cystic fibrosis.

 KEY POINTS

- Cystic fibrosis is a multisystem disease resulting from mutations of a gene that codes for a chloride channel on epithelial membranes.
- In the lungs viscid secretions predispose to infection and inflammation with progressive bronchiectasis.
- *Staphylococcus aureus*, *Pseudomonas aeruginosa* and *Burkholderia cepacia complex* are the main pathogens.
- Antibiotics, chest physiotherapy, nutritional support and anti-inflammatory drugs are key elements in treatment.
- Lung transplantation is the main option to be considered for patients with advanced lung disease.

 FURTHER READING

Bott J, Blumenthal S, Buxton M, et al. Guidelines for the physiotherapy management of the adult, medical, spontaneously breathing patient. *Thorax* 2009; **64** (suppl 1): 1–51.

Bourke SJ, Doe SJ, Gascoigne AD, et al. An integrated model of provision of palliative care to patients with cystic fibrosis. *Palliative Medicine* 2009; **23**: 512–7.

Cystic Fibrosis Foundation (USA): www.cff.org

Cystic Fibrosis Trust (UK): www.cftrust.org.uk/

Davis PB. Cystic fibrosis since 1938. *Am J Respir Crit Care Med* 2006; **173**: 475–82.

De Boeck K, Wilschanski M, Castellani C, et al. Cystic fibrosis:terminology and diagnostic algorithms. *Thorax* 2006; **61**: 627–35.

Dodge JA, Lewis PA, Stanton M, et al. Cystic fibrosis mortality and survival in the UK. *Eur Respir J* 2007: 522–6.

Elkins MR, Robinson M, Rose BR, et al. A controlled trial of long term inhaled hypertonic saline in patients with cystic fibrosis. *N Engl J Med* 2006; **354**: 229–40.

Farrell PM, Robenstein BJ, White TB, et al. Guidelines for diagnosis of cystic fibrosis in newborns through older adults: cystic fibrosis foundation consensus report. *J Pediatr* 2008; **153**: S4–14.

Flume PA, O'Sullivan BP, Robinson KA, et al. Cystic fibrosis pulmonary guidelines. *Am J Resp Crit Care Med* 2007; **176**: 957–69.

O'Sullivan BP, Freedman SD. Cystic Fibrosis. *Lancet* 2009: **373**: 1891–904.

10

Asthma

Definition

Asthma is a disease characterised by **airway inflammation** with **increased airway responsiveness** resulting in **airway obstruction**. The cardinal feature of the airway obstruction in asthma is **variability.** This can occur spontaneously over short periods of time or in response to treatment; when it is referred to as **reversibility**. Patients experience **symptoms** such as wheeze, cough and dyspnoea.

It is not a static uniform disease state but rather a **dynamic and heterogeneous clinical syndrome** that has a number of **different patterns** and which may progress through different stages so that not all features of the disease may be present in an individual patient at a particular point in time. For example, many patients with well-controlled asthma are asymptomatic with normal lung function between attacks although if further investigations were performed there would be evidence of airway inflammation and increased airway responsiveness. By contrast, in some patients with chronic asthma the disease may have progressed to a state of irreversible airways obstruction. Some patients with smoking-related chronic obstructive pulmonary disease (COPD), bronchiectasis or cystic fibrosis may demonstrate airways obstruction with a degree of reversibility but it is important to appreciate that these diseases are different from asthma with distinct aetiologies, pathologies, natural history and responses to treatment.

Prevalence

Asthma has been recognised since ancient times and it is now estimated that 300 million people worldwide have asthma. The reported prevalence of asthma greatly depends on the criteria used to define it and is confused by changes in diagnostic habit (**labelling shift**) whereby patients may now be diagnosed as having asthma whereas previously they were labelled as having 'wheezy bronchitis' in the case of children, or 'COPD' in the case of adults, for example. However, despite such labelling shifts there is a general consensus that the **prevalence of asthma has increased greatly in recent decades**. Studies using objective measures of reversible airways obstruction and airway hyper-responsiveness in combination with symptoms suggest that **about 7% of the adult population in the UK have asthma**. There is considerable interest in the reasons for the increased prevalence of asthma but no firm consensus on the environmental factors that underlie it.

Aetiology

Asthma is multifactorial in origin, arising from a complex interaction of **genetic** and **environmental** factors. It seems likely that airway inflammation occurs when genetically susceptible

Respiratory Medicine Lecture Notes, Eighth Edition. Stephen J. Bourke and Graham P. Burns.
© 2011 John Wiley & Sons, Ltd. Published 2011 by John Wiley & Sons, Ltd.

individuals are exposed to certain environmental factors but the exact processes underlying asthma may vary from patient to patient. In many cases the most important environmental factors are probably the intensity, timing and mode of exposure to **aeroallergens** that stimulate the production of IgE. However, it is often not possible in an individual case to identify a specific allergen that could be regarded as the cause of the asthma, let alone one for which exposure avoidance would bring about resolution or even an improvement of symptoms.

Genetic susceptibility

There is strong evidence of a hereditary contribution to the aetiology of asthma. It has long been known that asthma and atopy run in **families**. First-degree relatives of asthmatics have a significantly higher prevalence of asthma than relatives of non-asthmatic patients. It is important to appreciate, however, that families share environments as well as sharing genes, and that environmental factors are necessary for the expression of a genetic predisposition. **Atopy** is a constitutional tendency to produce significant amounts of IgE on exposure to small amounts of common antigens. Atopic individuals demonstrate positive reactions to antigens on skin prick tests and have a high prevalence of asthma, allergic rhinitis, urticaria and eczema. Several potential gene linkages (e.g. chromosome 11q13 location) to asthma and atopy have been suggested but it is clear that the genetic contribution to asthma is complex, possibly involving **polygenic inheritance** (several genes contributing to the asthmatic tendency in an individual) and **genetic heterogeneity** (different combinations of genes causing the asthmatic tendency in different individuals). The ADAM33 gene on chromosome 20p13, which is a disintegrin and metalloprotease gene, has been identified as being involved in the structural airway components of asthma, such as airway remodelling, which relates to the development of chronic persistent asthma with irreversible (fixed) airways obstruction and excess decline in FEV_1 over time.

Environmental factors

The importance of environmental factors in the aetiology of asthma has been particularly evident in studies of populations who have **migrated from one country to another**. For example, children from the Pacific atoll of Tokelau were found to have developed asthma with similar prevalence to native New Zealand children when they were evacuated to New Zealand following a typhoon that devastated the local economy, whereas children remaining in Tokelau had a significantly lesser prevalence. Similarly, movement of people from East to West Germany in the 1990s was associated with an increased incidence of asthma and atopy. There may be very many aspects of the environment that are important but a change to a **modern, urban, economically developed society seems to be particularly associated with the occurrence of asthma**.

Indoor environment

People spend at least 75% of their time indoors and overall exposure to air pollutants and allergens is determined more by concentrations indoors than outdoors. The indoor environment is particularly important in the case of young children because allergen exposure early in life may be particularly important in determining sensitisation. **House dust mites** (*Dermatophagoides pteronyssinus*) are found in high concentrations in carpets, soft furnishings and bedding. Exposure to high levels in early life is associated with an increased likelihood of sensitisation to house dust mites by 3 to 7 years of age. In one UK study environmental manipulation commenced in early pregnancy and focused mainly on house dust mite avoidance and showed some reduction in respiratory symptoms in the first year of life. However, subsequently there was a paradoxical effect of increased allergy but better lung function. **Pet-derived allergens** are widespread in homes where dogs, cats or budgerigars are kept. Epidemiological studies suggest that close contact with a cat or dog in early life may reduce subsequent prevalence of asthma and allergy, perhaps via the provocation of immune tolerance. In general, studies on domestic allergen avoidance are inconsistent and there is no clear strategy that can be recommended. Passive exposure to **cigarette smoke** in the home has an adverse effect on asthma and other respiratory diseases in children in particular.

Outdoor environment

Although there is a widespread view among the general public that the increasing prevalence of asthma is attributable to atmospheric pollution from motor vehicles, the balance of evidence suggests that any such influence on the *initiation* of asthma is small. Nevertheless, interactions between atmospheric pollutants, aeroallergens and climatic conditions plays an important, although complex and incompletely understood, part in *triggering exacerbations* of pre-existing asthma. **Climatic conditions** such as high pressure and humidity with calm still air can result in an accumulation of airborne pollutants (e.g. particulates, ozone) and of allergens (e.g. pollens, fungal spores). Several epidemics of acute asthma have been associated with thunderstorms, and these have particularly affected patients with pre-existing atopic asthma. Warm dry weather may cause a rapid rise in pollen concentrations and also in levels of ozone (O_3), nitrogen dioxide and sulphur dioxide because of atmospheric stability. Gusts of wind at the start of a thunderstorm lift allergens into the air. Rain disrupts pollen grains into a number of smaller allergenic particles. Under these circumstances atopic individuals with pre-existing asthma or hay fever are particularly vulnerable to the resultant allergen challenge.

Occupational environment

Many agents encountered in the workplace may induce **occupational asthma** (e.g. isocyanates, epoxyresins, persulphates, hard wood dusts (see Chapter 14)).

Pathogenesis and pathology (Fig. 10.1)

A series of factors combine to produce increasing airway inflammation and airway responsiveness, and when these features reach a sufficient level bronchoconstriction and asthma symptoms are triggered. In a sensitised atopic asthmatic, typically, the inhalation of an allergen results in a two-phase response consisting of an **early asthmatic reaction** reaching its maximum at about 20 minutes, and a **late asthmatic reaction** developing about 6–12 hours later. These atopic asthmatics have high levels of specific IgE that binds to receptors on inflammatory cells, most notably mast cells. Interaction of the IgE antibody and inhaled antigen results in the activation of these inflammatory cells and release of preformed mediators such as histamine, prostaglandins and leukotrienes that cause contraction of smooth muscle of the airways producing bronchoconstriction. The inflammatory response in asthma is highly complex involving the full **spectrum of inflammatory cells** including mast cells, eosinophils, B and T lymphocytes and neutrophils, which release an **array of mediators and cytokines**. These mediators regulate the response of other inflammatory cells, and have a number of effects resulting in **contraction of airway smooth muscle**, **increased vascular permeability** and stimulation of airway **mucus secretion**.

T-helper lymphocytes have an important role in the regulation of the inflammatory response. These cells may be divided into two main subsets on the basis of the profile of cytokines that they produce. **Th2 cells** produce pro-inflammatory interleukins and **up-regulate** the specific form of airway inflammation of asthma by enhancing IgE synthesis and eosinophil and mast-cell function. In contrast, **Th1 cells** produce cytokines that **down-regulate the atopic response**. In those who

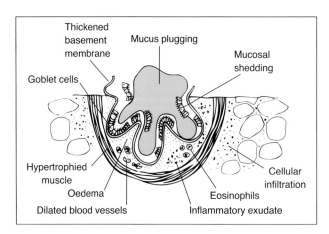

Figure 10.1 The pathogenesis and pathology of asthma. Asthma is characterised by a complex pattern of airway inflammation as a result of an interaction of genetic and environmental factors. Eosinophils, mast cells, neutrophils, B and T cells are all involved in the cellular infiltration. Mediators and cytokines regulate the inflammatory response and result in contraction of airway smooth muscle, increased permeability of blood vessels and mucus secretion. In chronic asthma airway remodelling results in structural changes and fixed airways obstruction.

are genetically susceptible to developing asthma, antigen presentation to T-helper cells leads to a Th2 response. Infection with respiratory syncytial virus augments a Th2 response, whereas some other microbial antigens lead to a Th1 response. It has been suggested that exposure to allergens and infections in early childhood is important in determining the pattern of immune response thereby modulating the genetic susceptibility to developing asthma. In affluent countries declining family size, improved household amenities and higher standards of cleanliness seem to be associated with an increased incidence of asthma. The **'hygiene hypothesis'** suggests that allergic diseases may be prevented by certain infections in early childhood. Thus, for example, children with older siblings are more likely to be exposed to childhood infections and have a lower incidence of asthma.

The wall of the airway in asthma is thickened by oedema, cellular infiltration, increased smooth-muscle mass and glands (Fig. 10.1). With increasing severity and chronicity of the disease **remodelling of the airway** occurs leading to fibrosis of the airway wall, fixed narrowing of the airway and a reduced response to bronchodilator medication. Mucus plugging of the lumen of the airway is a prominent feature of acute severe asthma. Although in clinical practice patients with asthma are sometimes classified as having atopic asthma (occurring in relation to inhalation of environmental antigens in a susceptible person) or non-atopic asthma (occurring without any definable relationship to an environmental antigen), the pathological features of the airway inflammation are identical. It is likely that the inflammatory cascade of asthma can be initiated by a variety of different factors in different patients.

Clinical features

The typical symptoms of asthma are **wheeze, dyspnoea, cough** and a sensation of **'chest tightness'**. These symptoms may occur for the first time at any age and may be episodic or persistent. In mild asthma the patient may be asymptomatic between episodes but experiences symptoms of asthma during viral respiratory tract infections or after exposure to certain allergens or other triggers. Sometimes the clinical pattern is of more persistent symptoms with chronic wheeze and dyspnoea. The variable nature of symptoms is a characteristic feature of asthma. Typically, there is a diurnal pattern with symptoms and peak expiratory flow (PEF) measurements being worse early in the morning – so-called **'morning dipping'**. Symptoms such as cough and wheeze often disturb sleep and the term **'nocturnal asthma'** emphasises this. In some asthmatics symptoms can be provoked by exercise (**'exercise induced asthma'**). This is different from normal exertional dyspnoea, the excess ventilation associated with exercise leads to measurable bronchoconstriction. Cough can sometimes be the predominant or only symptom and the lack of wheeze or dyspnoea may lead to a delay in making the diagnosis: so-called, **'cough variant asthma'**. Work in recent years has identified a condition termed: **eosinophilic bronchitis.** This is also a condition of airways inflammation, although the presence and activation of inflammatory cells is limited to the superficial layers of the airway walls rather than penetrating further to involve the airway smooth muscle. It usually presents as a chronic cough, perhaps displaying an asthmatic type of diurnal variability, although lung function is essentially normal. This feature may be the semantic divide that separates it from asthma although clearly the two conditions are very closely related. As with asthma inhaled corticosteroids are often a very effective treatment.

When assessing a patient presenting with breathlessness many of these clinical features can be vital clues to the diagnosis of asthma. A careful clinical history is therefore often the principal tool in diagnosis and should include the following.

- *Family history*: there is a significantly increased prevalence of asthma in relatives of patients with asthma or other atopic diseases (eczema, hay fever, allergic rhinitis).
- *Home environment*: smoking, or exposure to passive smoking in the home environment, is an adverse factor. Indoor allergens, particularly cat dander may be important in perpetuating asthma symptoms.
- *Occupational history*: it is important to identify if the patient's asthma could have been caused by exposure to asthmagenic agents at work, by enquiring about current and previous jobs, the tasks performed and materials used. Do symptoms improve away from work at weekends or on holidays? Are symptoms worse on return to work, particularly the evening or night after work? (See Chapter 14.)

- *Trigger factors*: are there any factors that precipitate symptoms?
  (a) exercise;
  (b) cold air;
  (c) viral respiratory infections;
  (d) allergen exposure (e.g. feather pillows, cat dander);
  (e) seasonal factors (e.g. grass pollen);
  (f) drugs (e.g. β-blockers, aspirin).
- *Response to treatment*: enquiry about the effectiveness of previous treatment with bronchodilator drugs or prednisolone yields clues to the reversibility of the disease and is particularly important in detecting asthma in older patients who may have been erroneously labelled as having COPD.

The characteristic features **on examination** of patients with asthma are diffuse bilateral **wheeze**, a **prolonged expiratory phase** to respiration and **lower costal margin paradox** (see Chapter 2) but there are often no signs detectable between episodes. There may be features of associated diseases such as allergic rhinitis, nasal polyps and eczema. It is essential to be alert for atypical features such as unilateral wheeze that suggests local bronchial obstruction by a foreign body (e.g. inhaled peanut) in a child or a carcinoma in an adult, for example. It is also important to ensure that there are no signs of cardiac or other respiratory disease. During acute attacks of asthma features such as tachycardia, tachypnoea, cyanosis, use of accessory muscles of respiration and features of anxiety and general distress indicate a severe episode. Chronic severe childhood asthma may cause chest deformity with the lower rib cage being pulled inwards (Harrison's sulcii) but these features are rarely seen nowadays.

Diagnosis

Although diagnosing asthma is straightforward when the patient presents with classic symptoms and evidence of variable or reversible airways obstruction, there are many pitfalls, and errors in diagnosis are common. **Failure to diagnose** asthma results in the patient being deprived of appropriate asthma treatment, for example a child with cough receiving recurrent courses of antibiotics for 'chest infections' when in fact he or she is suffering from asthma. Conversely, **incorrect diagnosis** of asthma might expose the patient to the risks of inappropriate treatment (e.g. recurrent courses of prednisolone) and delay appropriate management of other lung disease, e.g. inhaled foreign body in a child or tracheal tumour in an adult producing **wheeze simulating asthma**. On the one hand it is necessary to be alert to less well-recognised presentations of asthma, for example cough without wheeze, and on the other hand to be prepared to review the evidence for asthma if the response to treatment is poor or if unusual features emerge (e.g. could this child possibly have cystic fibrosis?). Evidence establishing the diagnosis of asthma and excluding other diseases often emerges over time and it is sometimes wise to use interim terms such as **'suspected asthma'** while gathering evidence of variable or reversible airways obstruction that allows a **firm diagnosis** of asthma to be established. Doubt may arise where it is difficult to obtain accurate peak flow or spirometry measurements as in the case of young children. Even when the diagnosis of asthma is established the diagnostic process should be taken further: **could this be occupational asthma?** Is there evidence of additional lung disease such as bronchiectasis or allergic bronchopulmonary aspergillosis? The doctor needs to exercise good clinical skills in applying two critical questions: **could this patient's symptoms be caused by asthma? Does this patient really have asthma?**

Investigations

In a straight forward case, a careful history and clinical assessment may strongly suggest the diagnosis of asthma. In such cases a trial of asthma treatment may be a reasonable next step. (Be prepared to be wrong; if there is not a clear response to treatment reconsider the diagnosis). In most cases however, given the likely need for treatment over many years it is important to try to gain objective support for the diagnosis.

Lung function tests

Confirmation of the diagnosis hinges on the demonstration of airflow obstruction that changes over short periods of time, either spontaneously (**variability**) or in response to treatment (**reversibility**).

  Spirometry allows clearer confirmation of airflow obstruction than the PEF rate (PEFR) and in that sense is preferable. A reduced FEV/VC ratio (usually taken to be < 0.7) confirms airway obstruction. However, the variability of asthma means that in some individuals (especially with relatively mild disease) spirometry may be normal between attacks.

- *Reversibility*: if airways obstruction is detected by spirometry the next step is to assess its reversibility to bronchodilator drugs. Typically, the patient is given 200 µg salbutamol and spirometry is repeated 15–20 minutes later. An alternative approach is to employ a 6-week trial of inhaled corticosteroid (e.g. 200 µg of beclometasone) or a 2-week trial of oral steroid (e.g. 30 mg/day of prednisolone). In each of these trials a >400 ml improvement in FEV_1 strongly suggests a diagnosis of asthma. Smaller improvements are more difficult to interpret and certainly do not exclude the diagnosis. In chronic severe asthma for example, the response to such treatments may become blunted over time. The diminution of response however does not alter the diagnosis. It remains asthma.
- *Variability:* in spirometry (irrespective of treatment) may be observed over a number of visits to the clinic for example. However, in the assessment of variability **PEFR** has the advantage of being measurable by a cheap, portable device that can be taken away from the clinic by the patient. In this way multiple measurements can be made with the potential for recording variability in relation to time of day or environment (in the of case asthma triggered by an occupational exposure for example). The patient needs to be taught how to use the device and record measurements in a **peak flow diary**. A characteristic pattern in asthma is **'morning dipping'** in which peak flow values are lowest in the morning, improving throughout the day. This diurnal variability is most marked in active, poorly controlled asthma. PEFR variability is calculated as the difference between the highest and lowest recording expressed as a percentage of the highest. A 20% or greater variability is highly suggestive of asthma.

Total lung capacity is usually increased in asthma as a manifestation of **hyperinflation**, and **residual volume** is elevated indicating **air trapping**. In contrast to patients with COPD (see Chapter 11), the airway obstruction of asthma is not associated with any impairment of gas diffusion so that transfer factor for carbon monoxide ($T_L$co) is characteristically normal and transfer coefficient (Kco) is often slightly elevated (see Chapter 3 for explanation). During an acute severe attack of asthma, **hypoxia** develops and is usually associated with increased ventilation and a reduced Pco$_2$. An elevated (or even normal) Pco$_2$ in a patient with acute severe asthma is a sign of a critically ill patient who is failing to maintain ventilation (see below).

Airway responsiveness is a measure of the general **'irritability' of the airways**, the degree to which **bronchoconstriction develops in response to physical or chemical stimuli**.

- *Exercise testing*: one of the most useful ways of demonstrating increased airway responsiveness or hyper-reactivity is to measure peak flow or spirometry before and after 5–10 minutes of vigorous exercise. A post-exercise fall in FEV_1 or peak flow of 20% is highly suggestive of asthma, as normal subjects usually show a degree of bronchodilatation, rather than bronchoconstriction, during exercise. An **exercise provocation test** is most useful if a patient with suspected asthma has normal peak flow or spirometry when seen in the clinic, such that reversibility testing may be of little use, and a 'provocation' test is more useful. The response is greater if exercise is performed in cold air.
- *Methacholine (or histamine) provocation tests*: the degree of airway responsiveness can be measured precisely in the laboratory. Under careful supervision, the patient inhales increasing doses of nebulised methacholine or histamine, starting at a very low dose, and serial spirometry is performed. By plotting the percentage fall in FEV_1 the concentration (C), or dose (D), of the chemical provoking (P) a 20% fall in FEV_1, can be calculated and expressed as a figure (e.g. PD_{20} methacholine 200 µg or PC_{20} histamine 4 mg/mL). Methacholine or histamine provocation tests are not usually required for the diagnosis of asthma in routine practice but are particularly useful in assessing changes in airway responsiveness in relation to exposure to environmental or occupational allergens (see Chapter 14) and in research studies.

Tests for hypersensitivity

Skin prick tests (Fig. 10.2) may be performed to identify atopy and to detect particular sensitivity to a specific antigen with a view to exclusion of exposure where possible (e.g. cat allergens). Drops of antigen extracts are placed on the flexor surface

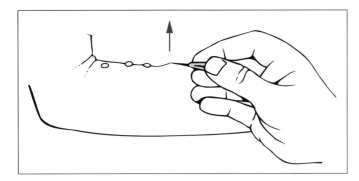

Figure 10.2 Skin prick test. Drops of antigen extracts and antigen-free control solution are placed on the flexor surface of the forearm. Each drop is pricked with a fine needle. The needle is held parallel to the skin surface, advanced slightly and a tiny fold of skin lifted briefly as shown. Deep stabs and bleeding should be avoided. Weal and flare are measured after 10–20 minutes.

of the forearm and the tip of a small stylet is pressed into the superficial epidermis through the drop of allergen. A positive reaction is manifest as a weal with a surrounding erythematous flare at about 15 minutes. The reaction to allergens should be compared with the reaction to a drop of histamine and to a drop of control solution containing no antigens. Total **IgE level** is often elevated in patients with atopic asthma and they sometimes have a mild peripheral blood **eosinophilia**.

Radioallergosorbent testing (RAST) is a means of measuring the level of circulating IgE specifically directed towards a particular antigen.

Some asthmatics develop an allergic reaction to *Aspergillus fumigatus*, a ubiquitous fungus which may colonise the airways. In these circumstances the asthma is typically severe and persistent requiring systemic steroid treatment. There is often associated severe airway inflammation and mucus plugging resulting in bronchiectasis (see Chapter 8). In addition to a positive skin prick test to *Aspergillus* these patients often have significant eosinophilia and **precipitating antibodies to *Aspergillus*** in their serum. Very rarely, asthma occurs as part of an eosinophilic vasculitis such as Churg–Strauss syndrome (see Chapter 15); in which case very high levels of blood eosinophilia occur.

General investigations

Further general investigations may be necessary to exclude other cardiorespiratory diseases. **Chest X-ray** is essential in older patients who have smoked, to exclude bronchial carcinoma, for example, and may be needed in children if there are any clinical features to suggest other diseases such as cystic fibrosis or bronchiectasis. **Bronchoscopy** is occasionally necessary to assess for vocal cord dysfunction, inhaled foreign bodies, bronchial carcinoma or rarer causes of

bronchial obstruction such as carcinoid tumours. **Exhaled nitric oxide** (NO) levels are increased in patients with asthma and this is a marker of airway inflammation that can be measured non-invasively. The equipment needed to measure exhaled NO is expensive and this test is mainly used in research studies rather than in routine clinical practice.

Management (Fig. 10.3)

Patient education

Asthma is frustrating, frightening and much misunderstood. Successful management of asthma requires that patients, or the parents of a child with asthma, understand the nature of the condition. The complexity of this explanation will of course vary with the background knowledge and character of the patient but it is a necessary foundation to an understanding of (and ultimately adherence to) treatment. When asthma has only recently developed, for example, the patient may be entirely focused on finding the once-and-for-all cure. Such a patient will not be receptive to the idea of finely tuning lifelong therapy to merely control the disease unless the practicality of the hoped for cure is discussed carefully. Time spent in discussion is very worthwhile. It is particularly important at the time of diagnosis, although education is an ongoing process and should play some part in most consultations.

At clinical review when attempting to assess the degree of symptom activity, general questions such as: 'How's your asthma?' are ineffective and should be avoided. They produce a reply rarely more informative than; 'Fine doctor'. Specifics, such as the Royal College of Physicians '3

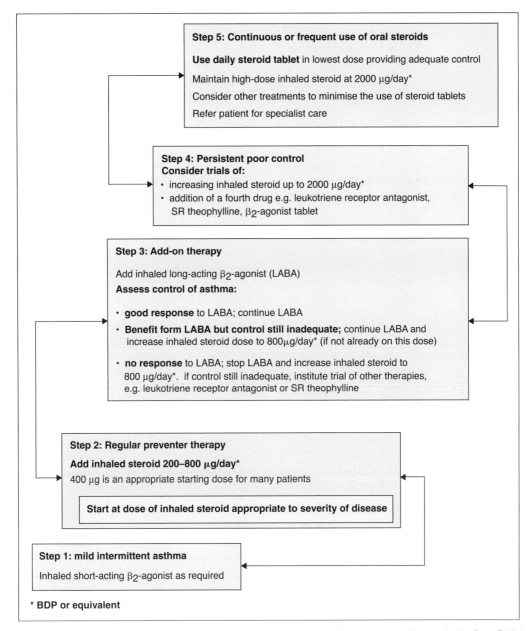

Step 5: Continuous or frequent use of oral steroids

Use daily steroid tablet in lowest dose providing adequate control

Maintain high-dose inhaled steroid at 2000 µg/day*

Consider other treatments to minimise the use of steroid tablets

Refer patient for specialist care

Step 4: Persistent poor control
Consider trials of:
- increasing inhaled steroid up to 2000 µg/day*
- addition of a fourth drug e.g. leukotriene receptor antagonist, SR theophylline, β2-agonist tablet

Step 3: Add-on therapy

Add inhaled long-acting β2-agonist (LABA)
Assess control of asthma:

- **good response** to LABA; continue LABA
- **Benefit form LABA but control still inadequate;** continue LABA and increase inhaled steroid dose to 800µg/day* (if not already on this dose)

- **no response** to LABA; stop LABA and increase inhaled steroid to 800 µg/day*. if control still inadequate, institute trial of other therapies, e.g. leukotriene receptor antagonist or SR theophylline

Step 2: Regular preventer therapy

Add inhaled steroid 200–800 µg/day*
400 µg is an appropriate starting dose for many patients

Start at dose of inhaled steroid appropriate to severity of disease

Step 1: mild intermittent asthma

Inhaled short-acting β2-agonist as required

* BDP or equivalent

Figure 10.3 Summary of the stepwise management of asthma in adults (Reproduced with permission from British Thoracic Society/Scottish Intercollegiate Guidelines Network. *British Guideline on the Management of Asthma 2009* (www.brit-thoracic.org.uk/).

Questions', are needed to gain a more accurate picture of asthma control.

1 In the last month/week have you had difficulty sleeping due to your asthma (including cough symptoms)?

2 Have you had your usual asthma symptoms (e.g. cough, wheeze, chest tightness, shortness of breath) during the day?

3 Has your asthma interfered with your usual daily activities (e.g. school, work, housework)?

The patients who reported their asthma to be 'fine', when asked if they wake at night may, after a brief pause to ensure they have heard you correctly, say: 'Of course I do doctor – I've got asthma!' This highlights another important issue that needs to be tackled. Many patients (indeed many doctors) have inappropriately low expectations of what can be achieved with appropriate use of modern inhaled medications. Although we are still some way from a cure, many people with asthma, particularly the young, should be able to achieve something close to, if not *complete* alleviation of day-to-day symptoms; **'total control'.** Time often needs to be spent in consultation raising expectations of what can be achieved. Many keen sports men and women have given up their sport, believing serious competition or even enjoyment of the sport is entirely precluded by asthma. This hardly ever need be the case. Clinical consultation then is as much about redefining goals as the practicalities of treatment regimens.

The practicalities must be addressed however. Good asthma control for most patients does not depend on the latest, expensive, high-tech treatment; it depends on getting the basics right. Unfortunately it is the basics that are so often neglected. Good inhaler technique is critical but disappointingly rare. The fault almost always lies with the clinician, not the patient. An inhaler should never be prescribed unless time is taken to coach (and then check) technique.

Most patients with asthma should be able to **monitor and manage** their own condition to a considerable degree and to recognise when medical advice is needed, in much the same way as patients with diabetes monitor their blood sugar levels and adjust insulin therapy.

The amount of information given to each patient needs to be varied in accordance with their needs and, indeed, wishes but all patients should know about features that indicate when their asthma is deteriorating and what action to take in these circumstances. Healthcare professionals should be aware that it is often those patients least interested in learning about their disease who are at greatest risk and that features such as depression, anxiety, denial of disease and non-adherence with treatment are strongly associated with asthma deaths. Particular effort is required to identify and target resources at such patients. Information conveyed in discussion with the patient should be supplemented by written information. Many organisations such as the British Lung Foundation and the National Asthma Campaign in the UK provide excellent literature for patient use. But a pre-printed leaflet may sometimes seem to be about 'someone else's asthma'. A few carefully selected notes including a **personalised asthma plan** *handwritten* in front of the patient can be a very powerful communication tool. Advice, so conveyed, is often highly valued by the patient as it is seen as being about them and their asthma.

Avoidance of precipitating factors

Most patients with atopic asthma react to many different antigens so that environmental control measures are generally not particularly helpful. The level of **house dust mite** can be reduced by encasing mattresses in occlusive covers and by frequent washing of blankets and duvets but the improvement in asthma control, even in those known to be sensitised, is usually disappointing. Avoidance of exposure to **pet allergens** from dogs or cats, for example, is more feasible but the result of these interventions is often not dramatic either. Similarly, it is difficult to avoid exposure to **outdoor allergens** although some patients benefit from precautions such as increasing asthma treatment or remaining indoors with closed windows when pollen counts are high.

Desensitisation (immunotherapy) is a highly specialised technique in which repeated injections of an allergen are given to a sensitised subject in an attempt to produce 'blocking antibody' of IgG type that prevents the allergen binding to specific IgE on mast cells. It is most commonly used in the treatment of well-documented life-threatening anaphylactic reactions to insect stings but there is no evidence of its benefit in asthma and there are major concerns about the risk of anaphylaxis.

Avoidance of irritants such as **cigarette smoke** or generally dusty environments is advisable. Avoidance of **β-blocker** drugs is important for all patients with asthma, and patients who are sensitive to **aspirin** should avoid all aspirin-containing products and non-steroidal anti-inflammatory drugs. **Viral infections** often precipitate attacks of asthma so that it is advisable for patients to monitor peak flow measurements or symptoms carefully during such infections and to intensify asthma treatment as required. Because influenza infection may precipitate severe exacerbations of asthma, annual **influenza vaccination** is recommended.

Exercise is a particular factor precipitating asthma. Bronchoconstriction may develop within minutes of onset of vigorous activity. This response usually resolves within 30 minutes and there then follows a refractory period of about 2 hours when further bronchoconstriction is more difficult to provoke. A warm-up period before the main exercise may help. It is important to remember that exercise induced asthma is indeed asthma. It responds as asthma does to all the standard therapies. Good overall asthma control is therefore probably more important than the 'quick fix' before the event.

Drug treatment

Short-acting bronchodilator drugs ('relievers') are used to relieve symptoms of bronchoconstriction. **Inhaled corticosteroids ('preventers')** treat the underlying chronic inflammatory process in asthma and are used either alone or in combination with a **long-acting bronchodilator** as maintenance therapy. Most patients with chronic asthma should be able to live perfectly normal lives on a combination of these treatments. The need for oral **prednisolone ('rescue medication')** should be rare indeed, although recognising when it is required is an important part of good asthma management.

Bronchodilators

- **Short-acting β_2-agonists**: (e.g. salbutamol, terbutaline) stimulate β-adrenoceptors in the smooth muscle of the airway, producing smooth-muscle relaxation and **bronchodilatation**. They have an onset of action within 15 minutes and a duration of action of 4–6 hours. Side-effects include tremor and palpitations but these are uncommon unless very high doses are used. The principal safety issue with bronchodilators (long acting, as well as short acting) is not one of side effects but of over-reliance at the expense of appropriate use of inhaled corticosteroids. The prompt relief they offer is seductive but they do nothing to control the underlying disease process; inflammation. Such symptomatic relief can disguise the severity of asthma and only delay its treatment. Anyone needing more than three doses of short-acting β_2-agonists per week should have their maintenance therapy increased. Increasing need for bronchodilator medication is a warning of declining control and should act as a prompt to action. As a group, patients consuming more than 10–12 puffs of β_2-agonists per day, have a recognised increased risk of fatal asthma.

- **Long-acting β_2-agonists**: (e.g. salmeterol, formoterol) have a duration of action of more than 12 hours. This gives them a convenient twice-daily dosing regime (which coincides nicely with the usual regimen employed for inhaled corticosteroids). Not long after their introduction there was concern about an increase in asthma deaths associated with their use. This, however, seems to have been as a result of a concomitant reduction in the use of corticosteroids rather that a direct pharmacological effect of the drugs themselves. Their use is only recommended as an adjunct to inhaled corticosteroids so that control of the airway inflammation is not neglected. **Combination inhalers**, which combine a long-acting β_2-agonist and a corticosteroid, are now very widely used in asthma management. They enjoy the benefits of simplicity and convenience (factors associated with better adherence to treatment). They are also a way of ensuring the improved symptom control brought about by the use of the long-acting β_2-agonist does not result in a neglect of corticosteroids. The particular combination inhaler Symbicort® contains formoterol as its long-acting β_2-agonist. Formoterol has the same duration of action as other long-acting β_2-agonists but also benefits from an onset of action as brisk as that seen with the short-acting β_2-agonists. **S**ymbicort can therefore be used, as both a **M**aintenance **A**nd **Re**liever **T**herapy. The rationale for the so-called **SMART** regimen is that it automatically delivers an increase in the corticosteroid treatment at times when declining control would naturally lead to increasing reliever usage. In selected patients this has proved to be a useful strategy but careful patient education about the **specific issues related** to this regimen is needed.

- **Anti-muscarinic bronchodilators**: (e.g. ipratropium or the long-acting tiotropium) produce bronchodilatation by blocking the bronchoconstrictor effect of vagal nerve stimulation on bronchial smooth muscle. They take about 1 hour to reach their maximum effect and have a duration of action of about 4–6 hours in the case of Ipratropium, >24 hours in the case of Tiotropium. Side-effects are uncommon but nebulised anticholinergic drugs may be deposited in the eyes, aggravating glaucoma. In most patients with asthma they are less effective than β_2-agonists. Inhaled preparations are therefore not used widely in chronic asthma management. Nebulised ipratropium, on the other hand, provides a useful adjunct to salbutamol in the treatment of acute severe asthma (see later).

- **Theophyllines**: increase cyclic adenosine monophosphate (cAMP) stimulation of β-adrenoceptors by **inhibiting the metabolism of cAMP** by the enzyme phosphodiesterase. They may also have other effects including some anti-inflammatory actions. They are not available in inhaler form and absorption from the gastrointestinal tract and clearance of the drug by the liver are variable so that the dose needs to be titrated carefully in accordance with blood levels. Side-effects such as nausea, vomiting, headache, tachycardia and malaise are common. Hepatic clearance of theophyllines is reduced by drugs such as cimetidine, ciprofloxacin and erythromycin, and toxicity can occur if these medications are prescribed without adjustment in the dose of theophylline. Aminophylline is an intravenous form of theophylline (combined with ethylenediamine for solubility) that may be used in severe attacks of asthma. It must be given slowly (over at least 20 minutes) with careful adjustment of dose in accordance with blood levels in order to avoid serious toxicity such as convulsions and cardiac arrhythmias. It does not usually result in any additional bronchodilatation compared with standard treatment with nebulised bronchodilators and systemic steroids, and side-effects are common so that its use is usually reserved for very severe asthma not responding to standard treatment.
- **Magnesium**: magnesium sulphate (1.2–2 g as an intravenous infusion over 20 minutes) acts as a smooth-muscle relaxant and is safe and effective in treating patients with acute severe asthma who have not had a satisfactory initial response to nebulised salbutamol.

Anti-inflammatory drugs

- **Inhaled corticosteroids**: (e.g. beclometasone, budesonide, fluticasone, mometasone, ciclesonide) are the mainstay of asthma treatment because they **counteract airway inflammation**; which is the key underlying process in asthma. It is essential that the patient understands that this is a **preventative treatment** that needs to be taken regularly. It is important to explain to patients that, in contrast to the short-acting β_2-agonists, these drugs provide no immediate relief of symptoms. Without proper patient education the

drugs may be neglected on the mistaken assumption that 'they're not working'. **Adherence** is improved by using a twice-daily regime whereby the patient's 'preventative' steroid inhaler is left at their bedside or by their toothbrush and taken regularly every night and morning. The dose is adjusted to give optimal control and varies greatly from patient to patient. The **potency** of the various available inhaled steroids differs; the same anti-inflammatory effect can be achieved with one drug at half the dose required with another. Clinical guidelines, in specifying steroid dosage, therefore refer to 'beclometasone equivalent'. This variation does NOT imply superiority of one steroid over another. The critical comparator is not potency but the efficacy to side-effect profile. In this regard there is no great difference between any of the available products. In choosing an inhaled steroid it is probably as wise to choose on the basis of the inhaler device the drug is available in. The device the patient can use is likely to be the most effective. Many adult patients with relatively mild asthma achieve good control with a dosage of about 400 µg/day beclometasone, but some patients with chronic severe asthma may require up to 2000 µg/day. In adult patients **'low-dose'** (below the equivalent of about 800 µg/day beclometasone) inhaled steroids are not usually associated with any significant adverse effects apart from oropharyngeal candidiasis or hoarseness of the voice, which can be reduced by using a spacer device in the case of metered dose inhalers or a dry powder device and gargling the throat with water after inhalation. With **'high-dose'** inhaled steroids (above about 800 µg/day beclometasone) biochemical evidence of suppression of adrenal function, and increased bone turnover are detectable in some patients. The clinical significance of such systemic effects needs to be considered in the context of the dangers of uncontrolled asthma and alternative therapies such as oral prednisolone. The dosage of inhaled steroids should be reviewed regularly to ensure that the patient is taking as much as is required to control their asthma ('step up') but, equally, as little as necessary ('step down') so as to minimise the risk of adverse effects with long-term usage. Patients taking high-dose inhaled corticosteroid should carry a steroid treatment card advising of the risk of adrenal suppression.

- **Sodium cromoglycate** is a preventative inhaled treatment that has a number of anti-inflammatory actions including stabilisation of mast cells. It is mainly used in children with mild asthma and it has no significant adverse effects. However, it is **less effective** than inhaled steroids. Nedocromil is another inhaled compound with similar properties to cromoglycate.

- *Oral steroid treatment*: **'rescue' courses** of oral steroids may be needed to control exacerbations of asthma. Typically, this consists of 30–40 mg/day of prednisolone for about 7 days in an adult. Treatment is continued until asthma control has been achieved. Most patients should be taught to start their own short course of oral prednisolone in accordance with a predetermined action plan (for example, when peak flow falls below 60% of the patient's best value). Patients should understand the potential adverse effects of long-term use of prednisolone and the difference between this and infrequent short-courses which (if truly infrequent) are safe. A very small number of patients require **long-term systemic prednisolone** to control severe asthma. These patients should be attending a hospital specialist and it should have been clearly established that their asthma cannot be controlled by other measures. The dosage of steroids needs to be kept as low as possible. All other effective therapies, particularly inhaled steroids, should be continued at full dose. In these circumstances the patient should be given a **'steroid treatment card'** documenting the dosage of steroids used, advising about adverse effects and warning patients that steroids should not be stopped suddenly because of the risk of adrenal insufficiency. Booster doses may be required during illnesses and patients may be particularly susceptible to infections such as chickenpox. Other **adverse effects** include peptic ulceration, myopathy, osteoporosis, growth suppression, depression, psychosis, cataracts and cushingoid features. Patients receiving long-term oral prednisolone should be considered for preventative treatment of osteoporosis such as smoking cessation, exercise, hormone replacement therapy, adequate dietary calcium intake and bisphosphonate treatment where appropriate.
- *Leukotriene receptor antagonists*: (e.g. montelukast, zafirlukast) block the effects of cysteinyl leukotrienes; which are metabolites of arachidonic acid with bronchoconstrictor and pro-inflammatory actions. Leukotriene antagonists are a modality of anti-inflammatory therapy in asthma, which are given orally in tablet form. Some patients report a clear improvement in symptoms although in many the response is disappointing. Their place is as add-on therapy (only to be used after inhaled steroids and a long-acting bronchodilator). As such they are a reasonable option to try. If no benefit can be discerned after 1 month however, they should be stopped.

- *Anti-IgE treatment* (**omalizumab**) is a monoclonal antibody that binds to IgE. It is a new form of add-on therapy for some patients with severe persistent IgE-mediated asthma to inhaled allergens, who are not controlled by high dose inhaled corticosteroid and long-acting β-agonist medication. It is administered by subcutaneous injection every 2–4 weeks and the dose depends on the baseline IgE level. Its use is currently restricted to hospital-based physicians who are experienced in the treatment of severe persistent asthma.

- *Bronchial thermoplasty* is a novel, still rather experimental, technique whereby heat is applied directly to the central airways via bronchoscopy. Thermal 'damage' to smooth muscle reduces its quantity and functionality and in one major study led to improved lung function and reduced need for reliever medication over a 22-week follow-up. More evidence of both safety and efficacy will be required before the technique could be established as a component of clinical practice.

Stepwise approach to treatment of asthma (Fig 10.3)

The British Thoracic Society guidelines on the management of asthma recommend a stepwise approach to treatment according to the severity of the asthma. The **aim of treatment** is to control the disease. **Control** is defined as:

- no daytime symptoms;
- no night-time wakening due to asthma;
- no need for reliever medication;
- no exacerbations;
- no limitations on activity including exercise;
- normal lung function (in practical terms FEV_1 and/or PEF >80% predicted or best);
- with minimal or no side-effects.

Patients should start treatment at the step most appropriate to the initial severity of their asthma and treatment is adjusted as appropriate thereafter. For the majority of patients, asthma is controlled by a combination of a regular inhaled steroid and use of an inhaled bronchodilator drug as required. Bronchodilator drugs are primarily intended to provide symptom relief whereas inhaled steroids are targeted at the underlying inflammatory process in the airways. Treatment should be **'stepped up' as much as necessary** to control the asthma; when control has been achieved treatment may be **'stepped down'** so that the patient is on **no more treatment than is necessary**.

Asthma is a dynamic condition changing over time and ongoing management requires an assessment of the level of control of the asthma that has been achieved and adjustment of medication to find the optimal balance between control of the asthma, use of medication and potential adverse effects of treatment.

Inhaler devices

The inhaled route is preferred for bronchodilator and corticosteroid drugs because it allows these drugs to be delivered directly to the airway reducing the risk of systemic adverse effects. A large number of different inhaler devices and drug formulations are available. Current evidence suggests that there is no major difference in the clinical effectiveness of the various devices **provided the patient is able to use the device appropriately**.

- *Metered-dose inhalers*: (Fig. 10.4) pressurised metered-dose inhalers use hydrofluoroalkane (HFA) as a propellant. It is essential to instruct the patient in the correct use of the inhaler and this should be rechecked frequently. About 10% of the drug is delivered to the lower airways and the remainder is mainly deposited in the oropharynx and swallowed, it is absorbed into the blood, but mostly metabolised by first-pass metabolism in the liver.
- *Spacer devices*: (e.g. Volumatic®, Nebuhaler®, Aerochamber®) (Fig. 10.5) Poor inhaler technique is a significant problem in the use of metered-dose inhalers. Large-volume spacer devices overcome some of these problems and improve deposition of the drugs in the lower airway to about 20% on average. The canister (cr) of pressurised aerosol is inserted into one end of the spacer device and the patient breathes through the other end via a one-way valve (v) that closes on expiration; (e) expiratory port. This **reduces the need for coordination of inspiration and actuation of the inhaler**. Distancing the inhaler from the mouth ('spacing') results in a fine aerosol of smaller particles **improving delivery of the drug to the lower airways**. Spacer devices should be cleaned monthly by washing in detergent and allowing them dry in air. They should be replaced at least every 12 months.
- *Breath-actuated aerosol inhalers*: (e.g. Autohaler®, Easi-breathe®) avoid the need for the patient to coordinate actuation of the inhaler and breathing. The valve on the inhaler is actuated as the patient breathes in, delivering the drug only during inspiration.

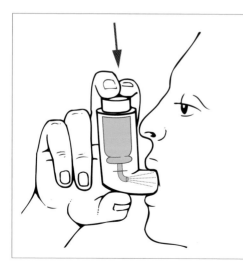

- Remove the cap and shake the inhaler
- Tilt the head back slightly and exhale
- Position the inhaler in the mouth (or preferably just in front of the open mouth)
- During a slow inspiration, press down the inhaler to release the medication
- Continue inhalation to full inspiration
- Hold breath for 10 seconds
- Actuate only one puff per inhalation

Figure 10.4 Pressurised metered-dose inhaler.

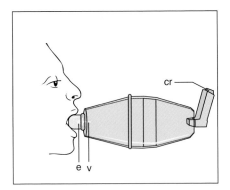

Figure 10.5 Example of a spacer device for use with metered-dose inhalers that allows the patient to inhale after discharge of the aerosol. The Volumatic® (Allen and Hanbury) is a large-volumed device, designed to allow free dispersal of the discharged material so that a high proportion of it forms particles small enough to be inhaled. It also allows large doses of aerosol to be inhaled relatively efficiently (see text). cr, canister of pressurised aerosol; e, expiratory port; v, valve that closes on expiration.

- **Dry-powder devices**: (Turbohaler®, Accuhaler®, Clickhaler®) (Fig. 10.6) in these devices the β-agonist or steroid drug is formulated as a dry powder without a propellant. Inspiratory airflow releases the powder from the device so that they are **breath actuated**, and this reduces the problem of coordination of inspiration and inhaler actuation. Some patients find dry-powder devices easier to use but they require an adequate inspiratory flow rate to achieve drug delivery.
- **Nebulisers**: (Fig. 10.7) in this form of inhaled therapy, oxygen or compressed air is directed through a narrow hole creating a local negative pressure (Venturi effect) that draws the drug solution into the air stream from a reservoir chamber. The droplets are then impacted against a small sphere, and small particles are carried as an aerosol, whereas larger particles hit the side wall of the chamber and fall back into the reservoir solution. The aerosol is administered by mask, or via a mouthpiece. Nebulisers are a convenient means of giving **high doses of bronchodilator drugs in acute attacks of asthma** where coordination of inhaler administration

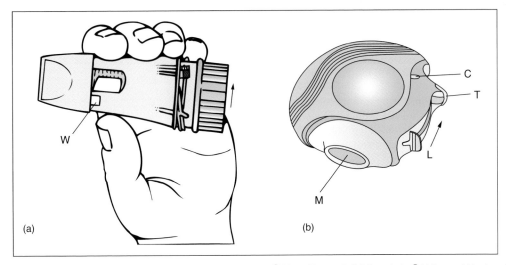

(a)

(b)

Figure 10.6 Examples of dry-powder inhalers: (a) Turbohaler® (AstraZeneca); (b) Accuhaler® (Allen and Hanbury). (a) Turbohaler®: the inhaler is shown with the cover removed, the mouthpiece is to the left. Up to 200 doses of the powdered drug are stored in a reservoir through which the air channel passes. A dose of the dry powder is rotated into the air channel by turning the distal section (arrow). The number of doses remaining is indicated in a small window (W). (b) Accuhaler®: the inhaler is opened by pushing the thumb grip (T) right around until it clicks. The inhaler is shown open. Sliding the lever (L) around as far as it will go pierces an individual blister and places a dose of the drug in the mouthpiece (M). There is a counter (C) indicating how many doses are left.

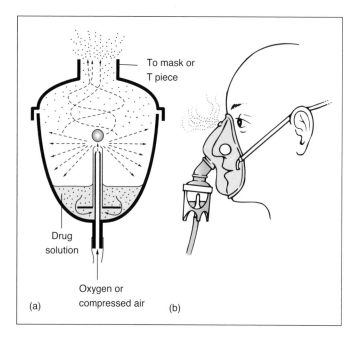

To mask or
T piece

Drug
solution

Oxygen or
compressed air

(a)   (b)

Figure 10.7 Nebuliser treatment. (a) Diagram of typical nebulisation mechanism. (b) Nebuliser mask for administration of high-dose bronchodilator (see text).

may be difficult in a distressed patient. They may also be used for delivering inhaled steroids (e.g. budesonide) in very young children although it is important to realise that properly used dry-powder devices, for example turbohaler, or metered-dose inhalers and spacer devices deliver a greater percentage of the administered dose to the lower airway and are therefore the devices of choice for routine long-term treatment. The danger of patients having nebulisers at home for administration of bronchodilators lies in the fact that they may over-rely on the temporary alleviation of symptoms by nebulised bronchodilators to the detriment of regular anti-inflammatory therapy. They may also lead to a delay in seeking urgent medical advice during acute severe asthma attacks.

Acute severe asthma

Some patients with asthma are particularly susceptible to recurrent sudden attacks of severe asthma but any patient with asthma may develop an acute attack under certain circumstances (e.g. viral infection, allergen exposure). It is crucial that all patients with asthma know how to recognise the features of a severe attack and know what action to take. Most of the people who die of acute asthma

do so because the severity of the attack was underestimated and not treated adequately or promptly. It is important therefore that doctors and patients recognise the features of worsening asthma control and a severe attack.

Signs of acute severe asthma

Any one of:

- PEF 33–50% of best or predicted;
- respiratory rate $\geq$25 /min;
- heart rate $\geq$110 bpm;
- inability to complete sentences in one breath.

Life-threatening asthma

Any one of the following in a patient with acute severe asthma:

- clinical signs:
  - altered conscious level
  - exhaustion
  - arrhythmia
  - hypotension
  - cyanosis
  - silent chest
  - poor respiratory effort
- measurements:
  - PEF $<$33% of best or predicted
  - O_2 saturation $<$92%
  - $P_aO_2 < 8$kPa
  - Normal P_aCO_2

Near-fatal asthma

Raised $P_a co_2$ and/or requiring mechanical ventilation with raised inflation pressures.

Immediate management

- *Oxygen*: the highest concentration available should be used. Masks delivering 24 or 28% are not appropriate. Aim for a saturation >94%.
- *High-dose nebulised β-agonist*, for example salbutamol 5 mg or terbutaline 10 mg. This may be repeated after 15–30 minutes if the patient's condition is not improving. Multiple doses from an inhaler should be given with a spacer device if a nebuliser is not available.
- *High-dose systemic steroid*, for example prednisolone 30–50 mg orally, or hydrocortisone 100 mg 6-hourly intravenously, or both, immediately.

If response to this initial therapy is poor add the following.

- *Nebulised ipratropium*: add ipratropium 0.5 mg to the nebulised β-agonist.
- *Intravenous magnesium sulphate*: 1.2–2 g infusion over 20 minutes.
- *Intravenous bronchodilators*: intravenous aminophylline is unlikely to result in any additional bronchodilatation compared with standard care. Side-effects such as arrhythmias may also be problematical. Some patients with near fatal or life threatening asthma may gain additional benefit from intravenous aminophylline (5 mg/kg loading dose over 20 minutes unless on maintenance oral therapy, then infusion of 0.5 mg/kg/hour) but such patients have been difficult to identify in trials and are probably rare.

- *Intravenous β₂-agonists:* are sometimes used (salbutamol or terbutaline 250 μg over 10 minutes, then infusion of 5 g/min) but they should be reserved for those patients in whom nebulised therapy cannot be used reliably.

Investigations

Arterial blood gases, urea and electrolyte concentrations, electrocardiogram in older patients, chest X-ray.

Monitoring treatment

Continued vigilance is required. The patient's condition may deteriorate some hours after an initial improvement (e.g. during the night after admission). Measure and record PEF 15–30 minutes after starting treatment and thereafter according to the response (at least 4 times daily measurements). Monitor respiratory rate, pulse, patient's general condition and oxygen saturation frequently. Nursing staff should be asked to call the doctor if there is a deterioration in these signs. Acute severe asthma usually acts as a powerful stimulus to ventilation resulting in a reduced $P co_2$. By the time of admission however, the patient may have had progressive symptoms over a few days with very little sleep. Fatigue and exhaustion are often present. Even a normal $P co_2$ (let alone an elevated value) in the context of acute severe asthma is therefore an ominous sign. Transfer of the patient to an intensive therapy unit (ITU) may be advisable so that their condition can be monitored more closely. Intermittent positive pressure ventilation is only rarely necessary but is used when the patient shows signs of exhaustion (rising $P co_2$),

---

Table 10.1 Diagnosing asthma. 'All that wheezes is not asthma and not all asthma wheezes'

Underdiagnosis: Could this patient's symptoms be caused by asthma?

Overdiagnosis: Does this patient really have asthma?

- Recognise **symptoms** suggestive of asthma (e.g. wheeze, cough, recurrent 'chest infections')
- Establish evidence of **airways obstruction** (e.g. ↓ peak flow, ↓ FEV_1, ↓ FEV_1/VC ratio)
- Assess **variability**, **reversibility**, **provocability** of airway obstruction: serial peak flow chart (e.g. morning dipping; response to bronchodilator and steroid trial; exercise-induced fall in peak flow)
- **Monitor** progress and **review diagnosis** (e.g. has 'wheezy bronchitis' of childhood evolved into established asthma or was it a result of viral bronchiolitis?)
- Consider **additional diagnoses** (e.g. occupational asthma, allergic bronchopulmonary aspergillosis)
- Exclude alternative diagnoses (e.g. cystic fibrosis, COPD, carcinoma, inhaled foreign body)

COPD, chronic obstructive pulmonary disease; FEV_1, forced expiratory volume in 1 second; VC, vital capacity.

failure to maintain oxygenation or deterioration in vital signs.

Management during recovery in hospital and following discharge

The opportunity should be taken to improve the patient's understanding of asthma and its management, and to provide written guidance on future management. Ways of improving the patient's response to worsening asthma should be identified. Most crises resulting in hospital admission are probably preventable. The importance of peak flow measurement in determining treatment changes should be explained. Possible precipitating factors should be identified. Inhaler technique should be checked and performance recorded. If necessary, alternative inhaler devices should be used. Specialist follow up is advisable.

 Respiratory emergencies **Asthma**

- **Oxygen**: high flow. Aim for a saturation >94%.
- **Nebulised β-agonist**: salbutamol 5 mg or terbutaline 10 mg. This may be repeated after 15–30 minutes if the patient's condition is not improving. Continue 4–6 hourly or more frequently, as required
- **High-dose systemic steroid**, for example prednisolone 30–50 mg orally, or hydrocortisone 100 mg 6-hourly intravenously, immediately.

If response to initial therapy is not adequate add the following.

- *Nebulised ipratropium.* 0.5 mg, 6-hourly
- *Intravenous magnesium sulphate.* 1.2–2 g infusion over 20 minutes.

Closely monitor: clinical condition, PEF and arterial blood gases. If poor response to treatment, fatigue, failure to achieve adequate oxygenation or $P\text{co}_2$ within normal range, discuss with ITU.

 KEY POINTS

- Asthma is a dynamic heterogenous clinical syndrome, characterised by chronic airway inflammation, airway hyper-responsiveness, symptoms and airways obstruction.
- Asthma is multifactorial in origin, arising from a complex interaction of genetic and environmental factors.
- The clinical diagnosis of asthma should be supported by evidence of variable or reversible airways obstruction on spirometry or peak flow measurements.
- Most patients with asthma can be managed perfectly well by proper attention to detail with the basic therapies (regular inhaled corticosteroids and an inhaled bronchodilator).
- Instruction in the correct use of an appropriate inhaler device is crucial in the treatment of asthma.
- Most patients (and many doctors) have inappropriately low expectations of disease control. Aim for 'total control'.

 FURTHER READING

Asthma UK: www.asthma.org.uk.

British Thoracic Society/Scottish Intercollegiate Guidelines Network. *British Guideline on the Management of Asthma 2009.* London: British Thoracic, 2009 (http://www.brit-thoracic.org.uk/).

Carlsen KH, Delgado L, DelGiacco S. Diagnosis, prevention and treatment of exercise-related asthma, respiratory and allergic disorders in sports. *Eur Respir Mon* 2005; **10**: 1–105.

Chu EK, Drazen JM. Asthma: one hundred years of treatment and onward. *Am J Respir Crit Care Med* 2005; **171**: 1202–8.

Dolovich MB, Ahrens RC, Hess DR, et al. Device selection and outcomes of aerosol therapy: evidence based guidelines of the American College of Chest Physicians/American College of Asthma, Allergy and Immunology. *Chest* 2005; **127**: 335–71.

Global Initiative for Asthma (GINA): www.ginasthma.com.

Holgate ST, Yang Y, Haitchi HM, et al. The genetics of asthma. *Proc Am Thorac Soc* 2006; **3**: 440–3.

Masoli M, Fabian D, Holt S, Beasley R. The global burden of asthma: executive summary of GINA Dissemination Committee report. *Allergy* 2004; **59**: 469–78.

Chronic obstructive pulmonary disease

Introduction

Chronic obstructive pulmonary disease (COPD) is a major cause of morbidity and mortality worldwide. It has a profound effect on both the quantity and quality of life. In the UK an estimated 3 million people have COPD yet more than 2 million of these remain undiagnosed. There are 110 000 admissions to hospital with exacerbations of COPD and 30 000 people die of the disease each year. Mortality has fallen in men but continues to rise in women, reflecting smoking patterns over the second half of the twentieth century. As the worldwide epidemic of smoking spreads, with increasing smoking rates in China, Africa and Asia it is predicted that COPD will become the third most common cause of death worldwide by 2020. There is an urgent need to improve awareness, prevention and treatment of this disease.

Definitions

Chronic obstructive pulmonary disease

COPD is defined as a chronic, slowly progressive disorder characterised by **airflow obstruction** that does not change markedly over several months. Although there is some overlap in the features of COPD and asthma, they are separate disorders with different aetiologies, pathologies, natural history and responses to treatment. In asthma, airway inflammation and hyper-reactivity are the key factors giving rise to bronchial muscle contraction and airways obstruction. In COPD, structural and pathological changes occur that manifest in the various facets of the condition: chronic bronchitis, airway obstruction and emphysema.

Chronic bronchitis

Chronic bronchitis is a hypersecretory disorder defined as the presence of **cough productive of sputum on most days for at least 3 months of 2 successive years** in a patient in whom other causes of a chronic cough have been excluded (e.g. tuberculosis, bronchiectasis). The diagnosis is made on the basis of symptoms. The airways of patients with chronic bronchitis show mucous gland hypertrophy and an increased number of goblet cells. Although chronic bronchitis and obstructive lung disease result from inhaling cigarette smoke, they do not show a clear relationship to each other and are distinct components of the spectrum of COPD. Mucus hypersecretion is mainly caused by changes in the central airways

Respiratory Medicine Lecture Notes, Eighth Edition. Stephen J. Bourke and Graham P. Burns.
© 2011 John Wiley & Sons, Ltd. Published 2011 by John Wiley & Sons, Ltd.

whereas progressive airways obstruction arises principally from damage to the peripheral airways and alveoli.

Airway obstruction (see Chapter 3)

Airway obstruction is an increased resistance to airflow caused by diffuse airway narrowing. The term denotes a disturbance of physiology as manifest by a **reduced forced expiratory volume in 1 second/vital capacity (FEV$_1$/VC) ratio**. From a practical perspective a FEV$_1$/VC ratio less than 0.7 is deemed to denote airway obstruction, though in truth the normal value of this ratio varies with age (see later). A number of factors contribute to airway obstruction in COPD: destruction of alveoli by emphysema leads to loss of elastic recoil and a loss of outward traction on the small airways such that they collapse on expiration (Figs. 11.1 and 11.2); airway inflammation with thickening of the airway wall (different to that seen in asthma and usually the result of tobacco smoke); accumulation of mucous secretions obstructing the airway lumen.

Emphysema

Emphysema is defined in terms of its pathological features that consist of **dilatation of the terminal air spaces of the lung distal to the terminal bronchiole with destruction of their walls**. Physiologically, emphysema is characterised by a reduction in the transfer factor for carbon monoxide and transfer coefficient (Chapter 3). High-resolution computed tomography (CT) scans can demonstrate the parenchymal lung destruction of emphysema. Two main patterns of emphysema are recognised (Fig. 11.1): **centriacinar** (centrilobular) emphysema involves damage around the respiratory bronchioles with preservation of the more distal alveolar ducts and alveoli. Characteristically, it affects the upper lobes and upper parts of the lower lobes of the lung. **Panacinar (panlobular) emphysema** results in distension and destruction of the whole of the acinus, and particularly affects the lower half of the lungs. Although both types of emphysema are related to smoking and may be present together, it is possible that they may arise by different mechanisms. Panacinar

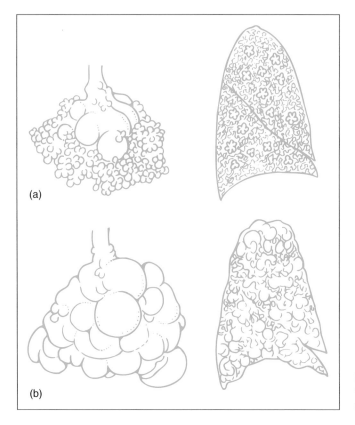

(a)

(b)

Figure 11.1 Emphysema. Diagrammatic view of lobule and whole lung section in (a) centrilobular and (b) panacinar emphysema.

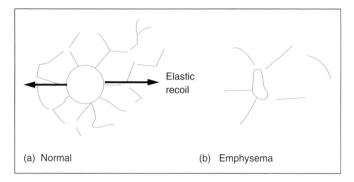

Elastic recoil

(a) Normal

(b) Emphysema

Figure 11.2 Emphysema consists of dilatation of the terminal air spaces of the lungs, distal to the terminal bronchiole with destruction of their walls. Small peripheral airways lack cartilage and depend on the support of the surrounding alveoli to maintain their patency (a). Alveolar destruction in emphysema results in a loss of elastic recoil and a loss of outward traction on the small airways such that they collapse on expiration contributing to the airways obstruction (b).

emphysema is the characteristic feature of patients with α_1-anti-trypsin enzyme deficiency.

Aetiology

Worldwide, a number of factors may be important in the development of COPD, the smoke from indoor cooking on open fires for example, but in the developed world **tobacco smoking** is far and away the most important cause. Even in the developing world smoking is of increasing importance. The total dose of tobacco inhaled is critical and depends on factors such as **age of starting** smoking, **depth of inhalation** and total **number of cigarettes** smoked (one 'pack year' is defined as the equivalent of 20 cigarettes per day for 1 year).

Although nearly all patients with COPD have smoked heavily, only about 15% of smokers develop COPD, suggesting that genetic susceptibility plays a part. There is a higher prevalence of COPD in **men** than in women, in patients of **lower socio-economic status** and in **urban** rather than rural areas.

There is evidence that COPD may be aggravated by **air pollution** but the role of pollution in the aetiology of COPD appears to be small when compared with that of cigarette smoking. Some dusty occupational environments are associated with the development of chronic bronchitis and COPD, for example those involving exposure to coal dust, cotton dust and grain (see Chapter 14). However, the contribution of occupation to the development of COPD is small when compared with the dominant effect of cigarette smoking.

A variety of **factors in early childhood** have an important influence on the development of obstructive airways disease in adulthood by determining the maximum lung function achieved in adolescence and possibly also the subsequent rate of decline in lung function. Such factors include **passive exposure** to **cigarette smoke** either transplacentally *in utero* or environmentally in the home. Some studies suggest that the presence of **airway responsiveness** predicts an accelerated rate of decline in lung function in smokers. The **genetic factors** that contribute to the differences between individuals in their susceptibility to developing COPD if they smoke are poorly defined except in the case of the inherited **deficiency of anti-protease enzymes**. It is thought that emphysema develops as a consequence of destruction of lung tissue by proteolytic digestion resulting from an imbalance between proteases and anti-proteases and between oxidants and anti-oxidants. Genetic deficiency of the principal anti-protease, α_1-anti-trypsin, is associated with the development of severe emphysema at a young age. α_1-anti-trypsin deficiency accounts for fewer than 1% of all cases of COPD but it is possible that other, unidentified proteases may be important.

Clinical features and progression

COPD has a wide spectrum of severity. The characteristic feature of the airway obstruction and emphysema of COPD is **gradually progressive breathlessness** sometimes associated with wheeze. Because of the large pulmonary reserve, patients with a sedentary lifestyle often do not notice breathlessness until a great deal of lung

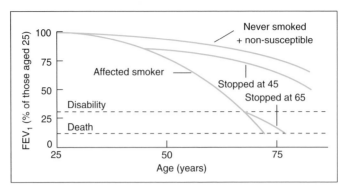

Figure 11.3 Change in FEV$_1$ with age: effect of smoking and stopping smoking. Non-smokers show a small progressive decline in function with age. Many smokers are unaffected by smoking and show the same decline as non-smokers. Some smokers are affected and show a steeper decline. By the time disability is noted, ventilatory function is seriously reduced to about one-third of predicted normal values. Those affected by smoking can be detected by measurement of FEV$_1$ many years before they become disabled. Stopping smoking slows the rate of decline. (From Fletcher & Peto, 1977.)

function has been permanently lost. Many people are in their fifties at the time of diagnosis and may have been smoking since their teens. Figure 11.3 illustrates the insidious progressive way in which lung function is lost in COPD. The graph also demonstrates the benefits of smoking cessation (see later).

Chronic **cough** and **sputum** production are the clinical manifestations of the mucus hypersecretion of chronic bronchitis that affects about 15% of men and 5% of women in the UK. **Infective exacerbations** of bronchitis are common and are characterised by an increased cough with purulent sputum. Non-typable unencapsulated strains of *Haemophilus influenzae* often colonise the normal upper respiratory tract. In chronic bronchitis disruption of the mucociliary defence mechanism facilitates spread of infection to the bronchial tree, where infection may provoke inflammation and a self-perpetuating vicious circle of inflammation and infection, further compromising pulmonary clearance mechanisms and aggravating airways obstruction. Extension of infection into the lung parenchyma, if it occurs, gives rise to **bronchopneumonia** (see Chapter 6).

Two main clinical patterns of disturbance may be discerned in patients with advanced COPD, which differ mainly in the extent to which ventilatory drive is preserved in the face of increasing airway obstruction: **'pink puffers'** and **'blue bloaters'** (Fig. 11.4). These represent two extremes of a spectrum and most patients do not fit either pattern completely, but have some features of both. 'Pink puffers' have well-preserved ventilatory drive even in the presence of severe airways obstruction. Dyspnoea is usually intense but P_{CO_2} is often maintained in the normal range at rest until the terminal stages of the disease. 'Blue bloaters' have poor ventilatory drive and easily drift into respiratory failure with hypercapnia, hypoxaemia and right heart failure, particularly during exacerbations.

Investigations

There is no single diagnostic test for COPD. Making a diagnosis relies on clinical judgement based on a combination of history, physical examination and confirmation of the presence of airflow obstruction using spirometry.

Lung function tests (Chapter 3)

Spirometry is the most accurate measure of airflow obstruction and is therefore crucial in the diagnosis of COPD. In the context of COPD, the diagnosis of airflow obstruction and the assessment of severity is based on **post-bronchodilator spirometry**.

The FEV$_1$/VC ratio declines naturally with age and the definition of airway obstruction should more correctly be defined by the lower limit of the normal range for the patient's age but for convenience a ratio: FEV$_1$/VC < 0.7 is generally taken to

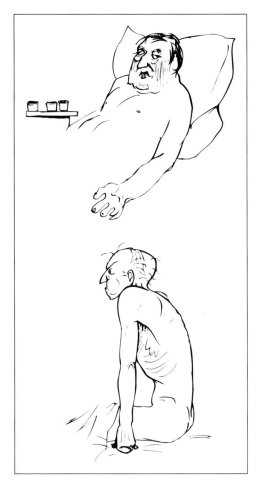

Figure 11.4 'Blue bloater' (above) and 'pink puffer' (below). (Original drawings reproduced by kind permission of Dr R.A.L. Brewis. From *Lecture Notes on Respiratory Disease*, 1st edn.)

performance of reversibility tests can be very useful in identifying an unsuspected case of asthma. Asthma and COPD are different conditions with different treatment algorithms. The two can co-exist. When they do, treatment strategies must deal with both conditions.

Total lung capacity and **residual volume** are often elevated signifying hyperinflation and air trapping. **Transfer factor for carbon monoxide** and **transfer coefficient** are typically reduced in emphysema.

Oximetry is useful in measuring oxygen saturation non-invasively but a sample of **arterial blood** is necessary to assess P_{O_2} and P_{CO_2} levels.

Radiology (Fig. 11.5)

The **chest X-ray** typically shows hyperinflation of the chest with flattened low hemidiaphragms, an increased retrosternal airspace and a long narrow cardiac shadow. The chest X-ray is also an important investigation in excluding additional diagnoses (e.g. lung cancer) and in detecting complications of COPD (e.g. pneumothorax, bronchopneumonia). **High-resolution CTscans** can demonstrate the extent of emphysema and the presence of bullae but are not required for the routine care of patients with COPD.

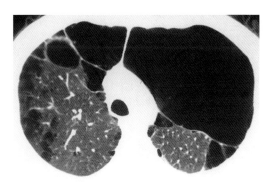

Figure 11.5 This 42-year-old man had smoked 20 cigarettes a day since the age of 14. He presented with a 5-year history of progressive breathlessness and could walk only 100 metres. He had severe airways obstruction with a FEV_1 of 0.5 L, and transfer factor for carbon monoxide and transfer coefficient were reduced to 30% of the predicted values. High-resolution computed tomography shows extensive emphysematous bullae with dilated distal airspaces, cysts and destruction of alveolar architecture. α_1-anti-trypsin levels were unrecordable.

define airway obstruction irrespective of age. The severity of airflow obstruction can be arbitrarily defined, as mild (FEV_1 >80% predicted), moderate (FEV_1 79–50% predicted), severe (FEV_1 49–30% predicted) and very severe (FEV_1 <30% predicted).

Spirometry can also be used to assess the degree of reversibility of the airways obstruction to bronchodilators or corticosteroids but this is a complex area. There is considerable variability in the change in FEV_1 in response to the same stimulus from day to day and the overall clinical usefulness of inhaled corticosteroids is generally not predicted by the response to a reversibility test (see management below). Nevertheless the

A multisystem disease

It is important to assess the full impact of the disease on all aspects of the patient's life. Breathlessness can be quantified using the **Medical Research Council Dyspnoea Scale**:

- grade 1: breathless only on strenuous exertion;
- grade 2: breathless when walking up a slight hill;
- grade 3: more breathless than contemporaries when walking on level ground;
- grade 4: breathless on walking about 100 metres;
- grade 5: breathless on dressing or undressing.

A number of questionnaires are available for assessing the overall function, **quality of life** and **impact** of the disease, such as the **COPD Assessment Test (CAT)**. Depression and anxiety are common and should be sought out (e.g. **Hospital Anxiety and Depression questionnaire**) and treated appropriately. Severe COPD can result in **cachexia** and **loss of muscle mass**; which reduces mobility and adds to the restriction on the patient's **social function**. **Nutritional** issues should also be identified and treated. The **BODE index** (body mass index, airflow obstruction, dyspnoea and exercise capacity) can be calculated to give an indication of prognosis. Some patients with chronic hypoxaemia develop **polycythaemia** with elevated haemoglobin levels. Patients with **cor pulmonale may show features** of right ventricular hypertrophy (right axis deviation, dominant R wave in V_1) on electrocardiography (**ECG**) and a dilated hypertrophied ventricle with tricuspid regurgitation on echocardiography (ECHO).

Management

For years COPD was dogged by a negative image. Being characterised by airway obstruction it fared poorly in its comparison with asthma. Airway obstruction in asthma is reversible, in COPD it is not in general. 'Non-reversible' was often confused with 'non-treatable'. It was the disease for which 'little could be done', indeed little was done. Over the last four decades of the twentieth century, as we began to get to grips with many diseases in the developed world, the age-adjusted death rate for coronary heart disease (CHD), for example, fell by almost 60%; a testament to what medicine and good public health measures can achieve. Over the same period of time, the age-adjusted death

rate for COPD, a disease in which the risk factors were just as well understood, rose by 163%. The reasons for this stark divergence in fortunes are manifold but it is noteworthy that, where CHD was a disease of the affluent and articulate in society, COPD has perhaps been, a disease of the 'disenfranchised'. The socioeconomic influence on COPD persists. Not only is there a higher prevalence of COPD in patients of **lower socioeconomic status,** this group also has the highest rate of underdiagnosis. COPD accounts for a considerable part of the **reduced life expectancy** in areas of deprivation compared with England as a whole.

In the past ten years there has been a revolution in our approach to COPD.

With the development of some new treatments, and indeed a fresh look at some of the old, we have managed to move beyond the nihilistic mindset. In COPD we now recognise that it is possible to have a very positive impact on a great number of clinically important outcomes, including: breathlessness, cough, sputum, exacerbation rate, hospital admission rate, disability, exercise endurance, quality of life, anxiety, depression, rate of progression of the disease and even mortality. The interventions that achieve these outcomes still do not have a great short-term impact on FEV_1, but in the face of such evidence it would be difficult to continue to view COPD as an 'untreatable' condition.

In managing patients with COPD we now have a great array of tools at our disposal including pharmacological, physical and psychological interventions. The appropriateness of each, needs to be considered carefully for every single patient and integrated into an overall comprehensive individualised management plan.

The first consideration in any patient still smoking has to be smoking cessation. If this can be achieved it will have a far greater impact on the long-term progression of the disease then any other intervention.

Smoking cessation

Figure 11.3 illustrates the decline in lung function seen in smokers with COPD. Many patients are well down the slippery slope before the diagnosis is established. The graph also demonstrates the effect of smoking cessation on disease progression. Although it is clear that the lung function lost is never regained (emphysema is permanent damage), smoking cessation changes the course of the disease. Indeed despite the vast sums of money spent on drug development, smoking cessation remains the only proven **disease-modifying** intervention for COPD. If smoking cessation occurs early enough in the course of the disease then the rate of decline in FEV_1 returns (approximately) to what it would have been had the patient never smoked – a natural age-related decline. Clearly the earlier smoking cessation can be achieved, the better the preservation of lung function. Although lung function never returns to normal it is clear that the patient will be far better off than if they had continued to smoke. Year on year they will experience fewer symptoms and a better quality of life as well, of course, as living longer. Smoking cessation therefore remains one of the most important components of management. Doctors need to do more than just pay lip service to smoking cessation. All patients still smoking, regardless of age, should be encouraged to stop, and offered help to do so, at every opportunity. The risks of lung cancer and heart disease are important issues to discuss of course but many patients are well aware of this increased 'risk' and have already rationalised the issue in their own mind. What many COPD patients are not aware of is the startling decline in quality of life that awaits them (not a risk, a certainty) if they continue to smoke. A description of the practical implications of declining lung function; a transition from mild breathlessness to being entirely housebound can have a powerful impact on a patient's determination to quit. Without this firm commitment by the individual, smoking cessations aids will achieve little. When used in conjunction with willpower, pharmacotherapy can improve quit rates.

Pharmacotherapy for smoking cessation

Small doses of nicotine produce predominantly stimulant effects such as arousal, whereas larger doses produce mainly depressant effects such as relaxation and relief of stress. **Nicotine withdrawal** can cause irritability, restlessness, anxiety, insomnia and a craving for cigarettes. Nicotine replacement therapy approximately doubles the success rates of attempts at smoking cessation and smokers should be encouraged to use it to avoid withdrawal symptoms. Typically, a heavy smoker is given **transdermal nicotine patches** 21 mg/day for 4 weeks, reducing to 14 mg/day for 2 weeks and then 7 mg/day for 2 weeks. Most withdrawal symptoms have resolved within that period of time. The patch is applied to the skin each morning and delivers a constant dose over 16–24 hours, but the onset of action is quite slow. Patients who experience marked cravings for cigarettes may benefit from using nicotine **chewing gum**, **lozenges**, **inhalator** or **nasal spray** that provide more rapid peak blood levels from absorption of the nicotine through the buccal or nasal mucosa. Nicotine replacement therapy is safe, but is not recommended in pregnancy. Addiction to nicotine replacement therapy can occur in a few patients who use it in the long term, but most patients can be weaned off treatment over a few weeks. **Bupropion (amfebutamone)** is a newer antidepressant drug that significantly improves the success of attempts at smoking cessation, although its mode of action is uncertain. It has some significant side-effects, most notably a 1 in 1000 risk of epileptic seizures such that it is contraindicated in patients with convulsive disorders, central nervous system disease, bulimia or anorexia nervosa, and in patients experiencing symptoms of withdrawal from alcohol or benzodiazepines. **Varenicline** is a nicotinic receptor partial agonist. As such, it both reduces cravings for and decreases the pleasurable effects of cigarettes, and through these mechanisms it can assist some patients to quit smoking. Side-effects include: nausea (common), headache, difficulty sleeping and abnormal dreams.

Pharmacological treatments in the management of stable COPD

Short-acting bronchodilators

Short-acting β_2-agonists, such as salbutamol and terbutaline, relax bronchial smooth muscle by stimulation of β-adrenoreceptors. **Short-acting anti-cholinergic drugs,** such as ipratropium, produce bronchodilatation by blocking the bronchoconstrictor effect of vagal nerve stimulation of bronchial smooth muscle. Although some bronchodilatation is in fact achievable it is the impact on breathlessness that is of most relevance. These old, long-established drugs are reasonably effective, short-term, symptom relievers and (β_2-agonists at least) remain first-line drugs, particularly in mild COPD.

Long-acting bronchodilators

Long-acting β_2-agonists, such as **salmeterol** and **formoterol**, give more prolonged relief of symptoms with a duration of action of about 12 hours and are a reasonable additional **maintenance therapy** when short-acting bronchodilators alone fail to provide adequate relief of symptoms.

Tiotropium is a **long-acting anti-cholinergic drug** that has greater affinity and a slower rate of dissociation from muscarinic receptors than ipratropium. It has a duration of action of at least 24 hours and therefore a convenient once daily dosage. As it also outperforms the short-acting ipratropium on all important indices, it has effectively superseded it. Tiotropium is a very good maintenance therapy. Although it can be used along side a long-acting β_2-agonists it cannot be used in conjunction with ipratropium. Ipratropium therefore, once a stalwart of COPD treatment, now has no real place in the management of chronic stable disease.

Although symptomatic relief of breathlessness is an important aim of treatment, COPD is a multifaceted disease and modern, comprehensive treatment strategies must therefore offer more than just short-term relief from this symptom.

Corticosteroids

COPD is a **chronic progressive condition**. In many other chronic progressive conditions 'disease modifying' drugs have been developed (disease-modifying antirheumatic drugs (DMARDs) in rheumatoid arthritis and statins in ischaemic heart disease for example). These drugs do not merely relieve symptoms at the time of use, they alter the long-term course of the disease. In COPD, disease progression is most commonly defined by the rate of decline in FEV_1. The drug that can halt or even slow that decline has long been sought. At the turn of the millennium two large international studies set out to determine if inhaled corticosteroids might be the disease modifying drug for COPD.

It transpired that corticosteroids are not that drug. Out of that investigation however, emerged evidence that inhaled corticosteroids could have a significant beneficial impact in the frequency of exacerbations; an outcome crucially important to many COPD patients. Subsequent studies have re-investigated this effect comparing it with the effect from long-acting β_2-agonists as well as the two drugs used together in a **combination inhaler** (e.g. Seretide® and Symbicort®). Although the individual components both have a positive impact, the greatest benefit is seen with the combination, which typically produces a 30% reduction in exacerbation frequency. There is also a positive knock on effect in reducing hospital admission rates. These important benefits are seen principally in moderate to severe disease; at the mild end of the spectrum the impact seems slight. The combination inhalers are now licensed for use with the indication of reducing exacerbation frequency in patients with an FEV_1 < 60% predicted. Inhaled corticosteroids alone are not licensed and have no place in the management of COPD.

Tiotropium

The symptomatic relief of breathlessness offered by tiotropium has already been discussed. In this sense tiotropium is effective in all grades of severity. In addition, as with the combination inhalers, in moderate to severe disease tiotropium has a beneficial impact on both exacerbation frequency and hospital admission rates.

Treatment strategy

In relation to the inhaled therapies the treatment strategy differs depending on the severity of the disease. In mild disease (other than smoking cessation support, for which the benefit is prognostic) treatment is principally aimed at short-term symptom control. Options such as tiotropium and long-acting β_2-agonists can be tried. They are usually effective but if not, it is likely to be evident within the first month and they should be stopped. In moderate and severe disease the situation is very different. Although symptom control remains important, there is, in addition, evidence of 'prognostic benefit' from certain treatments. Group mean data from very large studies tells us that the use of tiotropium and/or a combination inhaler will reduced the frequency of both exacerbations and hospitalisations. In contrast to the symptom controllers in mild disease, prognostic treatments should not be stopped if the patient reports no perceived benefit in the first month. This may seem obvious enough but the approach is quite a radical departure from traditional practice with inhaled therapies, where a 'try it and see' approach has been the norm. The principal of prognostic treatment is, of course, well understood and accepted in other clinical contexts such as: blood pressure control, hypercholesterolaemia and the use of β-blockers post myocardial infarction.

Inhaler technique

If you assume that **most people who have inhalers don't use them properly**, you'll not go far wrong! This is not usually the fault of the patient but of the prescriber who failed to spend time teaching and checking inhaler technique. There seems to be a general assumption that getting the inhaler technique 'about right' is good enough. It's not; lung delivery falls sharply if technique is not perfect and in many cases technique is so poor lung delivery is likely to be zero. Whenever an inhaler is prescribed care must be taken to coach (and then test) inhaler technique. This should, of course, be done by someone who understands it themselves. Technique should then be tested every time the patient is reviewed.

Oral medications

Methylxanthines such as aminophylline and theophyllines have a number of effects including cyclic adenosine monophosphate (cAMP) stimulation of β-adrenoceptors by inhibiting the metabolism of cAMP by the enzyme phosphodiesterase. Theophylline should only be used after a trial of short-acting bronchodilators and long-acting bronchodilators. Plasma levels need to be monitored as the therapeutic window is narrow. The dose should be reduced if a macrolide or fluroquinolone antibiotic is prescribed

A long-acting **PDE-4 inhibitor** roflumilast was launched in 2010. It has some benefit in reducing exacerbation frequency in patients at the severe end of the spectrum with the chronic bronchitis phenotype. It is licensed for use in Europe but not in the United States.

Mucolytics are drugs that increase the expectoration of sputum by reducing its viscosity. They were blacklisted in the NHS for a period of time; deemed not to work. The rational for this belief stemmed from the fact that they did not improve FEV_1. A reappraisal of the earlier studies rather than a rash of new studies led to a significant change in opinion. Although mucolytics do not have an impact on FEV_1, they can reduce the frequency of exacerbations in some patients with COPD who have a chronic productive cough. To most patients this would be a far more important outcome than a change in the result of a lung function test they barely understand. Doctors have finally recognised this priority too. The drugs are no longer banned, but recommended in patients with a chronic cough productive of sputum.

Psychological treatment

Anxiety and depression are common in COPD of all grades of severity and not just confined to severe disease. **Cognitive–behavioural therapy (CBT)** should be the first-line therapy although it is not yet widely available.

Pulmonary rehabilitation

Pulmonary rehabilitation is a multidisciplinary programme of care for patients with COPD that is individually tailored and designed to optimise the patient's physical and social performance and autonomy. Typically a pulmonary rehabilitation programme involves the skills of doctors, respiratory nurse specialists, physiotherapists, dieticians, social workers and occupational therapists. Many patients with COPD are in a vicious cycle of breathlessness, reduced physical activity and deconditioning of skeletal muscles, with resultant loss of social contact and autonomy. Pulmonary rehabilitation can break this vicious cycle and can **reduce dyspnoea, improve exercise tolerance and quality of life**. The key components of a rehabilitation programme need to be adjusted to meet the needs of the individual patient, but typically include the following.

- *Exercise training*: breathless patients often reduce their level of exercise and lose general fitness and muscle mass that causes a vicious cycle of deteriorating exercise capacity. Exercise training (e.g. walking, cycling) can counteract muscle atrophy and improve fitness. Improvement in lower limb function may help walking, and arm training improves performance of day-to-day tasks such as lifting, dressing, washing and brushing hair, for example. Typically an exercise training programme involves three supervised aerobic exercise sessions per week over a period of 8 weeks.
- *Smoking cessation*: advice, encouragement and support in achieving and maintaining smoking cessation.
- *Optimising drug treatment*: ensuring that the patient is taking a comprehensive treatment regimen, with a good inhaler technique.
- *Education* of the patient and family about the nature and cause of the disease and its management. The programme should include aspects such as how and when to take medications, the benefits of exercise, the importance of smoking cessation and the use of techniques such as breathing control, relaxation and anxiety management. Patients who are vulnerable to exacerbations can be taught to recognise the onset of symptoms of an exacerbation and instructed to

start a course of prednisolone and to increase their use of bronchodilator drugs, with an antibiotic for purulent sputum.

- *Breathing control techniques* involve pursed lip breathing, slower deeper respirations and better coordination of breathing patterns. Physiotherapy techniques such as active cycle breathing, chest percussion and forced expiratory techniques may be useful in patients who have difficulty expectorating secretions.
- *Social support:* patients with advanced disability may have difficulty in performing daily tasks such as climbing stairs, shopping and washing, and may benefit from assessment by an occupational therapist with regard to home aids such as stair lifts and bath aids. Assessment by a social worker allows the patient to obtain appropriate allowances, such as disability or mobility allowances, from government agencies.
- *Psychological support*: depression and social isolation are common and can be helped by psychological support focusing on restoring coping skills. Patient self-help groups may be useful. Some patients will require referral for more formal treatment such as CBT.
- *Nutrition*: poor nutrition is common in patients with advanced COPD and is associated with poor overall health status and an increased mortality. Patients with COPD are often underweight because of the increased work of breathing, the systemic effects of inflammatory cytokines and decreased food intake from anorexia and breathlessness. Some patients, in contrast, are overweight because of reduced activity and overeating. The patient's weight and body mass index should be measured and appropriate dietary advice given.

Pulmonary rehabilitation is an enormously valuable intervention but if the patient does not continue to exercise after completion of the formal programme the benefits in exercise performance are likely to be lost gradually over the following 6 months. Ideally patients should be encouraged to continue regular exercise and many such opportunities exists in local sports centres and gyms. Patients also benefit in this context from being on appropriate inhaled medication. The right symptom relievers are proven to both amplify the fitness benefits gained from pulmonary rehabilitation and slow the 'post programme' decline.

Oxygen therapy in stable disease

'Short of breath' does not imply 'short of oxygen'. It is important to understand that it is quite possible to experience breathlessness from a physiological cause without being hypoxic. In this context breathing supplemental oxygen will achieve nothing. As a simple analogy; imagine a car breaking down despite a full tank of petrol, in such circumstances supplying more petrol will do nothing to get the car re-started. Supplemental oxygen in a patient who is not hypoxic is similarly pointless.

Many breathless patients ask their doctor for oxygen therapy, many well-meaning doctors duly prescribe it. These prescriptions are costly and many are of no benefit to the patient whatsoever.

There are, nevertheless, a number of circumstances when oxygen therapy can not only improve symptoms but also extend life. Proper (specialist) assessment is required to ensure that the patients who need oxygen therapy receive it and those that do not, do not.

Long-term oxygen therapy

Hypoxia within the lung leads to pulmonary vasoconstriction that puts a strain on the right heart. The right heart struggles for a while, hypertrophies but eventually fails. Right heart failure caused by lung disease is known as **cor pulmonale**. The first sign is often ankle swelling. This is sometimes (incorrectly) perceived as a minor 'cosmetic' issue to be fixed with a small dose of diuretic. A moment's reflection however, would remind one that having half of the heart not working is likely to be a serious matter. It is. Cor pulmonale is a fatal disease. Patients with COPD and chronic hypoxia have a poor prognosis with a mortality rate of about 50% within 3 years.

The clinical features of hypoxia are non-specific, and periodic measurement of oxygen saturation by oximetry is useful in detecting these patients. In the early 1980s two major studies, the British Medical Research Council (MRC) Study and the American Nocturnal Oxygen Therapy Trial (NOTT), showed that the administration of oxygen for at least 15 hours/day (preferably longer) improved survival in patients with severe airflow obstruction (FEV_1 < 1.5 L) and hypoxia (Po_2 < 7.3 kPa (55 mmHg). It is important to understand that oxygen therapy has no impact on the progression of COPD (rate of decline of FEV_1); the improvement in survival is via the relaxation of pulmonary vasoconstriction and the alleviation of the strain on the right heart. It is the premature death from a complication of COPD, cor pulmonale, that is prevented.

Prescribing criteria

Long-term home oxygen therapy is indicated for **patients with severe COPD (FEV$_1$ < 1.5 L) and persistent hypoxia (Po$_2$ < 7.3 kPa (55 mmHg))**. Many patients who are hypoxic during an exacerbation will recover over a few weeks and will not require long-term oxygen. Arterial blood gases should therefore be measured on two occasions, at least 3 weeks apart, during a stable phase before diagnosing persistent hypoxia. Patients with more borderline oxygen levels (7.3–8.0 kPa (55–60 mmHg)) who have elevated haematocrit or already have features of cor pulmonale such as oedema are also likely to benefit from long-term oxygen. The oxygen is usually given via nasal cannulae at a flow rate of about 2 L/min but the dose required and mode of administration should be decided by a specialist in the context of the patient's arterial blood gas measurement.

Oxygen concentrator

Long-term home oxygen therapy is often provided from an oxygen concentrator. This is an electrically powered machine that separates oxygen from the ambient air using a molecular sieve. The machine is installed in the patient's house and plastic tubing relays oxygen to points such as the bedroom and living room. Providing oxygen cylinders to the patient's home for long-term oxygen therapy is impractical and much more expensive than installation of an oxygen concentrator. The patient and family should be warned not to smoke in the presence of oxygen because of the risk of causing a fire. It is essential that the patient understands that the main aim of long-term oxygen therapy is to improve prognosis (reduce mortality rate) rather than to alleviate symptoms and that it is necessary to comply with oxygen therapy for at least 15 hours/day. Patients often have to be reminded of this 15-hour rule as it runs counter to the instruction ('don't take more than...') that accompanies most other prescriptions.

When first advised of the need to spend so much of the day 'tied to an oxygen machine' patients are often visibly deflated. They imagine sitting next to a large oxygen cylinder, looking at the clock and waiting for 15 hours to pass. In fact the treatment can be accommodated far more easily than first imagined and time should be spent reassuring the patient on this matter. For a start, oxygen can be applied at night as the patient sleeps (that is 8 hours clocked up with no effort at all). Sufficient tubing around the home allows the patient to continue ordinary domestic activities during the day. A further 7 hours can therefore usually be clocked up without any limitation to lifestyle. Remind patients that the 15-hour rule still leaves them 9 hours in the day to be 'out and about'. Most patients find that if they simply use the oxygen whenever they are at home they can quite easily accumulate a sufficient number of hours with no deleterious effect on quality of life.

Ambulatory oxygen

Ambulatory oxygen may be appropriate for patients who are active enough to leave the home regularly, who demonstrate a fall in oxygen saturation to below 90% on exercise and who show symptomatic benefit from oxygen in terms of walking distance (assessed formally using a 6-minute walk test). It is given using a refillable portable container of liquid oxygen.

Short-burst oxygen is the use of oxygen for short periods to relieve dyspnoea after exercise. In these circumstances the patients typically breathes oxygen from a cylinder for a few minutes after exercise around the house. However, the benefit of this form of oxygen therapy is not clearly established. It is most commonly employed as a palliative measure in 'end-stage' disease.

Hypoxia during air travel

Patients with lung disease are vulnerable to developing hypoxia when travelling by plane. Commercial aircraft routinely fly at about 38 000 feet (11 400 m) and are pressurised to a cabin altitude of 8000 feet (2438 m) The reduced partial pressure of oxygen at this altitude is equivalent to breathing 15% oxygen at sea level, and causes the Po$_2$ of a healthy passenger to fall to between 7.0 and 8.5 kPa (52–64 mmHg). Although this does not usually cause symptoms or problems for most passengers it can produce critical hypoxia for patients with lung disease. Pre-flight assessment should include an overall assessment of the patient's condition and treatment with particular regard to dyspnoea, exercise capacity, previous flying experience, spirometry and oxygenation. If the oxygen saturation is >95% then in-flight oxygen is not required. If oxygen. saturation is < 92%

supplementary in-flight oxygen is usually prescribed at a rate of 2–4 L/min by nasal cannulae. If the oxygen saturation is between 92 and 95% then further assessment is recommended. This may include a **hypoxic challenge test** during which arterial blood gases are measured when the patient has been breathing 15% oxygen for 20 minutes, and in-flight oxygen is usually recommended if the P_{O_2} falls below 7.4 kPa (56 mmHg).

Surgery

A small number of patients with COPD may benefit from surgery. **Lung transplantation** is an option, although lack of donor organs severely limits the utilisation of this procedure. **Bullectomy** may be appropriate where a large bulla is compressing surrounding viable lung. **Lung volume reduction surgery** is an option for selected patients with severe disability. In emphysema, destruction of the alveoli results in a loss of elastic recoil with collapse of small airways on expiration and hyperinflation of the lungs with flattening of the diaphragm. Volume reduction surgery aims to resect functionally useless areas of lung thereby reducing the overall volume of the lungs in order to restore elastic recoil so that there is an increased outward traction on the small airways, relief of compression of normal lung and restoration of more normal diaphragmatic and thoracic contours allowing better respiratory motion during breathing. Patients whose emphysema preferentially affects the upper lobes may be the most suitable patients for this procedure. In certain patients lung function, exercise performance and quality of life are improved but the benefit tends to decline with time.

Emergency treatment

Exacerbations of COPD are characterised by an acute worsening of symptoms with increased breathlessness, sputum volume and sputum purulence. They may occur spontaneously or as a result of infections. There are associations between COPD admissions and the weather. The strongest relate to cold weather (admissions peak 12 days after a cold snap) and season (worse over the New Year).

Patients can be taught to recognise the onset of an exacerbation and to institute a **self-management plan** whereby they increase the dose and frequency of bronchodilator medication and start a course of oral prednisolone and an antibiotic, according to a predetermined plan. Mild exacerbations can be **managed at home** but patients with severe exacerbations require **admission to hospital**. Deciding whether a patient can be managed at home requires an overall assessment of the severity of the COPD (e.g. baseline FEV_1, oxygen saturation, exercise capacity), the home circumstances (e.g. family support, able to cope), and key adverse features that indicate a severe exacerbation (e.g. confusion, cyanosis, severe respiratory distress).

Patients admitted to hospital should have a chest x-ray, oximetry, arterial blood gas measurement, an ECG (to exclude comorbidities), full blood count and urea and electrolyte measurements. Culture of sputum is often performed but rarely produces a result in time to influence antibiotic prescribing. Blood cultures should be taken if the patient is pyrexial and a theophylline level should be measured in patients on theophylline therapy.

Bronchodilator therapy is usually given by nebuliser using a combination of **salbutamol** 2.5–5 mg and **ipratropium** 500 mcg with **prednisolone** 30 mg/day for 5–7 days.

Antibiotics

In some cases, exacerbations of COPD are associated with infections with viruses or with bacteria and antibiotics should be used to treat exacerbations of COPD associated with a history of more purulent sputum. Common bacteria include: *Haemophilus influenzae, Streptococcus pneumoniae* or *Moraxella catarrhalis*. Although **amoxicillin** has a reasonably good spectrum of activity against many of these organisms, 15–20% of *Haemophilus influenzae* and many strains of *Moraxella catarrhalis* are resistant to **amoxicillin** so that other antibiotics such as **co-amoxiclav** (amoxicillin and clavulanic acid), **trimethoprim**, **ciprofloxacin**, **tetracycline** or **clarithromycin** may be needed. In many cases exacerbations of COPD seem to arise as a result of a spontaneous worsening or are provoked by non-infectious events such as air pollution, smoking or adverse weather conditions. Patients with exacerbations without more purulent sputum do not need antibiotic therapy unless there is consolidation on a chest radiograph or clinical signs of pneumonia.

Pneumococcal vaccination and annual **influenza vaccination** are recommended for patients with COPD.

Emergency oxygen

Oxygen is delivered in most emergency situations with the aim of achieving a near normal saturation (94–98%). However, for some patients such levels are dangerous and may be life threatening.

Patients with established respiratory failure who have chronically raised P_{CO_2} (type 2 respiratory failure) become unresponsive to the carbon dioxide stimulus to ventilation and rely increasingly on hypoxaemia to maintain the drive to breathe. If they are given high concentrations of oxygen they breathe less and underbreathing results in increasing hypercapnia, acidosis, narcosis, respiratory depression and ultimately death. Uncontrolled oxygen therapy poses a risk to this subset of patients with COPD. The risk of course, must be balanced against the threat of hypoxia. Because of the shape of the oxyhaemoglobin dissociation curve, there is little benefit in increasing the patient's oxygen saturation above about 90% (P_{O_2} above about 8 kPa (60 mmHg)).

In patients at risk of hypercapnic respiratory failure (which unless proven otherwise includes any patient with an exacerbation of COPD) treatment should be commenced using a 28% Venturi mask (Fig. 11.6) in pre-hospital care or a 24% Venturi mask in the hospital settings with an initial target saturation of 88–92% pending urgent blood gas assessment to determine the patient's ventilatory status (pH and P_{CO_2}) (Chapter 3).

It is essential to document carefully the amount of oxygen being breathed when measuring arterial gases. Avoid measuring gases immediately after the patient has received nebulised drugs using high-flow oxygen.

Sometimes there is concern about using high-flow oxygen (e.g. 6–8 L/min) to nebulise bronchodilator drugs in patients with hypercapnia and occasionally air is used to nebulise these drugs. However, nebulising drugs using air during acute exacerbations of COPD may leave the patient dangerously hypoxic. One option it to deliver concomitant supplemental oxygen via nasal cannulae. Alternatively it is safe to use oxygen to nebulise the drug provided the nebulisation time can be strictly limited to 10 minutes. The patient is then not exposed to the risk of either hypoxia or prolonged high-concentration oxygen.

Ventilatory support

At times despite the best efforts of doctors acute respiratory acidosis supervenes (when high-flow

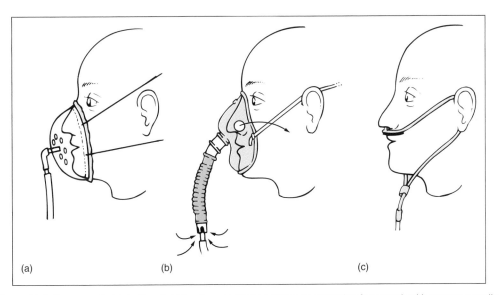

(a)　　　　　　　(b)　　　　　　　　　　　　　(c)

Figure 11.6 Oxygen administration. (a) Simple uncontrolled high-concentration face mask with oxygen supplied directly to the mask space. (b) Fixed performance Venturi mask delivering a controlled (fixed) dose of low-concentration oxygen. (c) Nasal cannulae delivering an uncontrolled level of oxygen in a convenient continuous manner.

oxygen is inappropriately delivered it may occur *because* of the efforts of doctors). It is crucially important to recognise respiratory acidosis when present and blood gas analysis is essential to the management of acute exacerbations of COPD in hospital.

After initial management with nebulised bronchodilators and appropriate oxygen therapy if the pH is below the normal range (<7.35) then **Non-Invasive Ventilation(NIV)** should be employed (unless there is a specific contraindication (rare) or the patient declines it). It should be delivered in a dedicated setting with staff who have been trained in its application and there should be a clear plan covering what to do in the event of deterioration.

When used in this context, NIV not only reduces the likelihood that the patient will progress to need intubation and invasive ventilation, it has also been demonstrated to **reduce inpatient mortality by 50%**. Despite the overwhelming evidence of such substantial clinical benefit, a number of national audits have demonstrated that NIV is not utilised as often as it should be. This seems to be as a result of both a lack of knowledge of the specific indication and a failure to appreciate the magnitude of the benefit. A rather laissez faire and fatalistic approach is still worryingly common. In the light of current evidence such an approach is frankly wrong.

Practical application

NIV is delivered via a tight-fitting mask strapped in place over the nose and mouth and connected to a specifically designed ventilating machine. The spontaneous respiratory efforts of the patient are used to trigger the ventilator to deliver additional tidal volume under positive pressure. Lack of familiarity with the technical aspects of NIV may be what deters many doctors from employing this therapy. Yet in most UK hospitals the practical aspects of NIV use are handled by the on-call physiotherapy team or specialist nurses. All the doctor really needs to know is the arterial pH and how to pick up a telephone.

Prior to the advent of NIV, the intravenous respiratory stimulant **doxapram** was used in a similar context. This option may still be useful for those few patients unable to tolerate NIV but **invasive ventilation** (i.e. endotracheal intubation and ventilation on ITU) should be considered.

Admission avoidance and early supported discharge for COPD

Novel ways of managing patients with acute exacerbations of COPD are being developed. In some cases admission to hospital can be avoided by undertaking an initial assessment, in the patient's home, usually by a specialist nurse according to an agreed protocol with the back up of a respiratory specialist and admission to hospital if needed. Easy access to such a reassuring review can often prevent patients calling an ambulance unnecessarily. Such schemes are being increasingly adopted, although they are perhaps still rather probationary with, as yet, no proven model firmly established.

For other patients **early supported discharge** is more appropriate whereby after initial treatment and stabilisation in hospital ongoing care is provided to the patient in their own home. This model of care is now well established. It is safe, effective and very popular with patients.

 Respiratory emergencies COPD

Tests

Chest X-ray, oximetry, arterial blood gases, ECG, sputum culture, blood count, urea, electrolytes

Treatment

- Bronchodilators, for example nebulised **salbutamol** 2.5–5 mg and **ipratropium** 500 mcg; repeat as needed and continue 4–6 hourly.
- Steroids: **prednisolone** 30 mg/day orally for 5–7 days.
- Antibiotics, for example **amoxicillin** 500 mg t.i.d. orally or intravenously. Check previous sputum microbiology and consider doxycycline, ciprofloxacin, clarithromycin, co-amoxiclav if needed.
- Oxygen: aim for O_2 saturation 88–92% unless and until hypercapnia is excluded on arterial blood gases.
- Ventilatory support: **non-invasive ventilation** if hypercapnic with pH <7.35 or endotracheal ventilation in ITU if appropriate

Both of these models of care are very cost-effective compared with a standard, prolonged hospital admission. Their safety and success however, is entirely dependant on the expertise and experience of the staff delivering them.

 KEY POINTS

- Smoking-related COPD is a major cause of morbidity and mortality worldwide.
- Spirometry is essential in assessing airways obstruction (FEV_1/FVC ratio < 0.7) in COPD.
- Smoking cessation is the most important intervention in reducing the rate of progression of COPD.
- COPD is an eminently treatable condition.
- Inhaled β_2-agonist and anti-cholinergic bronchodilators improve: symptoms, exercise capacity and quality of life.
- Combination inhalers and tiotropium can reduce exacerbations and hospitalisations in moderate to severe disease.
- During exacerbations of COPD patients who remain hypercapnic and acidotic (pH < 7.35) despite nebulised bronchodilators, systemic steroids, antibiotics and controlled oxygen therapy should be treated with NIV.
- Pulmonary rehabilitation improves the patient's physical and social performance and quality of life.
- Long-term oxygen therapy at home improves the prognosis of patients with COPD who have persistent hypoxia ($Po_2 < 7.3$ kPa (55 mmHg)).

 FURTHER READING

British Thoracic Society Standards of Care Committee. Guideline for Emergency Oxygen Use in Adult Patients. *Thorax* 2008; **63** (suppl VI): 1–81 (www.brit-thoracic.org.uk).

British Thoracic Society Standards of Care Committee Intermediate Care. Hospital-at-Home in Chronic Obstructive Pulmonary Disease Guideline. *Thorax* 2007; **63** (suppl 3): 200–10 (www.brit-thoracic.org.uk).

British Thoracic Society Standards of Care Committee. Non-invasive ventilation in acute respiratory failure. *Thorax* 2002; **57**: 192–211 (www.brit-thoracic.org.uk).

British Thoracic Society Standards of Care Committee. Managing passengers with respiratory disease planning air travel. *Thorax* 2002; **57**: 289–304 (2010 update available www.brit-thoracic.org.uk).

Celli BR, MacNee W. Standards for the diagnosis and treatment of patients with COPD: a summary of the ATS/ERS position paper. *Eur Respir J* 2004; **23**: 932–46.

Department of Health Home Oxygen Service: http://www.homeoxygen.nhs.uk/2.php

Fletcher C, Peto R. The natural history of chronic airflow obstruction. *BMJ* 1977; **1**: 1645.

National Institute for Health and Clinical Excellence. *Chronic Obstructive Pulmonary Disease: Management of Chronic Obstructive Pulmonary Disease in Adults in Primary and Secondary Care (2010)*. NICE, 2010 (http://guidance.nice.org.uk/CG101/Guidance/pdf/English).

Ram FSF, Wedzicha JA, Wright J, Greenstone M. Hospital at home for patients with acute exacerbations of chronic obstructive pulmonary disease: systematic review of evidence. *BMJ* 2004; **329**: 315.

Royal College of Physicians, British Thoracic Society, Intensive Care Society. The Guideline Development Group. *Non-Invasive Ventilation in Chronic Obstructive Pulmonary Disease: Management of Acute Type 2 Respiratory Failure*. Concise Guidance to Good Practice Series No 11. London: Royal College of Physicians, 2008 (http://bookshop.rcplondon.ac.uk/).

12

Carcinoma of the lung

Introduction

Lung cancer is the most common cause of cancer death in the world with more than one million deaths occurring yearly. In the UK it kills about 34 000 people each year and it has overtaken breast cancer as the leading cause of cancer deaths in women. It is a lethal disease with only 25% of patients surviving 1 year, and only 7% surviving 5 years from diagnosis. About 90% of lung cancers are caused by smoking, and smoking prevention and smoking cessation are the crucial issues in dealing with this major public health problem.

Aetiology (Table 12.1)

The epidemic spread of lung cancer in the twentieth century followed about 20 years after increases in **tobacco-smoking** habits (Fig. 12.1). The commercial manufacture of cigarettes started around 1900 and smoking soon became popular among men. At that time lung cancer was a very rare disease. By the end of the 1940s about 70% of men and 40% of women smoked. Doctors then started to be aware of an increasing incidence of lung cancer and noticed that the patients were smokers. By 1950 an epidemic of lung cancer had become apparent and studies, such as those of Doll and Hill in the 1950s, established the causative link

between smoking and lung cancer. Doll and Hill studied the smoking habits and cause of death of UK doctors and showed a significant and steadily rising incidence of deaths from lung cancer as the amount of tobacco smoked increased. At that time 83% of doctors had smoked but thereafter the medical profession were the first to put research into practice, by stopping smoking! In the early 1960s the Royal College of Physicians of London and the Surgeon General of the USA published their landmark reports documenting the causal relationship between smoking and lung cancer. The risk of death from bronchial carcinoma increases by a factor roughly equal to the number of cigarettes smoked per day. For example, a man smoking 30 cigarettes/day has over 30 times the risk of dying from lung cancer than a man who has never smoked. On stopping smoking, excess risk is approximately halved every 5 years thereafter. Smoking has decreased in popularity such that now in the UK about 29% of men and 28% of women smoke. Reflecting these changes, lung cancer mortality rates have begun to decline in men and in younger women, although rates in older women are still rising. Although smoking in the UK is declining, it is increasing in developing countries so that the epidemic of smoking-related mortality and morbidity that has dominated health trends in the Western world in the twentieth century may be repeated in the developing world in the next hundred years.

Breathing other people's tobacco smoke – **passive or environmental smoke** – is also a cause

Respiratory Medicine Lecture Notes, Eighth Edition. Stephen J. Bourke and Graham P. Burns.
© 2011 John Wiley & Sons, Ltd. Published 2011 by John Wiley & Sons, Ltd.

Table 12.1 Aetiology of carcinoma of the lung

- Tobacco smoking
- Passive smoking
- Genetic factors
- Ionising radiation (e.g. radon gas)
- Asbestos exposure
- Diffuse lung fibrosis (e.g. fibrosing alveolitis)
- Lack of dietary fruit and vegetables

of lung cancer. For example, a woman who has never smoked has an estimated 24% greater risk of developing lung cancer if she lives with a smoker. Genetic factors may be important in determining the way individuals metabolise inhaled carcinogens or in the expression of oncogenes or tumour-suppressor genes, and a **family history** of lung cancer is a risk factor for the development of the disease. There is an increased incidence of lung cancer in patients with **diffuse lung fibrosis** such as idiopathic pulmonary fibrosis and so-called **'scar carcinomas'** may occur in areas of focal fibrosis resulting from previous tuberculosis. The male to female ratio for lung cancer is approximately 1.5:1 reflecting past smoking differences. Smoking and lung cancer are both associated with **social deprivation**. Some studies suggest that a high dietary intake of fruit and vegetables containing β-carotene reduces the risk of lung cancer. Exposure to **ionising radiation** such as from radon gas arising from the ground and building materials in some homes may be important and accounts for a proportion of lung cancers in non-smokers. Occupational exposure to **asbestos** is associated

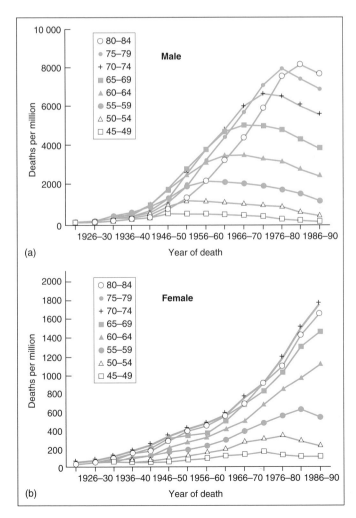

Figure 12.1 (a) Male and (b) female mortality from lung cancer by age and year of death, England and Wales, 1921–90. (Reproduced with permission from the Lung and Asthma Information Agency. From *Trends in Lung Cancer and Smoking*. Factsheet 93/1 www.laia.ac.uk).

with an increased risk of lung cancer with an approximately linear relationship between the dose of asbestos and the occurrence of lung cancer. The interaction between asbestos and smoking is multiplicative.

Pathology (Fig. 12.2)

Although the pathology of lung cancer is complex, for clinical purposes the disease is classified into two groups:

1 **Small-cell carcinoma** (20% of lung cancer).
2 **Non-small-cell carcinoma** (80%), comprising **squamous-cell carcinoma** (45%), **adenocarcinoma** (20%) and **large-cell (undifferentiated) carcinoma** (15%).

Small-cell (oat-cell) carcinoma arises from neuroendocrine cells of the bronchial tree and its endocrine potential is sometimes manifest clinically by ectopic hormone production. This is a highly malignant cancer that grows rapidly and metastasises early. Squamous-cell carcinoma is the most common type of lung cancer and shows the greatest tendency to cavitate. The incidence of adenocarcinomas seems to be rising and is currently about 20%. These tumours often arise in the periphery of the lung, sometimes as 'scar carcinomas' and show the least relationship to smoking.

About 15% of lung cancers do not show squamous or glandular differentiation and are classified as large-cell undifferentiated carcinomas.

Diagnosis

Lung cancers arising centrally in the bronchial tree often present with **chest symptoms** (e.g. haemoptysis) whereas peripheral tumours may grow silently without causing local symptoms until late in the course of the disease (Fig. 12.3). Such tumours may be found coincidentally on a **chest X-ray** or present with non-specific **general symptoms** (e.g. weight loss), with effects of **metastases** (e.g. to brain, bone) or with non-metastatic **paraneoplastic syndromes**.

Paraneoplastic syndromes arise at sites distant from the tumour or its metastases and result from the production of hormones, peptides, antibodies, prostaglandins or cytokines by the tumour. The **syndrome of inappropriate anti-diuretic hormone** (ADH) secretion is most common with small-cell cancer and results in a low serum sodium, potassium and urea, a serum osmolarity below 280 mosmol/L and a urine osmolarity greater than 500 mosmol/L. Treatment consists of restriction of fluid intake, and drugs such as tolvaptan (a vasopressin receptor antagonist) 15–60 mg/day or demeclocycline (which competes for ADH

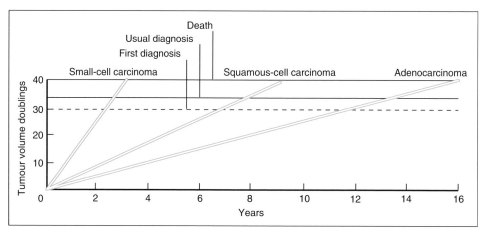

Figure 12.2 Lung cancer growth rates. As a rough approximation, small-cell carcinomas double monthly, squamous-cell carcinomas 3 monthly and some adenocarcinomas 6 monthly. A tumour typically becomes evident on a chest X-ray when it reaches about 1 cm in diameter, corresponding to about 30 doubling volumes. Symptoms usually arise later than this. By 40 doublings death will usually have occurred. Diagnosis occurs late in the course of the disease and most of the tumour's life history is subclinical.

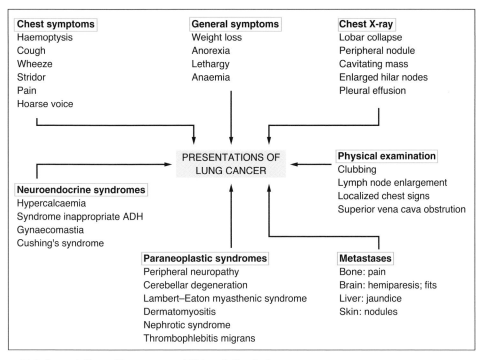

Figure 12.3 Presentations of lung cancer. ADH, anti-diuretic hormone.

renal tubular binding sites) 600–1200 mg/day. **Hypercalcaemia** in patients with lung cancer may be indicative of bone metastases but squamous-cell carcinomas sometimes secrete a parathyroid hormone-related protein that causes non-metastatic hypercalcaemia. Clearly, some patients will present primarily with chest symptoms, often against a background of pre-existing smoking-related lung disease (e.g. chronic obstructive pulmonary disease (COPD)). Equally, a diagnosis of lung cancer must be considered in patients presenting with a variety of medical problems.

Tumours in certain specific locations may cause problems by direct invasion of adjacent structures. Direct invasion of the mediastinum may cause paralysis of the **phrenic nerve**, manifest by elevation of the hemidiaphragm, or of the **recurrent laryngeal nerve**, particularly on the left side where it passes around the aortic arch to the superior mediastinum, causing vocal cord palsy with hoarseness and diminished cough reflex. Injection of Teflon® or Bioplastique® into the paralysed vocal cord under general anaesthesia can improve voice quality by building up the volume of the vocal cord enabling better apposition. **Obstruction of**

the superior vena cava causes venous engorgement of the upper body with facial oedema, headache, distended pulseless jugular veins and enlarged collateral veins over the chest and arms. These symptoms require urgent treatment by chemotherapy in the case of small-cell cancer or radiotherapy in the case of other tumours. Insertion of an expandable metallic wire stent into the strictured vein under radiological guidance can give rapid relief of symptoms in severe cases. A **Pancoast tumour** (Fig. 12.4) is a carcinoma situated in the superior sulcus of the lung where the subclavian artery forms a groove over the lung apex. Because of its particular anatomical location a tumour here gives rise to a characteristic syndrome: ipsilateral Horner's syndrome (ptosis, meiosis, enophthalmos, anhydrosis) because of stellate ganglion involvement; pain caused by erosion of the posterior first and second ribs, and wasting of the small muscles of the hand as a result of brachial plexus invasion. The tumour may invade a vertebral foramen giving spinal cord compression. These tumours are notoriously difficult to detect on a chest X-ray and the cause of the patient's pain is often misdiagnosed initially.

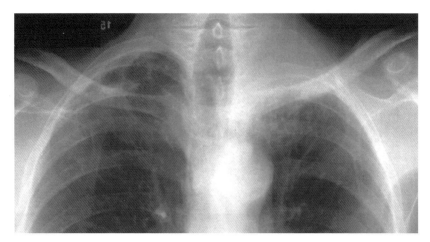

Figure 12.4 Pancoast tumour. This 68-year-old man presented with a 3-month history of left shoulder pain. On examination he had features of a left Horner's syndrome (ptosis, meiosis, enophthalmos, anhydrosis). Chest X-ray shows a mass at the apex of the left lung eroding the first and second ribs posteriorly. Percutaneous biopsy showed squamous-cell carcinoma. He was treated with palliative radiotherapy.

The chest X-ray plays a pivotal role in the investigation of lung cancer, and a range of abnormalities may be apparent. A peripheral tumour may be seen as a small nodule or mass in the lung. A cavitating mass is characteristic of squamous-cell carcinoma (Fig. 4.7). Central tumours may cause bronchial obstruction typically giving rise to atelectatic collapse of a lung or lobe of a lung (Fig. 12.5), or to pneumonic consolidation distal to the obstruction. Thus, 'loss of volume' of a lobe (atelectatic collapse) on a chest X-ray in a patient with apparent pneumonia is a sinister feature suggesting bronchial obstruction by a carcinoma. The chest X-ray may show evidence of spread of the tumour to bone (e.g. rib or vertebral destruction), pleura (e.g. effusion), hilar or mediastinal structures. **Computed tomography (CT) scanning** is the next key investigation in defining the extent and spread of the tumour and in planning the best approach to obtaining histological diagnosis.

Histological–cytological diagnosis should be obtained wherever possible. **Sputum cytology** is positive in about 40% of cases, and is particularly useful in patients unfit for invasive tests. **Bronchoscopy** allows direct visualisation and biopsy of central tumours. Peripheral tumours seen on chest X-ray may not be accessible to bronchoscopy and **percutaneous needle biopsy** of these lesions under radiological guidance is a useful technique (Fig. 12.6). Small peripheral cancers need to be distinguished from rare benign tumours (e.g. hamartomas) and from granulomas resulting from

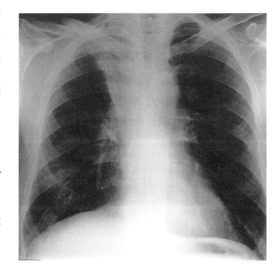

Figure 12.5 Right upper lobe collapse. This 65-year-old smoker presented with haemoptysis. Chest X-ray shows a triangular-shaped opacity in the right upper zone indicating collapse of the right upper lobe. Bronchoscopy showed a tumour occluding the orifice to the right upper lobe and biopsy showed a large-cell undifferentiated carcinoma. Computed tomography showed that the tumour was confined to the right upper lobe without mediastinal invasion or metastases. He was treated by right upper lobectomy. Coincidentally the X-ray also shows an old un-united fracture of the right clavicle.

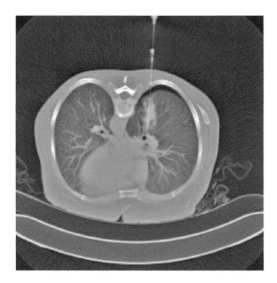

Figure 12.6 This 66-year-old smoker was found to have a mass in the periphery of the lung when an X-ray was performed during an exacerbation of COPD. Percutaneous fine needle aspiration of the lesion was performed under computed tomography guidance and showed adenocarcinoma on cytology. The procedure has caused a small pneumothorax that resolved spontaneously without the need for intervention.

previous tuberculosis, but it may be advisable to proceed to surgical resection without histological confirmation of the diagnosis if the risk of cancer is high. Diagnosis may also be achieved by obtaining material from a site of metastasis (e.g. lymph node, skin, pleural effusion).

Bronchoscopy

Flexible fibreoptic bronchoscopy is usually performed as an outpatient procedure under sedation (e.g. midazolam) and topical anaesthesia (e.g. lidocaine to the vocal cords and airways). The bronchoscope is usually passed through the nose into the orophayrynx, and then through the vocal cords into the trachea and bronchial tree to the subsegmental level. The bronchial tree is illuminated by light transmitted from a light source to the tip of the bronchoscope and the image is transmitted to the eyepiece or displayed on a screen. About two-thirds of lung cancers are visible through the bronchoscope, and therefore bronchoscopy is a key investigation for lung cancer or haemoptysis. A biopsy forceps or cytology brush may be passed through the channel to obtain

samples from a tumour and saline washings can be aspirated for cytology or microbiology tests (Fig. 13.1). Bronchoscopy is a very safe procedure but is contraindicated in patients with uncontrolled angina or recent myocardial infarction. Sedation should be avoided or used with particular caution in patients with respiratory depression. Pulse oximetry is used to monitor oxygen saturation and supplemental oxygen is given. The bronchoscope is carefully cleaned with detergent and immersed in glutaraldehyde to prevent transmission of infection between patients. It is recommended that the bronchoscopist and nurses should wear masks, goggles and gowns to prevent contracting infections (e.g. tuberculosis) from the patient by aerosols generated by coughing.

Endobronchial ultrasound(EBUS) is a newer technique that allows needle aspiration to be performed, under ultrasound guidance via a specially designed bronchoscope, of mediastinal lymph nodes (e.g. subcarinal, paratracheal nodes) and of tumours causing extrinsic compression of bronchi. It is a very useful technique in the diagnosis and staging of lung cancer. Ultrasound needle biopsy of small supraclavicular nodes is also a useful, minimally invasive, method of obtaining cytology. About 50% of patients with mediastinal adenopathy on CT scan will also have small pathological supraclavicular nodes that can be detected and aspirated using ultrasound.

Communicating the diagnosis

Telling a patient of the diagnosis of lung cancer is a difficult clinical skill that needs to be developed by training and experience. Patients want to talk honestly about what is happening to them and to know more about the way ahead. The patient's awareness of the diagnosis often emerges over a number of consultations and the time that elapses between initial suspicion of tumour and histological confirmation of the diagnosis is often useful in allowing the patient an opportunity to come to terms with the situation. When discussing the diagnosis it is essential to allow adequate time for questions, to ensure privacy during the interview, to encourage a relative or friend to accompany the patient for support and to have further counselling available for the patient from skilled nurses. Some patients may find written information about lung cancer and its treatment useful.

Inevitably, patients will experience emotions such as shock, anger and denial and the doctor must work through these emotions with the patient. It is useful to be able to bring the interview to a conclusion on a more positive note by discussing a management plan. Many patients will initially be too shocked to understand the information given and it is often useful to arrange a further interview either with the hospital doctor, nurse or general practitioner to answer the patient's questions. Rapid communication between all members of the medical team is crucial in these circumstances.

Treatment (Fig. 12.7)

Treatment depends on the histological **cell type**, the **stage** of the disease and the **fitness** of the patient. The management plan is discussed by the **multidisciplinary team** following a review of the patient's radiological, histopathological and clinical details.

Small-cell carcinoma (20%)

Small-cell carcinoma is a highly malignant cancer that has usually disseminated widely by the time of diagnosis such that systemic treatment in the form of **chemotherapy** is required. On rare occasions when small-cell carcinoma is diagnosed by surgical resection of a peripheral nodule, adjuvant chemotherapy is given post-operatively. Various combinations of chemotherapeutic agents are available using drugs such as carboplatin, cisplatin, etoposide, cyclophosphamide, doxorubicin, vincristine, gemcitabine, vinorelbine, irinotecan and taxanes (paclitaxel, docetaxel). Combinations of these drugs (e.g. carboplatin and etoposide) are usually given as a day treatment in pulses at intervals of about 4 weeks for up to six cycles of treatment. Untreated patients with small-cell carcinoma are usually very symptomatic with a median survival of only 3 months. Combination chemotherapy achieves a symptom-relieving remission of the cancer in about 70% of patients with reduction in tumour size and prolongation of survival. Small-cell cancer is staged as **limited disease** when it can be encompassed within a 'tolerable' radiotherapy port (involving one hemithorax, including ipsiplateral mediastinal, subcarinal and supraclavicular nodes or contralateral hilar nodes), or **extensive disease** when it has spread beyond a radiotherapy port (distant metastases or spread beyond one hemithorax). In limited stage disease chemotherapy improves survival from an average of 3 months without treatment to 12 months with treatment, and 5–10% of patients achieve a 5-year survival. In extensive stage disease chemotherapy improves survival from an average of 6 weeks to 8 months. **Consolidation radiotherapy** is usually given to the site of the tumour and mediastinal nodes. Cerebral metastases are common so that prophylactic cranial radiotherapy is also given to patients with limited disease who have responded to chemotherapy. Patients receiving chemotherapy require careful monitoring of their full blood count to avoid problems arising from bone marrow suppression such as anaemia, haemorrhage or infection. Hair loss occurs with some drugs and patients may choose to wear a wig. Careful attention to anti-emetic medications (e.g. ondansetron, domperidone, metoclopramide) can usually prevent nausea and vomiting.

Non-small-cell cancer (80%)

Surgical resection of the tumour offers the best chance of cure in non-small-cell carcinoma but is only possible if the patient is fit for surgery and if the tumour has not already metastasised. **Staging** (Table 12.2) is the assessment of the extent and spread of the disease and is important in determining the potential resectability of the tumour and the prognosis of the patient. The TNM system is the most widely used and is based upon the size, location and degree of invasion of the tumour (T), the presence of regional lymph node involvement (N) and distant metastases (M). The accuracy of staging depends on the degree of assessment, for example staging at thoracotomy may show more advanced disease than was apparent on CT scanning.

When staging a tumour the patient's **symptoms** should be carefully reviewed for any indication of metastatic disease (e.g. bone pain). Clinical **examination** may show evidence of tumour spread to lymph nodes or reveal features of distant metastases. **Bronchoscopy** allows direct visualisation of many tumours and may show features of inoperability (e.g. vocal cord palsy, splaying of the carina by subcarinal lymphadenopathy or extension of the tumour to within 2 cm of the main carina). Elevated liver function tests or bone **biochemistry**

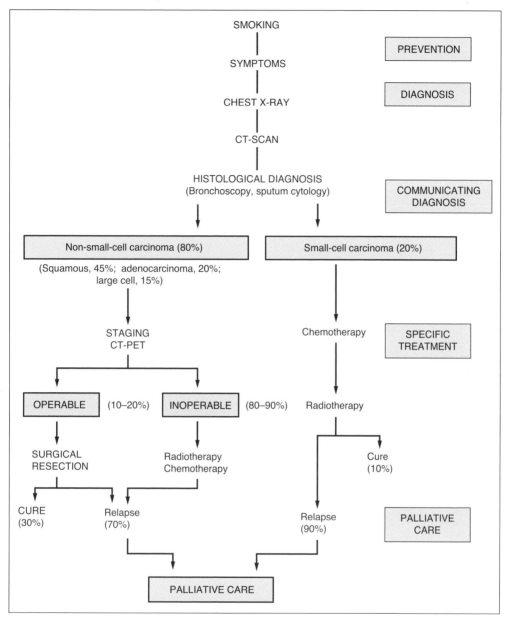

Figure 12.7 The 5-year mortality rate of lung cancer is about 93%, emphasising the fact that the disease is usually disseminated at the time of presentation. Prevention of lung cancer by avoidance of smoking is the most important strategy in the fight against this disease. Choice of treatment depends on cell type and stage of disease. About 20% of lung cancers are small-cell carcinomas and are best treated by chemotherapy followed by radiotherapy. There is usually a good response to chemotherapy but relapse is likely. About 80% are non-small-cell carcinomas and require careful staging and assessment for potential operability. About 10–20% of non-small-cell carcinomas are suitable for surgery but only 30% of patients undergoing resection will be alive in 5 years. A judicious plan of assessment allows careful selection of the best choice of specific anti-cancer treatment with either curative or palliative intent. Symptom relief and palliative care are crucial aspects in the overall management, and the communication of information between doctor and patient at all stages of the disease is of paramount importance. CT, computed tomography; PET, positron emission tomography.

Table 12.2 Outline of the main examples of TNM staging of non-small-cell lung cancer

Stage	TNM			Operability	5-year survival (%)
IA	$T_{1a,b}$	N_0	M_0		70%
IB	T_{2a}	N_0	M_0		50%
IIA	$T_{1a,b}$	N_1	M_0	Resectable	
	T_{2a}	N_1	M_0		45%
	T_{2b}	N_0	M_0		
IIB	T_{2b}	N_1	M_0	Resectable	30%
IIB	T_3	N_0	M_0		
IIIA	T_1,T_2	N_2	M_0		
	T_3	N_1	M_0	Not-resectable	$< 10\%$
	T_4	N_0,N_1	M_0	(chemo/radiotherapy)	
IIIB	T_4	N_2	M_0		
	Any T	N_3	M_0		
IV	Any T	Any N	M_1		0%

Tumour (T)

T_1 Tumour < 3 cm without invasion more proximal than a lobar bronchus

T_{1a} Tumour < 2 cm

T_{1b} Tumour > 2 cm < 3 cm

T_2 Tumour > 3 cm < 7 cm, or tumour involving main bronchus (but more than 2 cm away from carina), or invading visceral pleura

T_{2a} Tumour > 3 cm < 5 cm

T_{2b} Tumour > 5 cm < 7 cm

T_3 Tumour > 7 cm or invading chest wall, diaphragm, phrenic nerve, mediastinal pleura or within 2cm of carina or separate tumour nodule in same lobe

T_4 Tumour of any size invading mediastinum, heart, great vessels, trachea, recurrent laryngeal nerve, oesophagus, vertebrae, carina; separate tumour nodule in different ipsilateral lobe

Nodes (N)

N_0 No node metastasis

N_1 Metastasis in ipsilateral bronchial or hilar nodes

N_2 Metastasis in ipsilateral mediastinal or subcarinal nodes

N_3 Metastasis in contralateral mediastinal, hilar or supraclavicular nodes

Metastasis (M)

M_0 No distant metastasis

M_1 Distant metastasis

Carcinomas that are stage I or IIA are treated by surgical resection with curative intent, if the patient is fit for surgery. Some tumours that are Stage IIb have poor results when surgery is attempted. Sometimes the tumour is up-staged after surgery when histology shows more extensive disease, and adjuvant chemotherapy may be used. Carcinomas that are stage III or IV are not suitable for surgery, but may be suitable for treatment with chemotherapy and radiotherapy with palliative intent.

are indications for imaging of the liver by ultrasound or CT scans, and bone by isotope scans. CT scanning is the key investigation in staging lung cancer particularly in assessing mediastinal invasion by the tumour and involvement of hilar and mediastinal nodes. Enlarged (>1 cm) lymph nodes are suggestive of malignant involvement, but if the tumour otherwise appears operable **positron emission tomography** (see Chapter 4) is undertaken to assess active disease in mediastinal nodes and to detect distant metastases. Biopsy of the mediastinal nodes may then be undertaken by **mediastinosopy** or **endobronchial ultrasound**-guided needle aspiration.

- **Surgery**: unfortunately only about 10–20% of non-small cell carcinomas are suitable for surgical resection because of the advanced stage of the disease at diagnosis. The decision about the **patient's fitness** to undergo resection of the tumour is based particularly upon the lung function tests and the patient's general fitness. Unfortunately, these patients often have substantial cardiovascular disease and smoking-related COPD. No single test predicts feasibility of surgical resection and greater risks may be justified for a tumour that is otherwise curable by resection, but a forced expiratory volume in 1 second (FEV1) $<50\%$ of predicted or the presence of hypoxaemia (P_{O_2} $<8\,\text{kPa}$ (60 mmHg)) would suggest that the patient is not fit for thoracotomy. Lobectomy has a 30-day mortality of about 3%, compared to 8% for pneumonectomy. Mortality and morbidity increase with age. Surgery typically achieves a 70% 5-year survival in patients with stage IA ($T_1N_0M_0$) disease, a 40% 5-year survival in stage IB ($T_2N_0M_0$) disease, and 25% 5-year survival in stage 2 (T_{1-2},N_1M_0) disease. **Adjuvant chemotherapy** (i.e. post surgery) can improve survival rates by about 4% at 5 years in selected patients.
- **Radiotherapy** is chiefly undertaken for the relief of symptoms. Superior vena caval obstruction, lobar collapse from bronchial obstruction, haemoptysis or chest wall pain usually respond well to radiotherapy. Radical radiotherapy, using larger doses, is occasionally used with curative intent for small localised tumours that are not treatable by surgery because of poor patient fitness. This sometimes involves continuous hyperfractionated accelerated radiotherapy (**CHART**) with fractions of radiotherapy being given at 8 hour intervals in a concentrated fashion.
- **Chemotherapy** can improve the survival and quality of life of some patients with advanced non-small-cell lung cancer. First-line chemotherapy typically consists of cisplatin or carboplatin combined with gemcitabine, paclitaxel or vinorelbine. Docetaxel may be used as second-line therapy when relapse occurs after previous chemotherapy, although a variety of regimens are available. For patients with advanced

Table 12.3 World Health Organization performance status scale. Patients with performance status 3 or 4 are usually regarded as not being fit enough to tolerate chemotherapy

WHO Performance Status

0: Fully active

1: Restricted on strenuous activity but ambulatory and able to do light work

2: Ambulatory for >50% of day, able to self-care but unable to work

3: In bed or chair >50% of day, unable to care for self

4: Confined to bed or chair, unable to self-care

(stage III or IV) non-small cell cancer, who are fit to undergo chemotherapy (Table 12.3), treatment on average extends survival by about 2 months, improving 1-year survival from 5% to 25%. The role of chemotherapy before (neoadjuvant) or after (adjuvant) surgery is being studied in ongoing clinical trials.

Advances in the understanding of cancer cell biology has led to new treatments. Over-expression of the **epidermal growth factor receptor** (EGFR) is a feature of non-small-cell lung cancer. Two oral EGFR inhibitors, geftinib and erlotinib have demonstrated anti-tumour activity in patients with non-small-cell lung cancer who have failed to respond to chemotherapy. Bevacizumab is a monoclonal antibody that binds vascular endothelial growth factor, which is being evaluated in the treatment of advanced disease.

Palliative care

Palliative care focuses on improving the patient's functioning and psychosocial well-being with relief of symptoms. Even when the disease cannot be cured, rapid assessment and diagnosis is important in addressing the patient's symptoms and anxieties. Regular review of patients with lung cancer is essential in providing support for the patient and his or her family and in identifying the nature and origin of symptoms as they arise.

When dealing with a symptom such as pain, specific anti-cancer treatment (e.g. radiotherapy) is often the most effective method of symptom relief. Where there is persistent pain, analgesics need to be given regularly and prophylactically in advance of the return of pain. Mild pain may be treated by a **non-opioid analgesic** (e.g. a non-steroidal anti-inflammatory drug (NSAID) or paracetamol). More severe pain may be treated by a combination of a **weak opioid** (e.g. codeine) and a non-opioid (e.g. naproxen) drug. **Strong opioids** should be used immediately for any severe pain. Often pain control is achieved by use of slow-release morphine tablets 12 hourly combined with a NSAID, with additional use of morphine solution for any breakthrough pain. Certain types of pain may benefit from use of **co-analgesics** such as steroids (e.g. dexamethasone for nerve compression), benzodiazepines (anxiolytic), tricyclic antidepressants or anti-epileptics (e.g. gabapentin or pregabalin for neuropathic pain). Whenever opiates are prescribed it is necessary to prescribe a laxative (e.g. co-danthramer) to prevent constipation and an anti-emetic (e.g. metoclopramide) may be required initially.

Anorexia, weight loss, fatigue and general debility are common in the advanced stages of lung cancer. It is important to check for conditions requiring specific treatment such as anaemia (blood transfusion) or hypercalcaemia (pamidronate). Prednisolone may be useful in boosting appetite, and nutritional supplements may be helpful. Attention needs to be given to the patient's level of social support and help often needs to be given with tasks of daily living. If control of symptoms is not being achieved, help should be sought from a specialist in palliative care.

Other thoracic neoplasms

Alveolar cell carcinoma

This is a rare malignant tumour that arises in the alveoli of the lung and spreads along the alveolar and bronchiolar epithelium. Histologically, it resembles adenocarcinoma. Occasionally, this tumour produces large amounts of mucin causing copious sputum production (bronchorrhoea). On chest X-ray it may appear as more diffuse shadowing, resembling pneumonic consolidation, rather than as a discrete mass, and it is sometimes multifocal in origin. A transbronchial biopsy of alveolar tissue is often necessary for diagnosis. When the tumour is confined to one lobe surgical resection is the treatment of choice.

Carcinoid tumour

This rare tumour is less malignant than bronchial carcinomas in that it rarely metastasises and is often slow growing, although it may invade locally. It is not related to smoking and often affects younger patients. Most arise in the main bronchi and present with haemoptysis and wheeze. At bronchoscopy the tumour often has a smooth rounded appearance resembling a cherry and it may bleed profusely on biopsy because of its vascularity. Most can be cured by surgical resection. Very rarely, a carcinoid tumour of lung metastasises to the liver where secretion of substances such as 5-hydroxy indoleacetic acid (5-HIAA) produces the carcinoid syndrome of flushing, diarrhoea and wheeze.

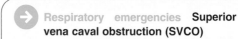

> **Respiratory emergencies** **Superior vena caval obstruction (SVCO)**
>
> - SVCO presents with headache, **distended neck veins** that are non-pulsatile, **oedema of the face** and arms, and dilated collateral veins over the chest.
> - **Lung cancer** is the most common cause of SVCO. Lymphoma, metastatic carcinoma, mediastinal tumours and thrombosis of central veins can also cause SVCO.
> - Urgent diagnosis of the underlying cause is needed to allow specific treatment. Chest x-ray and **urgent CTscan** allows a decision as to the best method of obtaining histological diagnosis.
> - A short tapering course of **dexamethasone** (initially 16 mg/day) may be useful in reducing oedema and inflammation around a tumour.
> - Insertion of a **metallic stent** into the compressed vein under radiological guidance can provide rapid relief of symptoms.
> - Urgent **chemotherapy** for small-cell carcinoma or **radiotherapy** for non-small-cell carcinoma are likely to achieve tumour shrinkage with relief of SVCO
> - **Anticoagulation** is sometimes used to reduce thrombosis but carries an increased risk of haemorrhage., and is usually only indicated if there is associated thrombosis in the compressed vein.

KEY POINTS

- Lung cancer is the most common cause of cancer death, killing about 34000 each year in the UK.
- Cigarette smoking is the main cause of lung cancer.
- Non-small-cell cancer accounts for 80% of lung cancer and is suitable for surgical resection in 10–20% of cases.
- Chemotherapy and radiotherapy improve survival and quality of life when surgery is not feasible.
- Small-cell cancer accounts for 20% of lung cancers and is treated by chemotherapy followed by radiotherapy.

 ## FURTHER READING

Auvinen A, Pershagen G. Indoor radon and deaths from lung cancer. *BMJ* 2009; **338**: 184–5.

British Thoracic Society Lung Cancer and Mesothelioma Specialty Advisory Group. Giving information to lung cancer patients. London: British Thoracic Society, 2008 (http://www.brit-thoracic.org.uk).

British Thoracic Society. Guidelines on the selection of patients with lung cancer for surgery. *Thorax* 2001; **36**: 89–108.

Demedts IK, Vermaelan KY, Van Meerbeeck JP. Treatment of extensive stage small cell lung carcinoma. Current status and future prospects. *Eur Respir J* 2010; **35**: 202–15.

Detterbeck FC, Boffa DJ, Tanoue LT. The new lung cancer staging system. *Chest* 2009; **136**: 260–71.

Doll R, Hill AB. The mortality of doctors in relation to their smoking habits. *BMJ* 1954; **i**: 1451–5.

Macmillan Cancer Support: http://www.macmillan.org.uk/

National Institute for Health and Clinical Excellence. *The Diagnosis and Treatment of Lung Cancer. Clinical Guideline 24*. London: NICE, 2005 (http://guidance.nice.org.uk/CG24/Guidance/pdf/English).

Price A. State of the art radiotherapy for lung cancer. *Thorax* 2003; **58**: 447–52.

Sculier J.P., Moro-Sibilot D. First and second-line therapy for advanced nonsmall cell lung cancer. *Eur Respir J* 2009; **33**: 915–30.

Silvestri GA, Rivera MP. Targeted therapy for the treatment of advanced non-small cell lung cancer: a review of the epidermal growth factor receptor antagonists. *Chest* 2005; **128**: 3975–84.

Interstitial lung disease

Introduction

Clinical presentation

The terms 'interstitial lung disease' and 'diffuse parenchymal lung disease' are imprecise clinical terms used to refer to a diverse range of diseases that result in inflammation and fibrosis of the alveoli, distal airways and septal interstitium of the lung. Patients with these diseases typically present with progressive **breathlessness**, a dry cough, lung **crackles** and diffuse **infiltrates on chest X-ray**. Lung function tests usually show a restrictive defect (reduced total lung capacity and vital capacity (VC)), with normal forced expiratory volume in 1 second/VC (FEV_1/VC) ratio, **impaired gas diffusion** (reduced transfer factor) and **hypoxaemia** with hypocapnia.

Differential diagnosis

At presentation the differential diagnosis includes a number of other diseases such as infective pneumonia, pulmonary oedema, bronchiectasis and malignancy (e.g. alveolar cell carcinoma). The overall context of the disease is important and exclusion of other diseases may require further investigations (e.g. echocardiography) or observing the response to treatments (e.g. antibiotics, diuretics). Once the clinical features suggest interstitial lung disease a careful search for potential causes is undertaken. Particular attention is paid to any environmental **antigens** (e.g. budgerigar), **toxins** (e.g. paraquat) or **dusts** (e.g. asbestos) that patients encounter in their **occupational** or **home environments**. **Systemic diseases** (e.g. rheumatoid disease) commonly involve the lung parenchyma and many **drugs** can cause lung fibrosis (e.g. amiodarone, nitrofurantoin, bleomycin) or eosinophilic reactions in the alveoli (e.g. sulphonamides, naproxen).

Investigations

After a detailed clinical assessment, chest X-ray and lung function tests, the next key investigation is high-resolution computed tomography (CT) that gives precise information about the extent and pattern of the disease. In some cases this allows a diagnosis to be made with reasonable certainty but it may be useful to proceed to biopsy of the lung parenchyma to study the histological pattern of the disease. Small samples can be obtained by **transbronchial biopsy** of the lung parenchyma through a flexible bronchoscope (Fig. 13.1). Larger samples can be obtained by **surgical biopsy** under general anaesthesia by **video-assisted thoracoscopy**. In many cases the histological features are characteristic of a particular disease (e.g. granulomas in sarcoidosis or extrinsic allergic alveolitis; tumour cells in lymphangitis carcinomatosa), but in advanced disease the histology may show non-specific lung fibrosis without clues to its aetiology. **Bronchoalveolar lavage** may be performed through the bronchoscope at the same

Respiratory Medicine Lecture Notes, Eighth Edition. Stephen J. Bourke and Graham P. Burns.
© 2011 John Wiley & Sons, Ltd. Published 2011 by John Wiley & Sons, Ltd.

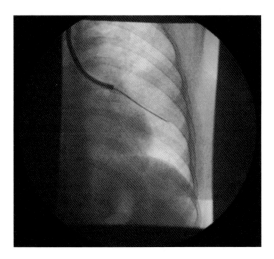

Figure 13.1 **Transbronchial lung biopsy**. A small specimen of lung parenchyma can be obtained by passing a biopsy forceps through a flexible bronchoscope, usually under radiological guidance, into the lung periphery. A sample of lung tissue is obtained by biopsying between two limbs in a branching small bronchus. There is a small risk of causing haemorrhage or pneumothorax, so the patient's condition and lung function should be adequate to tolerate these complications.

time as transbronchial biopsy. Aliquots of saline are instilled via the bronchoscope, which is held in a wedged position in a subsegmental bronchus, and fluid is then aspirated for cell analysis. A lymphocytic alveolitis is characteristic of sarcoidosis, for example. Many of these diseases are characterised in their early stages by an inflammatory alveolitis, which is responsive to corticosteroids, whereas in the later stages there may be irreversible lung fibrosis. Careful clinical investigation of patients presenting with features of interstitial lung disease aims to move from this imprecise clinical label to a diagnosis of a specific disease process (Fig. 13.2).

is more common in men (**male/female ratio 2:1**) and in the older age groups (**mean age 70 years**). It presents with the typical features of an interstitial lung disease as progressive dyspnoea, dry cough, crackles, restrictive defect in lung function and reticulonodular **infiltrates on chest X-ray** (Fig. 13.3). About 60–70% have clubbing. The aetiology is unknown but it appears to be the result of a failure of repair of lung tissue, whereby epithelial injury culminates in fibrosis rather than a controlled inflammatory and healing process. A possible association with previous exposure to environmental dusts (e.g. metal or wood dust) has been found in some epidemiological studies, cigarette smoking may be a co-factor for the initiation of the disease, and about 30% of patients have autoantibodies (e.g. rheumatoid factor, antinuclear factor) in their serum, suggesting that in some cases it may be a form of connective tissue disease primarily affecting the lungs. Lung biopsy shows a characteristic pattern of '**usual interstitial pneumonia**' with a heterogenous appearance such that there are alternating areas of normal lung, interstitial inflammation, fibrosis and honeycombing. The changes are more severe subpleurally. **High-resolution CT** scan typically shows evidence of advanced fibrosis with extensive areas of **reticulation and honeycombing** in a predominantly lower zone, subpleural distribution with minimal evidence of inflammation as **ground-glass opacities** (Fig. 13.4). Patients are usually treated with a combination of low-dose prednisolone, azathioprine and N-acetyl cysteine but unfortunately the response to treatment is poor and about 50% of patients die within 3 years of diagnosis. For younger patients lung transplantation may be an option (see Chapter 19). N-acetyl cysteine is an antioxidant that has been shown to slow the rate of decline in lung function, suggesting that the aberrant fibrosis may involve imbalances in the oxidant–antioxidant and protease–antiprotease systems of the lung.

Idiopathic pulmonary fibrosis

Idiopathic pulmonary fibrosis (IPF) (cryptogenic fibrosing alveolitis) is the classic example of a diffuse fibrotic lung disease. It is a serious disease that kills about 2500 people each year in the UK. It

Idiopathic interstitial pneumonias

The broad term 'idiopathic interstitial pneumonias' is used to describe a spectrum of inflammatory and fibrotic lung diseases of unknown cause, including IPF.

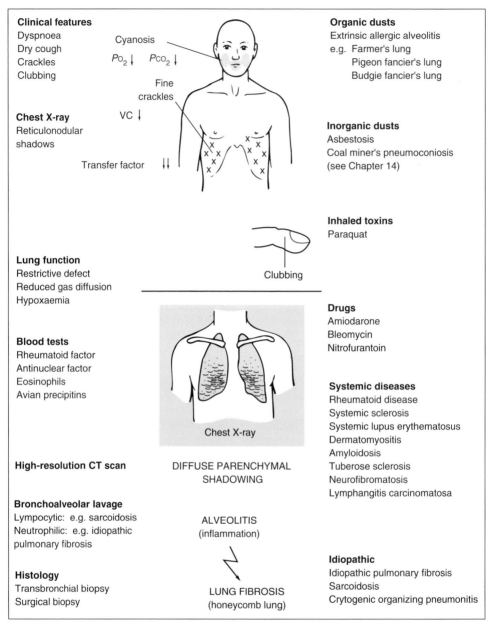

Clinical features
Dyspnoea
Dry cough
Crackles
Clubbing

Cyanosis
$Po_2\downarrow$ $Pco_2\downarrow$

Fine crackles

Chest X-ray
Reticulonodular shadows

VC $\downarrow$

Transfer factor $\downarrow\downarrow$

Lung function
Restrictive defect
Reduced gas diffusion
Hypoxaemia

Clubbing

Blood tests
Rheumatoid factor
Antinuclear factor
Eosinophils
Avian precipitins

High-resolution CT scan

DIFFUSE PARENCHYMAL SHADOWING

Bronchoalveolar lavage
Lympocytic: e.g. sarcoidosis
Neutrophilic: e.g. idiopathic pulmonary fibrosis

ALVEOLITIS
(inflammation)

Histology
Transbronchial biopsy
Surgical biopsy

LUNG FIBROSIS
(honeycomb lung)

Chest X-ray

Organic dusts
Extrinsic allergic alveolitis
e.g. Farmer's lung
    Pigeon fancier's lung
    Budgie fancier's lung

Inorganic dusts
Asbestosis
Coal miner's pneumoconiosis
(see Chapter 14)

Inhaled toxins
Paraquat

Drugs
Amiodarone
Bleomycin
Nitrofurantoin

Systemic diseases
Rheumatoid disease
Systemic sclerosis
Systemic lupus erythematosus
Dermatomyositis
Amyloidosis
Tuberose sclerosis
Neurofibromatosis
Lymphangitis carcinomatosa

Idiopathic
Idiopathic pulmonary fibrosis
Sarcoidosis
Crytogenic organizing pneumonitis

Figure 13.2 Summary of the clinical investigations and differential diagnosis of interstitial lung disease. CT, computed tomography; VC, vital capacity.

Non-specific interstitial pneumonia is characterised by more uniform inflammatory changes and less fibrosis on lung biopsy with correspondingly more ground-glass opacification on CT, a better response to corticosteroids and a more favourable prognosis than IPF. In **cryptogenic organising pneumonia** histology shows intra-alveolar buds of organising fibrosis. This seems to be a pattern of response in the lungs to a variety of insults. It particularly occurs in association with some drugs (e.g. amiodarone), connective tissue diseases (e.g. rheumatoid disease) or ulcerative colitis but often no cause is identifiable. Clinically, patients often have cough, malaise,

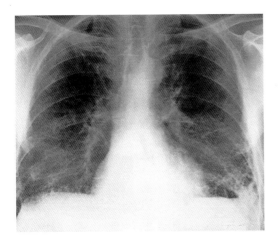

Figure 13.3 This 70-year-old man presented with a 6-month history of progressive breathlessness, crackles and clubbing with reduced lung volumes and impaired gas diffusion. The chest X-ray shows small lung volumes with reticular shadowing particularly affecting the lung peripheries and bases suggesting idiopathic pulmonary fibrosis. He failed to respond to prednisolone and died 1 year later of respiratory failure.

fever, dyspnoea with chest X-ray infiltrates and an elevated erythrocyte sedimentation rate (ESR). Often the patient is thought to have infective pneumonia but the differential diagnosis is widened when no pathogen is identified and the patient fails to respond to antibiotics. There is typically a dramatic response to corticosteroids although relapse may occur as the dose is reduced.

Desquamative interstitial pneumonia and **respiratory bronchiolitis–interstitial lung disease** are relatively rare forms of interstitial lung disease that affect smokers. They have particular features of desquamation of alveolar macrophages or bronchiolitis on biopsy. They respond well to smoking cessation and corticosteroids. **Lymphoid interstitial pneumonia** is characterised by the presence of lymphoid cells in the interstitium. It may occur as a complication of human immuno-deficiency virus (HIV) infection or connective tissue diseases. **Acute interstitial pneumonia** is a very aggressive form of interstitial lung disease characterised by rapidly progressive diffuse alveolar damage.

The idiopathic interstitial pneumonias, therefore, are a complex array of inflammatory and fibrotic lung diseases. The lungs may respond to different insults with a similar pattern of inflammation and fibrosis, and conversely a single agent, such as amiodarone, may produce a range of reactions within the lung. The overall clinical management requires the integration of clinical, radiological and histological features.

Connective tissue diseases

The typical clinical features of IPF with the histopathological pattern of usual interstitial pneumonia can occur in association with a connective tissue disease. When a patient presents with interstitial lung disease a careful search should be undertaken for features of connective tissue diseases e.g. Raynaud's phenomenon, inflammatory arthritis, sicca syndrome (dry eyes, dry mouth), myositis and skin changes. These diseases have a number of other lung complications.

Rheumatoid disease (Fig. 13.5)

Involvement of the **crico-arytenoid joint** causes hoarseness and sometimes stridor. **Obliterative bronchiolitis** results in progressive peripheral airways obstruction. **Pleural effusions** are common and analysis of the pleural fluid characteristically shows a high protein level (exudate) with a low glucose concentration and a high titre of rheumatoid factor. **Rheumatoid nodules** may develop in

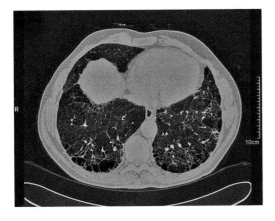

Figure 13.4 High-resolution computed tomography scan of a 70-year-old man with idiopathic pulmonary fibrosis showing 'honeycombing' that is a cluster or row of cysts due to advanced fibrosis in the subpleural area.

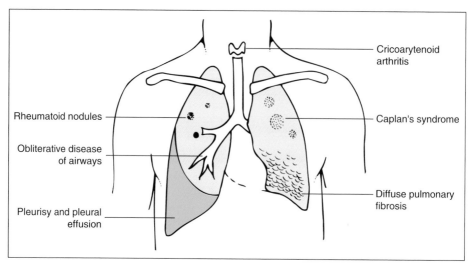

Figure 13.5 Summary of pulmonary complications of rheumatoid disease.

the lung parenchyma and show the same histological features as the rheumatoid subcutaneous nodules. When rheumatoid disease occurs in association with coalworker's pneumoconiosis, large cavitating pulmonary nodules may develop (**Caplan's syndrome**). Fibrotic lung diseases complicating rheumatoid disease is managed in the same way as IPF, but the prognosis is generally better. Drugs (e.g. methotrexate, infliximab) used to treat rheumatoid disease may cause inflammatory reactions within the lung and may also give rise to lung infections. In these circumstances diffuse infiltrates on chest X-ray could be as a result of infection, a drug reaction, lung involvement by the connective tissue disease or co-incidental lung disease (see Table 6.1). Bronchoalveolar lavage is useful in detecting infection. Where a drug reaction is suspected information is available on a website (http://www.pneumotox.com) and prompt cessation of the drug and treatment with corticosteroids are important.

Systemic sclerosis (scleroderma)

Diffuse lung fibrosis is the most common complication. **Chest wall restriction** by contraction of the skin is rare. **Aspiration pneumonia** may occur because of oesophageal dysmotility in the CREST variant of the disease: calcinosis, Raynaud's phenomenon, oesophageal dysfunction, sclerodactyly and telangiectasia. **Pulmonary hypertension** may also develop in patients with the CREST syndrome as a primary vascular phenomenon, often in the absence of significant pulmonary fibrosis (see Chapter 15).

Systemic lupus erythematosus

Pleural effusions are common and may cause **pleural thickening**. The phenomenon of 'shrinking lungs', in which the chest X-ray shows high hemidiaphragms with small lungs, is probably caused by myopathy of the diaphragm. Lung fibrosis may occur. Immunosuppressive treatments predispose to **opportunistic infections** (e.g. *Pneumocystis* pneumonia).

Extrinsic allergic alveolitis

Extrinsic allergic alveolitis (hypersensitivity pneumonitis) is an **immunologically mediated lung disease** in which a hypersensitivity response occurs in a **sensitised individual** to an **inhaled antigen**. Typical examples of this disease are **farmer's lung** and **bird fancier's lung**. When hay is harvested and stored in damp conditions it becomes mouldy, generating heat that encourages growth of fungi such as *Thermoactinomyces vulgaris* or *Saccharoployspora rectivirgula*. When the hay is subsequently used for foddering cattle, fungal spores may be inhaled. Avian antigens are inhaled by people who participate in the sport of pigeon racing or who keep pet birds such as budgerigars. Various water systems in the home or work environment can be contaminated by fungi or mycobacteria giving rise to extrinsic allergic alveolitis. Metalworking fluid alveolitis, for example, has been described in workers in car manufacturing from contamination of fluid used to cool and lubricate metals. The inhalation of these antigens provokes a complex immune response in susceptible individuals involving antibody reactions, immune-complex formation, complement activation and cellular responses, resulting in alveolitis. These diseases are less common in smokers, probably because of the immunosuppressive effects of cigarette smoke..

In the **acute form** of the disease the patient typically experiences recurrent episodes of dyspnoea, dry cough, pyrexia, myalgia and a flu-like sensation, occurring about 4–8 hours after antigen exposure. During such an episode lung function tests may show a reduction in lung volumes and gas diffusion, and chest X-ray may show diffuse shadowing. Sometimes the chest X-ray may be normal and CT is more sensitive in detecting the changes of extrinsic allergic alveolitis (Fig. 13.6). The acute illness is often misdiagnosed as pneumonia. The **chronic form** is characterised by the insidious development of dyspnoea and lung fibrosis. Lung biopsies show features of fibrosis,

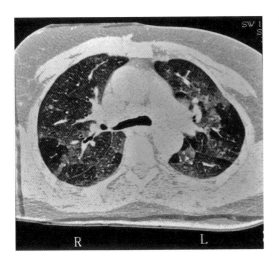

Figure 13.6 This 65-year-old man who kept 150 racing pigeons presented with recurrent episodes of dyspnoea, cough, fever and 'flu'. Computed tomography scan shows a characteristic pattern for extrinsic allergic alveolitis of 'ground-glass' shadowing with areas of decreased attenuation and air trapping on expiratory scans.

alveolitis and granuloma formation. Bronchoalveolar lavage typically shows evidence of a lymphocytic alveolitis with a predominance of T-suppressor lymphocytes. Precipitating antibodies to avian or fungal antigens can be detected in serum but are also found in many asymptomatic individuals so that they are not diagnostic.

Complete **cessation of exposure to the provoking antigen** is the main treatment. However, pigeon fanciers, for example, are very committed to their sport and will often wish to continue keeping pigeons. They can reduce antigen contact by wearing a mask and a loft-coat and hat (so as to avoid carrying antigen on their clothing or hair). **Steroids** (e.g. prednisolone 40 mg/day) hasten the resolution of the alveolitis and are often used during severe acute episodes. The immune response in extrinsic allergic alveolitis is complex and a variety of modulating factors influence the interaction of antigenic stimulus and host response so that the longitudinal course of the disease is variable with some patients developing lung fibrosis and others showing spontaneous improvement despite continued antigen exposure.

Sarcoidosis

Sarcoidosis is a mysterious **multisystem disease** characterised by the occurrence in affected organs of **non-caseating granulomatous lesions** that may progress to cause fibrosis. The aetiology is unknown but the accumulation of CD4 lymphocytes at disease sites is suggestive of an immunological reaction to an unidentified poorly degradable antigen. The frequent involvement of the lungs raises the possibility that such a putative antigen enters the body via the lungs. The compartmentalisation of CD4 lymphocytes in affected tissues is associated with a corresponding depletion of CD4 cells in other tissues and depression of some delayed-type hypersensitivity responses such that patients with sarcoidosis often demonstrate negative reactions to tuberculin (i.e. negative Heaf or Mantoux tests despite previous bacillus Calmette–Guérin (BCG) vaccination). Serum immunoglobulin levels are usually elevated and immune complexes are often present in acute sarcoidosis.

The clinical features of sarcoidosis are very varied but it is useful to consider two broad categories of disease: an acute form that is usually transient and often resolves spontaneously; and a chronic

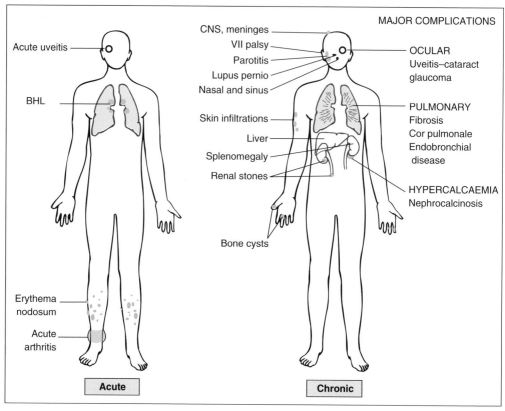

Figure 13.7 Principal clinical features of sarcoidosis. BHL, bilateral hilar lymphadenopathy.

form that is persistent and may cause fibrosis (Fig. 13.7).

Acute sarcoidosis

The acute form typically develops abruptly in young adults with **erythema nodosum** and **bilateral hilar lymphadenopathy(BHL)**, sometimes with **uveitis**, **arthritis** and **parotitis**.

Erythema nodosum

This appears as **round red raised nodules**, typically over the shins. It is a manifestation of hypersensitivity and is also found in other diseases such as streptococcal infection, tuberculosis, ulcerative colitis and Crohn's disease, and with drugs (e.g. sulphonamides, contraceptive pill), but in many cases no cause is identified.

Bilateral hilar lymphadenopathy

BHL is not associated with any signs on examination of the chest or with any loss of lung function

and is often found incidentally on a **chest X-ray**, but often the X-ray was taken in a patient with other features suggestive of sarcoidosis (Fig. 13.8). Although sarcoidosis is the most common cause of BHL, other causes include lymphoma, metastatic carcinoma, tuberculosis, fungal infections such as coccidioidomycosis and histoplasmosis in endemic areas (e.g. North America); and, in the past, berylliosis (e.g. beryllium used in fluorescent lighting).

Chronic sarcoidosis

The chronic form of sarcoidosis pursues a more indolent course, often in an older age group, with involvement of many tissues of the body.

Chronic pulmonary sarcoidosis

This involves the lung parenchyma with **reticular shadowing** often distributed in a perihilar fashion on chest X-ray (Fig. 13.9). There are often remarkably few signs on examination of the chest, and

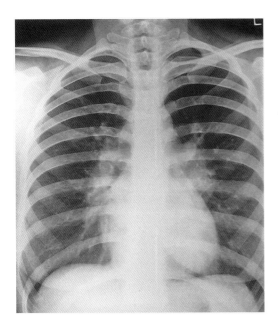

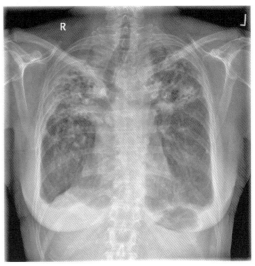

Figure 13.9 This 60-year-old woman presented with cough and progressive breathlessness. There were no crackles on auscultation of her chest but transfer factor for carbon monoxide and transfer coefficient were reduced to 60% of the predicted values. The chest X-ray shows extensive upper lobe fibrosis. Transbronchial lung biopsy showed non-caseating granulomas and lung fibrosis. Tests for tuberculosis were negative. She was treated with prednisolone with some improvement in lung function.

Figure 13.8 This 25-year-old woman presented with uveitis, arthralgia and erythema nodosum of her shins. The chest X-ray shows bilateral hilar lymphadenopathy. She was otherwise well and lung function tests were normal. A diagnosis of probable acute sarcoidosis was made. The disease resolved spontaneously without the need for any medical intervention.

lung function may be well maintained but the disease may progress in some patients causing **progressive fibrosis** and loss of lung function with impairment of gas diffusion, reduction in lung volumes and sometimes airways obstruction with air trapping and bulla formation.

Chronic extrapulmonary sarcoidosis

Sarcoidosis may affect virtually any organ in the body. **Ocular sarcoidosis** often presents as pain and redness of the eye as a result of anterior uveitis. Chorioretinitis, keratoconjunctivitis sicca and lacrimal gland enlargement may complicate chronic sarcoidosis. **Parotid gland enlargement** may be painful and sometimes causes facial nerve palsy. **Central nervous system** involvement may cause cranial nerve palsies, chronic meningitis, obstructive hydrocephalus and a variety of neurological syndromes. **Posterior pituitary** involvement may rarely cause diabetes insipidus. **Cutaneous sarcoidosis** may cause maculopapular eruptions, plaques, nodules and lupus pernio

(a violaceous chronic skin lesion particularly affecting the nose and cheeks). **Bone** cysts are sometimes found and are often asymptomatic. **Cardiac** sarcoid may cause conduction system damage and arrhythmias. **Hypercalcaemia** may result from increased bone resorption, and nephrocalcinosis, hypercalcuria and renal calculi may occur. Sarcoid granulomas and fibrosis may also be found in the liver, spleen, lymph nodes and muscle, for example.

Diagnosis

The diagnosis of sarcoidosis can often be made on **clinical** grounds, particularly when a young adult presents with classic features such as erythema nodosum and BHL. In less typical cases it is helpful to obtain **biopsy of an affected organ**. **Bronchial and transbronchial biopsies** are particularly useful and may be combined with **bronchoalveolar lavage**, which typically demonstrates evidence of a CD4 lymphocyte alveolitis. **Mediastinoscopy** and biopsy of hilar lymph nodes is sometimes indicated to exclude other diagnoses such as lymphoma. The histological appearances must be considered in the clinical context because they are not in themselves diagnostic, and other granulomatous disease (e.g. tuberculosis) must be excluded. Serum angiotensin-converting enzyme (ACE) levels are elevated in about two-thirds of patients with active sarcoidosis but this test lacks sensitivity and specificity and is therefore of limited value in diagnosis or in monitoring the course of the disease.

Treatment

In most patients sarcoidosis is a **self-limiting disease** that **resolves spontaneously** without treatment. However, a minority of patients with chronic sarcoidosis develop progressive fibrosis. Because the cause of sarcoidosis is unknown no specific treatment is available but **corticosteroids** suppress inflammation in the affected organs, frequently improving local and systemic symptoms. Their effect on the long-term natural history of sarcoidosis is less clear. They are usually used in patients with progressive disease and studies suggest some benefit from steroid therapy at the cost of adverse effects (e.g. osteoporosis, Cushing's syndrome). A short course of prednisolone is

---

sometimes used for particularly troublesome acute symptoms such as parotitis, arthritis or erythema nodosum if non-steroidal anti-inflammatory drugs are not sufficient. Uveitis may be treated by topical steroids, and skin manifestations may be amenable to steroid creams or steroid injections. Inhaled steroids have been tried for pulmonary disease but evidence of efficacy is lacking. In chronic sarcoidosis deciding who to treat and when to treat requires **careful judgement to balance the benefit and risks of chronic steroid therapy**.

 FURTHER READING

American Thoracic Society and European Respiratory Society. International multidisciplinary consensus classification of the idiopathic interstitial pneumonias. *Am J Respir Crit Care Med* 2002; **165**: 277–304.

American Thoracic Society and European Respiratory Society. Idiopathic pulmonary fibrosis: diagnosis and treatment: international consensus statement. *Am J Respir Crit Care Med* 2000; **161**: 646–64.

Bourke SJ, Dalphin JC, Boyd G, McSharry C, Baldwin CI, Calvert JE. Hypersensitivity pneumonitis: current concepts. *Eur Respir J* 2001; **18** (suppl 32): 81–92.

British Thoracic Society Interstitial Lung Disease Guideline Group. Interstitial lung disease guideline. *Thorax* 2008; **63** (suppl V): 1–58.

Demedts M, Behr J, Buhl R, et al. High-dose acetylcysteine in idiopathic pulmonary fibrosis. *N Engl J Med* 2005; **353**: 2229–42.

Fischer A, West SG, Swigris JJ, Brown KK, DuBois RM. Connective tissue disease-associated interstitial lung disease. *Chest* 2010; **138**: 251–6.

Martin W, Iannuzzi MC, Gail DB, Peavy HH. Future directions in sarcoidosis research. *Am J Respir Crit Care Med* 2004; **170**: 567–72.

Pneumotox-drug reactions: www.pneumotox.com

Strieter RM, Mehrad B. New mechanisms of pulmonary fibrosis. *Chest* 2009; **136**: 1364–70.

Westhovens R, DeKeyser F, Van den Hoogen FH, et al. The clinical spectrum and pathogenesis of pulmonary manifestations in connective tissue diseases. *Eur Respir Mon* 2006; **34**: 1–26.

 KEY POINTS

- Interstitial lung disease typically presents with breathlessness, crackles, reduced gas diffusion and VC and diffuse infiltrates on chest X-ray.
- Exclude other diagnoses, e.g. pulmonary oedema, bronchiectasis, pneumonia, alveolar cell carcinoma.
- Seek potential causes such as drugs (e.g. amiodarone), antigens (e.g. pet birds), occupational dust exposure (e.g. asbestos) and systemic diseases (e.g. rheumatoid disease).
- High-resolution CT shows the pattern and extent of fibrosis and alveolitis and lung biopsy may be needed to determine the histopathological pattern.
- Treatments such as prednisolone and azathioprine should be used judiciously assessing the benefits and adverse effects carefully.

Occupational lung disease

Introduction

The importance of the work environment as a cause of lung disease has been recognised since ancient times. Hippocrates (460–377 BC) taught his pupils to observe the environment of their patients. Ramazzini urged physicians to ask patients what work they did and to visit the workplace. In 1713 he published a treatise on work-related diseases (*De Morbis Artificium*) which included descriptions of baker's asthma and what is now known as extrinsic allergic alveolitis.

Occupational lung diseases result from the inhalation of dusts, gases, fumes or vapours encountered in the workplace, and the hazards of the work environment are constantly changing as old industries are replaced by new ones. The effects of inhaled substances depend on many factors including particle size, physical characteristics (e.g. solubility), toxicity, the intensity and duration of exposures and the person's susceptibility. Particles >10μm in diameter are usually filtered out of the inhaled airstream in the nose; particles of 1–10μm are mainly deposited in the bronchi; and particles < 1μm penetrate to the alveoli. Inhaled substances may exert their effects in various ways, and in many circumstances the precise mechanisms involved are incompletely understood. Some substances exert a non-specific **irritant** effect (e.g. generally dusty environment) or are **toxic** to the airways (e.g. chlorine, ammonia) with all workers exposed being similarly affected. Other substances induce **hypersensitivity** or allergic reactions in susceptible individuals giving rise to asthma or extrinsic allergic alveolitis (see Chapter 13), for example. Some inhaled dusts **promote fibrosis** in the lung parenchyma (e.g. silica, asbestos, coal dust) and some are **carcinogenic** (e.g. cigarette smoke, asbestos). Occasionally, **infective organisms** are inhaled (e.g. *Mycobacterium tuberculosis* in healthcare workers, *Chlamydophila psittaci* in bird handlers). Occupational exposure to **tobacco smoke** is a hazard to those working in places such as bars, restaurants and nightclubs and smoking bans are being introduced in many places as part of the requirements to provide a safe working environment.

Occupational asthma

Asthma is now the most common type of occupational lung disease. In the UK approximately 3000 new cases are diagnosed each year. Occupational asthma may be defined as **variable airways obstruction caused by workplace exposures**. In most cases it is the result of a **hypersensitivity reaction** to a substance at work but it may result from an **irritant effect** after high exposure to a gas, fume or vapour at work. This definition excludes the triggering of episodes of wheezing in patients with pre-existing asthma by mechanisms such as cold air or exercise at work. Occupational

Respiratory Medicine Lecture Notes, Eighth Edition. Stephen J. Bourke and Graham P. Burns.
© 2011 John Wiley & Sons, Ltd. Published 2011 by John Wiley & Sons, Ltd.

Table 14.1 Common causes of occupational asthma

Agent	Occupational exposure
Isocyanates	Spray paints, varnishes, adhesives, polyurethane foam manufacture
Flour	Bakers
Colophony	Electronic soldering flux
Epoxy resins	Hardening agents, adhesives
Animals (rats, mice)	Laboratory workers
Wood dusts	Sawmill workers, joiners
Azodicarbonamide	Polyvinyl plastics manufacture
Persulphate salts	Hairdressers
Latex	Healthcare workers
Drugs (penicillin, cephalosporins)	Pharmaceutical industry
Grain dust (mites, moulds)	Farmers, millers, bakers

asthma accounts for about 10–15% of cases of asthma in adults. The list of causes of occupational asthma is long and new agents are being continuously added. Some of the most common causes are shown in Table 14.1. Occupational asthma is rare among library, professional and clerical workers but is common among spray painters (isocyanates), bakers (flour), hairdressers (persulphates), cleaners and workers in the plastics and chemical industries (epoxy resins, azodicarbonamide), for example.

Diagnosis

To establish a diagnosis of occupational asthma it is first necessary to **confirm the presence of asthma** and, secondly, to show a **causal relationship between the asthma and the work environment**. Although the suspicion of occupational asthma is often based upon the **patient's history**, the diagnosis should be confirmed by **objective tests** wherever possible because of the importance of the diagnosis in terms of managing the patient, identifying the causative agent, reducing the risk to other workers and addressing the medicolegal and compensation aspects of the diagnosis. Characteristically, there is an initial latent interval of

asymptomatic exposure to the agent before symptoms develop. This **latent interval** varies from a few weeks to several years. Once the worker has developed sensitisation to the agent further exposure may provoke an **early asthmatic response** (reaching a peak within 30 minutes), a **late asthmatic response** (occurring 4–12 hours later) or a **dual response**. If an early response occurs, the relationship of symptoms to the work environment is usually apparent. Late responses typically develop the evening after exposure, disturbing sleep and causing cough and wheeze the following morning. Initially, symptoms **improve away from work** on holidays or at weekends and **deteriorate on return to work**. Once asthma becomes established symptoms may persist even when away from the work environment and are then also triggered by other factors such as exercise or cold air. Sometimes the sensitising agent also causes rhinitis and dermatitis. Occupational asthma may develop in workers with pre-existing asthma and this may lead to a delay in diagnosis if the relationship of symptoms to the work environment is not recognised. The patient may be exposed to a known inducer of asthma (e.g. paint sprayers using isocyanates) but doctors need to be constantly alert to new causes of occupational asthma. Atopy increases the risk of developing occupational asthma and smoking increases the risk of occupational asthma in workers exposed to isocyanates, for example.

Serial measurement of **peak expiratory flow** or **spirometry** over several days at work and away from work will usually show evidence of variable airways obstruction (the hallmark of asthma) and may demonstrate a relationship between symptoms, airways obstruction and the work environment. Lung function tests may be normal when the patient is seen away from the work environment. Assessment and management of occupational asthma is notoriously difficult as some workers may be reluctant to admit to symptoms in case this jeopardises their employment. Conversely, others may exaggerate symptoms in an attempt to gain compensation. Patients with suspected occupational asthma should therefore be referred for specialist assessment. One of the best ways of showing a relationship between asthma and the work environment is to perform a carefully supervised **workplace challenge study**. In this the patient is removed from the work environment for about 2 weeks and then returned to work under supervision. Serial measurements of spirometry or peak expiratory flow are performed on control days away from work and then over about 3 days on return to the patient's normal work environment. Serial measurements of **airway responsiveness** to methacholine or histamine (see Chapter 10) typically show sequential improvement away from work and rapid deterioration on return to work. Fig. 14.1 shows a typical late asthmatic reaction occurring during a workplace challenge study in a worker in a biocide manufacturing plant. The agent inducing the patient's asthma can often be identified with reasonable confidence by a **visit to the workplace** and an assessment of the materials used. However, workers may be exposed to many agents and it may be difficult to know which agent is causing asthma. **Laboratory challenge studies** involve the patient inhaling the specific suspect agent under double-blind, carefully controlled circumstances with serial measurements of spirometry and airway responsiveness. These studies are particularly useful in identifying previously unrecognised causes of occupational asthma but they should only be undertaken in specialist units, as they are potentially hazardous. In some cases of occupational asthma it is possible to demonstrate a positive skin prick test or circulating antibodies to the agent but such immunological reactions are often present in asymptomatic workers also.

Management

Treatment of occupational asthma involves management of both the **affected individual** and the **affected industry**. Early cessation of exposure to the inducing agent may result in complete resolution of the patient's asthma. The key factor in the patient's treatment is therefore not the institution of bronchodilator and steroid treatments as in conventional asthma but the **avoidance of exposure** to the inducing agent. This may be achieved in a number of ways but often involves moving the patient to a different job within the factory. Where there has been a delay in recognising the nature of the patient's asthma and in ceasing exposure chronic asthma may develop that persists even after cessation of contact with the inducing agent, and long-term inhaled steroid and bronchodilator drugs are then required.

Substitution of an alternative non-asthmagenic substance in the industrial process is the ideal solution as this also removes the risk to other workers. Where this is not possible, **enclosure** of

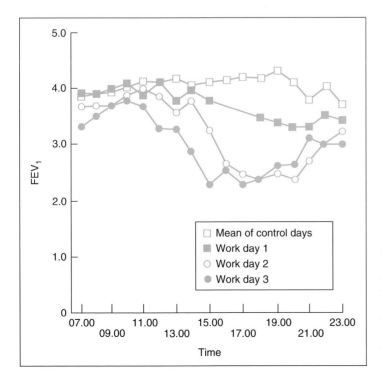

Figure 14.1 Workplace challenge study showing the mean forced expiratory volume in 1 second (FEV_1) on control days away from the workplace and progressive falls in FEV_1 over 3 days at work indicating late asthmatic reactions of increasing severity occurring in relation to exposure to a biocide in the workplace.

the process in a confined booth with **exhaust ventilation** may be possible. **Segregation** of the hazardous process may be useful in limiting the exposure to a small group of workers who are then provided with appropriate personal **protective devices** such as respirator masks. **Surveillance** of other workers should be undertaken where a work environment has been shown to cause asthma. This typically involves a pre-employment medical examination combined with periodic assessment of asthma symptoms, spirometry and, ideally, serial measurements of airway responsiveness. Institution of these measures in the workplace requires the cooperation of the factory safety officer, management, occupational health department and industrial hygienist. Hazards within the workplace fall within the remit of governmental agencies such as the Employment Medical Advisory Service (EMAS) of the Health and Safety Executive in the UK. Workers suffering disability as a result of their employment are entitled to **compensation** from the Department of Social Security in the UK, and may also wish to pursue legal action against their employer where there has been negligence in causing the disease.

Byssinosis

Byssinosis is a particular type of occupational asthma caused by the inhalation of **cotton** or **flax** dust. Symptoms typically arise after several years of working in the industry and show a characteristic pattern different from that seen in typical occupational asthma. Characteristically, workers complain of **chest tightness**, **cough** and **dyspnoea** on Mondays (or the first shift of the week) and, peculiarly, symptoms **improve throughout the working week**. There is sometimes a fall in forced expiratory volume in 1 second (FEV$_1$) during the working day but there is often a poor correlation between symptoms and FEV$_1$. Chronic productive cough and irreversible airways obstruction sometimes develop. It is difficult to understand what mechanisms give rise to the pattern of symptoms being worse at the start of the week and improving thereafter. It has been suggested that cotton particles may cause direct release of histamine and that symptoms resolve as histamine stores are depleted. However, the pathogenesis of byssinosis is uncertain, and alternative theories suggest that symptoms may be related to contamination of cotton by Gram-negative bacteria and endotoxins, or that immunological mechanisms may be important.

Popcorn worker's lung

Recently cases of severe **obliterative bronchiolitis** have been reported in workers in popcorn production plants due to inhalation of diacetyl, a ketone with butter-flavour characteristics. The patients developed progressive cough, breathlessness and wheeze with fixed airways obstruction. Computed tomography (CT) scans showed bronchial wall thickening and air trapping, and lung biopsies showed inflammation and occlusion of the small airways in the form of obliterative bronchiolitis. Further cases of **'food flavourer's lung'** have been identified in other areas of the food industry. Doctors need to be vigilant in order to detect new causes of occupational lung disease.

Pneumoconiosis

Pneumoconiosis is a general term used to describe lung fibrosis resulting from inhalation of dusts such as coal, silica or asbestos.

Coalworker's pneumoconiosis

The development of pneumoconiosis is directly related to the total exposure to coal dust. Dust exposure varies in different parts of the coalmine and is heaviest at the coalface. Improvements in ventilation and working conditions have considerably reduced the level of dust in modern coalmines. In many countries there has been a decline in the coal industry with increased use of alternative sources of energy. Coal dust inhaled into the alveoli is taken up by macrophages that are then cleared via the lymphatic drainage system or via the mucociliary escalator of the bronchial tree. If there is heavy prolonged exposure to dust the clearance mechanisms are overwhelmed and dust macules arise particularly in the region of the respiratory bronchioles. Release of dust from dying macrophages induces fibroblast proliferation and fibrosis. There is an important distinction to be made between the two major categories of coalworker's pneumoconiosis.

• *Simple coalworker's pneumoconiosis*: it consists of the accumulation, within the lung tissue, of small (< 5 mm) aggregations of coal particles that are uniformly dispersed and evident on chest X-ray as a delicate micronodular mottling. **Simple pneumoconiosis is not associated with any significant symptoms, signs, impairment of lung function or alteration to prognosis, for example life expectancy**. The size and extent of the nodules can be categorised for research and classification purposes by comparing the patient's X-ray with standard films published by the International Labour Office. The benign nature of simple pneumoconiosis is sometimes not appreciated and there is often a tendency to attribute any respiratory symptoms to the pneumoconiosis, whereas alternative explanations such as chronic obstructive pulmonary disease (COPD), asthma or heart disease are more likely to account for the patient's symptoms.
• *Complicated coalworker's pneumoconiosis* (progressive massive fibrosis): it is characterised by the occurrence of large black fibrotic masses in the lung parenchyma, consisting of coal dust and bundles of collagen. These are typically situated in the upper zones and appear as rather **bizarre opacities on chest X-ray** against the background of simple pneumoconiosis (Fig. 14.2). **Cavitation** of these lesions may occur and may result in the expectoration of black sputum (melanoptysis). Complicated pneumoconiosis often results in dyspnoea, a **restrictive ventilatory defect** (reduced lung volumes) and **impaired gas diffusion** (reduced transfer factor for carbon monoxide), and **reduced life expectancy**.

Caplan's syndrome (rheumatoid pneumoconiosis)

Coalworkers with **rheumatoid arthritis** may develop **multiple nodules** of about 0.5–2 cm in diameter in the lungs. These lung nodules are often accompanied by the occurrence of subcutaneous rheumatoid nodules.

Coalworker's bronchitis and emphysema

Coalminers have a high prevalence of **bronchitis**, **airways obstruction** and **emphysema** and since

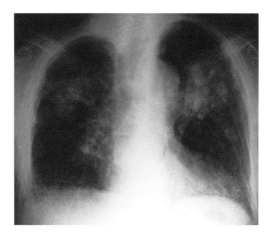

Figure 14.2 This 78-year-old man, who had been a faceworker in a coalmine for 40 years, presented with progressive breathlessness. Chest X-ray shows irregular opacities of progressive massive fibrosis in both upper lobes with extensive background nodular shadowing of coalworker's pneumoconiosis.

1993 they have been eligible for compensation from the Department of Social Security in the UK if they have worked underground in coal mines for at least 20 years and have reduced FEV_1.

Silicosis

This is a form of pneumoconiosis resulting from the inhalation of free silica (silicon dioxide). It is now less common in developed countries because of widespread recognition and control of the hazards of respirable silica dust in the mining and quarrying industries. There is a risk of silicosis in workers involved in: **quarrying**, grinding and dressing of sandstone, granite and slate; developing **tunnels** and sinking shafts (e.g. coalmines); **boiler scaling**; **sandblasting** of castings in iron and steel foundries; and the **pottery** industry where silica may be used in the lining of kilns and the dry-grinding of ceramic products. The use of handheld, high-speed tools on construction sites has also given rise to silicosis.

Simple nodular silicosis, like simple coalworker's pneumoconiosis, causes no symptoms and is an X-ray phenomenon. Complicated silicosis, however, results in **progressive fibrosis**, loss of lung function and breathlessness. The silicotic nodule

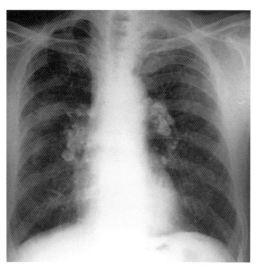

Figure 14.3 This 65-year-old man had had extensive exposure to silica when working in a stone quarry. Chest X-ray shows eggshell calcification (a rim of calcification around the outer margin) of the hilar lymph nodes with upper lobe fibrosis. Tests for tuberculosis were negative.

consists of concentric layers of collagen surrounding a central area of dust including quartz crystals and dying macrophages. There is a significantly increased risk of **tuberculosis** in patients with silicosis as silica interferes with the ability of macrophages to kill tubercle bacilli. Patients with silicosis are also at increased risk of developing **lung cancer**.

A chest X-ray typically shows **nodular opacities** particularly affecting the **upper lobes**. The nodules are usually denser and larger than those seen in simple coalworker's pneumoconiosis. **Eggshell calcification** of **hilar lymph nodes** is a particularly characteristic feature (Fig. 14.3). **Pleural thickening** may also occur.

Siderosis

Dust containing **iron** and its oxides is encountered at various stages in the iron and steel industry and in welding. It gives rise to a simple pneumoconiosis (siderosis) that produces a striking mottled appearance on the chest X-ray because of the high radiodensity of iron, but which is not accompanied by symptoms, signs or any physiological defect.

Other metals such as antimony and tin may produce a similar picture.

Asbestos-related lung disease

Asbestos is a collective term for a number of naturally occurring fibrous mineral silicates that are widely used because of their fire-resistant and insulation properties. Asbestos fibres are of two main types that have different physical and chemical properties: *serpentine asbestos fibres* (**chrysotile–white asbestos**) are wispy, flexible and relatively long, such that they are less easily inhaled to the periphery of the lung; *amphibole asbestos fibres* (e.g. **crocidolite–blue asbestos, amosite–brown asbestos, tremolite**) are straighter, stiffer and more brittle, and penetrate more deeply into the lung. They are also more resistant to breakdown within the lung.

Workers may be exposed to asbestos in many different settings so that it is important to take a detailed history of all the patient's occupations over the years and of the tasks undertaken. **Pipe laggers** and industrial **plumbers** often have had heavy exposure to asbestos because it is widely used for **thermal insulation** in **ships**, **power stations** and factories. Many workers in the **shipbuilding** industry were heavily exposed to asbestos when they worked alongside pipe laggers in confined spaces such as the engine rooms of ships. Sometimes housewives washing their husbands' work overalls inhaled significant amounts of asbestos. Workers in the **insulation industry** and those producing **asbestos products** may have been heavily exposed. Chrysotile asbestos is used in **brake-pad linings**, in **cement products**, in **pipes**, **tiles** and **roofing** materials. In many circumstances the asbestos is safely bound within composite materials but respirable dust may be produced by the **cutting of asbestos sheets**, or in demolition work involving the removal, or **stripping-off**, of asbestos insulation from pipes or boilers.

Strict precautions were eventually widely introduced in the 1970s to restrict exposure to asbestos with the use of protective respirators and exhaust ventilation, and the substitution of other materials where possible. However, the long lag interval between the inhalation of asbestos and the

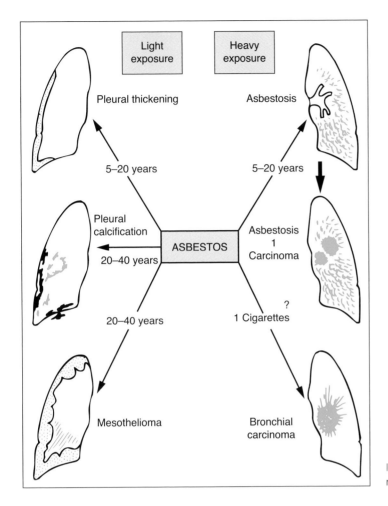

Figure 14.4 Pulmonary diseases relating to exposure to asbestos.

development of disease means that asbestos-related lung disease is still all too common. There are several different diseases related to asbestos exposure (Fig. 14.4) and they each have very different manifestations and prognosis.

- *Asbestosis:* asbestosis is a pneumoconiosis in which **diffuse parenchymal lung fibrosis** develops as a result of heavy prolonged exposure to asbestos. The lag interval between exposure and the onset of the disease is typically 10–25 years, and is shorter the more intense the exposure. The clinical features are similar to those of other interstitial lung diseases such as idiopathic pulmonary fibrosis, with **cough**, progressive **dyspnoea**, bibasal **crackles**, frequently **clubbing** and a **restrictive ventilatory defect** (reduced lung volumes) with **impaired gas diffusion** (reduced transfer factor for carbon monoxide). Chest X-ray

shows bilateral **reticulonodular shadowing**. CT is more sensitive in detecting early changes. Fibrosis is usually first evident around the respiratory bronchioles at the lung bases, becoming more diffuse as the disease progresses. **Asbestos bodies**, consisting of an asbestos fibre coated with an iron-containing protein, are usually seen within areas of fibrosis on light or electron microscopy. The disease is usually slowly progressive even after exposure has ceased, and is not usually responsive to corticosteroids. Patients with asbestosis are at substantial risk of developing lung cancer. It seems likely that some individuals have an increased susceptibility to developing asbestosis, although the nature of this susceptibility is unknown.
- *Pleural plaques:* pleural plaques are often visible as an incidental finding on chest X-rays of workers who have been exposed to asbestos.

They are often calcified and appear as **dense white lines** on the pleura of the chest wall, diaphragm, pericardium and mediastinum. When seen face-on they form an irregular '**holly leaf**' **pattern** (Fig. 14.5). They consist of white fibrous tissue usually situated on the parietal pleura. They **do not give rise to any impairment** of lung function or disability.

- *Asbestos pleurisy and pleural effusions:* many years after first exposure to asbestos, patients may develop episodes of pleurisy with **pleuritic pain** and **pleural effusions**. The pleural fluid is an **exudate** that is often **bloodstained** even in the absence of malignancy. There is sometimes associated elevation of erythrocyte sedimentation rate (ESR). Other causes of pleural effusion need to be excluded. Pleural biopsy shows evidence of inflammation and fibrosis without any specific diagnostic features. There is usually spontaneous resolution but recurrent episodes affecting both sides may occur and may lead to pleural thickening.

- *Pleural thickening:* localised or diffuse thickening and fibrosis of the pleura may develop as a result of asbestos exposure. There may be a history of recurrent episodes of acute pleurisy although these are often subclinical. The pleural

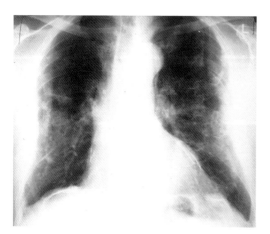

Figure 14.5 This 70-year-old man had had extensive exposure to asbestos when he worked as a pipe lagger in shipyards. His chest X-ray shows extensive calcified pleural plaques seen as dense white lines over the diaphragm and pericardium, and demonstrating a 'holly leaf' pattern when seen face-on over the mid zones of the lungs. There is pleural thickening in both mid zones with some blunting of the costophrenic angles.

thickening is usually most marked at the lung bases with **obliteration of the costophrenic angles**. It may initially be unilateral but often becomes bilateral. Areas of fibrous strands extending from the thickened pleura may give the appearance of '**crow's feet**' on X-ray and **rolled atelectasis** may appear as a rounded opacity caused by puckering of the lung by the thickened pleura. When the pleural thickening is extensive it causes **dyspnoea** and a **restrictive ventilatory defect**.

- *Asbestos-related lung cancer:* epidemiology studies show an increased risk of lung cancer in workers in the asbestos industry with an approximately linear relationship between the dose of asbestos and the occurrence of lung cancer. The interaction between **asbestos** and **smoking** is multiplicative. The clinical features, distribution of cell type, investigation and treatment of asbestos-related lung cancers are the same as for those not associated with asbestos exposure (see Chapter 12) but impairment of lung function as a result of asbestosis may preclude surgery. In the UK, workers are entitled to compensation from the Department of Social Security for asbestos-related lung cancer if it occurs in association with asbestosis or if they have had at least 1 year of heavy exposure or 5 years of moderate exposure to asbestos in certain occupations.

- *Mesothelioma:* it is a **malignant tumour of the pleura** that is associated with a history of asbestos exposure in at least 90% of cases. The risk is greatest in those exposed to **crocidolite (blue asbestos)**. Sometimes the period of exposure to asbestos may have been as short as a few months. At present there are about 2000 deaths each year in the UK from mesothelioma and the incidence is expected to continue to rise until about the year 2020 because effective controls on asbestos exposure were only widely introduced in the 1970s and there is an average **lag interval of 20–40 years** between exposure to asbestos and the development of mesothelioma. It usually presents with **pain, dyspnoea, weight loss** and **lethargy**, and features of a **pleural effusion** sometimes associated with a lobulated pleural mass on X-ray (Fig. 14.6). **CT scan** typically shows nodular pleural thickening encasing the lung and involving the mediastinal pleura. Video-assisted thoracoscopic **pleural biopsy** may be needed for definitive histopathological diagnosis and pleurodesis can be

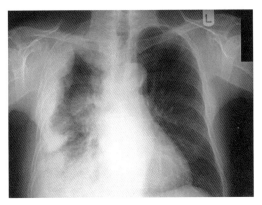

Figure 14.6 This 74-year-old man presented with right-sided chest pain and progressive breathlessness. He had been exposed to asbestos 40 years previously in his job as a plumber. His chest X-ray shows extensive lobulated pleural masses encasing the right lung. Percutaneous pleural biopsy showed malignant mesothelioma.

performed at the same time for control of a pleural effusion. As the tumour progresses it encases the lung and may involve the pericardium and peritoneum, and give rise to blood-borne metastases. Radical surgery in the form of **extrapleural pneumonectomy** can be attempted in only a small percentage of patients and has a poor success rate. **Radiotherapy** can reduce the risk of spread of the tumour through biopsy tracks and may relieve pain. **Chemotherapy**, using drugs such as pemetrexed and cisplatin, results in tumour shrinkage in about 40% of patients, with a small improvement in survival rates. Unfortunately prognosis is poor, with most patients **dying within 2 years** of diagnosis.

Patients who have suffered disability as a result of occupational lung disease have a statutory right to receive **compensation** from governmental agencies such as the Department of Social Security in the UK. In some cases they may wish to pursue **litigation** against their employer. The death of a patient with a suspected occupational lung disease should be reported to the relevant authority, such as the **coroner**, who may wish to undertake a **post-mortem examination**.

 KEY POINTS

- Asthma is the commonest type of occupational lung disease.
- Occupational asthma accounts for 10–15% of all cases of asthma in adults.
- Avoidance of exposure to the inducing agent is the main treatment of occupational asthma.
- Pneumoconiosis is a form of lung fibrosis due to inhalation of dusts such as asbestos, coal and silica.
- Mesothelioma is a malignant tumour of the pleura due to inhalation of asbestos 20–40 years previously.

 FURTHER READING

British Lung Foundation: Information on Asbestos and Mesothelioma: www.lunguk.org.

British Thoracic Society. Statement on malignant mesothelioma in the United Kingdom. *Thorax* 2007; **62** (suppl II): 1–19.

Edwards PR, Van Tongeren M, Watson A, Gee I, Edwards RE. Environmental tobacco smoke. *Occup Environ Med* 2004; **61**: 385–6.

Fishwick D, Barber CM, Bradshaw LM, et al. Standards of care for occupational asthma. *Thorax* 2008; **63**: 240–50.

Hendrick DJ. Popcorn worker's lung in Britain in a man making potato crisp flavouring. *Thorax* 2008; **63**: 267–8.

McDonald JC, Chen Y, Zekveld C, Cherry NM. Incidence by occupation and industry of acute work related respiratory diseases in the UK, 1992–2001. *Occup Environ Med* 2005; **62**: 836–42.

Nicholson PJ, Cullinan P, Newman Taylor AJ, Burge PS, Boyle C. Evidence based guidelines for the prevention, identification, and management of occupational asthma. *Occup Environ Med* 2005; **62**: 290–9.

OASYS. Occupational asthma causative agents/sensitizers: www.occupationalasthma.com/causative_agents.aspx.

Sigsgaard T, Nowak D, Annesi-Maesano I, et al. European Respiratory Society position paper: work-related respiratory diseases in the EU. *Eur Resp J* 2010; **35**: 234–8.

15

Pulmonary vascular disease

Pulmonary embolism

It is estimated that pulmonary emboli occur in about 1% of patients admitted to hospital and are directly responsible for about 5% of all deaths in hospital. The thrombus typically develops in the deep veins of the legs and then travels to the lungs causing obstruction of the pulmonary vasculature. Patients who are immobilised in the community or in hospital are particularly vulnerable to developing deep vein thrombosis (DVT) and then pulmonary embolism. It is the commonest cause of death after elective surgery and is one of the leading causes of maternal death in the UK. Strategies to defend against this killer rely on widespread use of subcutaneous heparin prophylaxis against DVT and rapid resort to full anti-coagulation pending definitive investigations in patients showing features suggesting DVT or pulmonary embolism.

Deep vein thrombosis

Factors predisposing to venous thrombosis were described by Virchow as a triad of venous stasis, damage to the wall of the vein and hypercoagulable states:

- *Venous stasis* occurs as a result of **immobility** (e.g. bed-bound patients on medical, surgical or obstetric wards, airplane flights), **local pressure** (e.g. tight plaster of Paris), **venous obstruction** (e.g. pressure of a pelvic tumour, pregnancy, obesity, varicose veins), congestive **cardiac failure** and **dehydration**.
- *Damage to a vein* occurs from local **trauma** to the vein, **previous thrombosis** and **inflammation** (phlebitis).
- *Hypercoagulable states* arise as part of the body's response to **surgery**, **trauma** and **childbirth**, and are found in association with **malignancy** and use of **oral oestrogen contraceptives**. Recurrent thrombosis is particularly likely to occur where there are specific inherited abnormalities of the clotting system such as **factor V Leiden gene mutation**, **anti-thrombin III**, **protein S** or **protein C deficiencies** and in **anti-cardiolipin antibody** disease. Patients with recurrent or unexplained thromboembolic disease should have specific tests for these conditions because long-term anti-coagulation is advisable.

Pulmonary embolism is particularly common when thrombosis occurs in the proximal femoral or iliac veins and is less likely to occur when thrombosis is confined to the calf veins. Most pulmonary emboli arise in the deep veins of the legs but they may occasionally arise from thrombus in the inferior vena cava, the right side of the

Respiratory Medicine Lecture Notes, Eighth Edition. Stephen J. Bourke and Graham P. Burns.
© 2011 John Wiley & Sons, Ltd. Published 2011 by John Wiley & Sons, Ltd.

heart or from indwelling catheters in the subclavian or jugular veins. DVT may cause permanent damage to the vein with impairment of venous drainage, oedema, pigmentation, ulceration and an increased risk of further thrombosis.

The classic signs of DVT are oedema of the leg with tenderness, erythema and pain on flexing the ankle (Homan's sign). However, thrombosis in the deep veins of the leg, pelvis or abdomen may be completely silent. DVT must be distinguished from other conditions such as cellulitis, muscle injury or ruptured cysts of the knee and **compression ultrasound** of the leg veins is the usual investigation used to confirm or exclude the diagnosis. Other investigations for detecting DVT include **venography** whereby injection of radiocontrast material outlines thrombus and ^{125}**I-fibrinogen isotope scan** that demonstrates incorporation of radiolabelled fibrinogen into the thrombus.

Clinical features

The clinical features of pulmonary embolism depend upon the size and severity of the embolism, as summarised in Fig. 15.1, although there is overlap between the different presentations. In **acute massive pulmonary embolism** the picture is often that of a patient recovering from recent surgery who collapses. Attempts at resuscitation are often unsuccessful and there is a rapid high mortality, with very limited opportunity for intervention. Occlusion of a large part of the pulmonary circulation produces a catastrophic drop in cardiac output and the patient collapses with hypotension, cyanosis, tachypnoea and engorged neck veins. Sometimes the presentation is more **subacute**, as a series of emboli progressively occlude the pulmonary circulation over a longer period of time, with the patient developing progressive dyspnoea, tachypnoea and hypoxaemia. **Acute minor pulmonary embolism** presents as dyspnoea, typically accompanied by pleuritic pain, haemoptysis and fever if there is associated **pulmonary infarction**. Prompt recognition and treatment of an acute minor embolism may prevent the occurrence of a massive embolism. **Chronic thromboembolic pulmonary hypertension** is a condition in which recurrent emboli progressively occlude the pulmonary circulation giving rise to progressive dyspnoea, pulmonary hypertension and right heart failure.

Pulmonary embolism is both under- and overdiagnosed in clinical practice leading to some patients failing to receive treatment for a potentially life-threatening condition and others being subjected to the risks of anti-coagulant therapy unnecessarily. Although it is crucial to confirm a clinical suspicion of pulmonary embolism by a definitive test, it is also important to avoid subjecting large numbers of patients to unnecessary and expensive investigations. Dyspnoea, tachypnoea (respiratory rate >20/min) and pleuritic pain are the three cardinal features of pulmonary embolism. If none of these features is present a diagnosis of pulmonary embolism is very unlikely.

Investigations

General investigations

General investigations may yield clues that point towards a diagnosis of pulmonary embolism and are particularly useful in excluding alternative diagnoses:

- *Chest X-ray* is often normal but **elevation of a hemidiaphragm** and areas of **linear atelectasis** are suggestive of pulmonary emboli. A small **pleural effusion** with **wedge-shaped peripheral opacities** may occur in association with pulmonary infarction, and rarely an area of lung infarction undergoes cavitation. In massive embolism an **area of underperfusion** with few vascular markings may be apparent. **Enlarged pulmonary** arteries are a feature of pulmonary hypertension in chronic thromboembolic disease. The chest X-ray helps exclude alternative diagnoses such as pneumothorax, pneumonia and pulmonary oedema.
- *Electrocardiogram* (ECG) is often normal apart from showing a **sinus tachycardia**. In major pulmonary embolism there may be features of **right heart strain** with depression of the ST segment and T wave in leads V_1–V_3, and evidence of right axis deviation with an **S1 Q3 T3** pattern. The ECG helps exclude myocardial infarction and cardiac arrhythmias.
- *Arterial blood gases*: characteristically pulmonary embolism is associated with ventilation of underperfused areas of lung resulting in hypoxaemia and hyperventilation so that arterial blood gases show a reduced Po_2 and Pco_2.
- *Lung function tests* are not usually helpful in the acute situation but in patients with dyspnoea caused by chronic or subacute pulmonary emboli there is reduced gas diffusion with

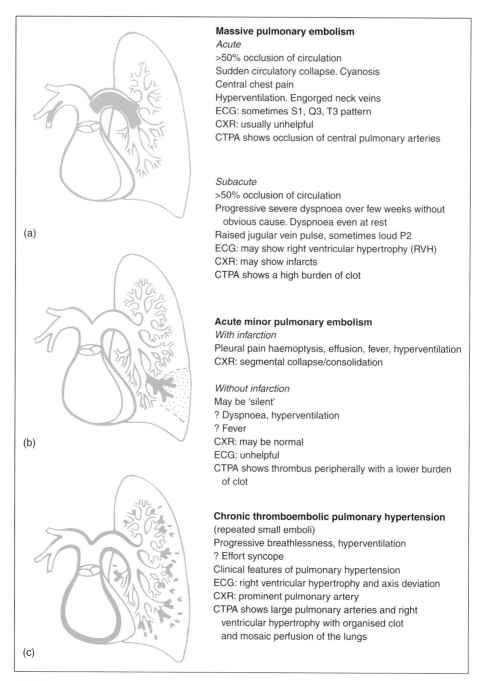

Massive pulmonary embolism
Acute
>50% occlusion of circulation
Sudden circulatory collapse. Cyanosis
Central chest pain
Hyperventilation. Engorged neck veins
ECG: sometimes S1, Q3, T3 pattern
CXR: usually unhelpful
CTPA shows occlusion of central pulmonary arteries

Subacute
>50% occlusion of circulation
Progressive severe dyspnoea over few weeks without
    obvious cause. Dyspnoea even at rest
Raised jugular vein pulse, sometimes loud P2
ECG: may show right ventricular hypertrophy (RVH)
CXR: may show infarcts
CTPA shows a high burden of clot

(a)

Acute minor pulmonary embolism
With infarction
Pleural pain haemoptysis, effusion, fever, hyperventilation
CXR: segmental collapse/consolidation

Without infarction
May be 'silent'
? Dyspnoea, hyperventilation
? Fever
CXR: may be normal
ECG: unhelpful
CTPA shows thrombus peripherally with a lower burden
    of clot

(b)

Chronic thromboembolic pulmonary hypertension
(repeated small emboli)
Progressive breathlessness, hyperventilation
? Effort syncope
Clinical features of pulmonary hypertension
ECG: right ventricular hypertrophy and axis deviation
CXR: prominent pulmonary artery
CTPA shows large pulmonary arteries and right
    ventricular hypertrophy with organised clot
    and mosaic perfusion of the lungs

(c)

Figure 15.1 Synopsis of pulmonary embolism. CTPA, Computed tomography pulmonary angiography; CXR, chest X-ray; ECG, electrocardiogram.

a reduction in the transfer factor for carbon monoxide. Lung function tests may also help identify other lung diseases (e.g. chronic obstructive pulmonary disease (COPD) and emphysema).

- *Blood tests*: There may be evidence of intravascular thrombosis (thrombin–anti-thrombin III complex assay) and fibrinolysis (fibrin degradation products). D-**dimer** is a breakdown product of cross-linked fibrin and levels are elevated in patients with thromboembolism. However, levels are also often elevated in other hospitalised patients so that D-**dimer assays can be used to exclude, but not to confirm venous thromboembolism**. A normal D-dimer level can be particularly useful in certain clinical settings. For example, a young woman on oral contraception who presents with isolated pleuritic pain is very unlikely to have pulmonary embolism if the respiratory rate is below 20/min and chest X-ray, arterial blood gases and D-dimer are normal. She can be reassured without the need for admission to hospital or further investigation.

Specific investigations

- *Pulmonary angiography* is the definitive test for diagnosing pulmonary embolism but it is an invasive test requiring specialist expertise and equipment that are not widely available, and it is associated with a small risk, particularly in critically ill patients. A catheter is passed from a peripheral vein (e.g. femoral vein), through the right side of the heart into the pulmonary arteries, and radiocontrast material is injected and a rapid sequence of X-rays is taken. The angiographic features of embolism are intraluminal filling defects, abrupt cut-off of vessels, peripheral pruning of vessels and areas of reduced perfusion.
- *Computed tomography pulmonary angiography* (**CTPA**) (Fig. 15.2) is increasingly being used as the definitive initial non-invasive imaging modality for pulmonary embolism. Very rapid spiral images are obtained during the injection of iodinated contrast medium into a peripheral vein. It has better specificity than ventilation–perfusion isotope scanning in the diagnosis of pulmonary embolism although it does involve a higher radiation dose. It also provides information on a potential alternative diagnosis when pulmonary embolism is excluded.

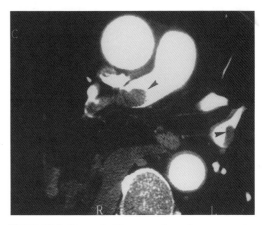

Figure 15.2 Computed tomography pulmonary angiogram showing clot in the main pulmonary artery of the right lung (upper arrow) and the lower lobe pulmonary artery of the left lung (lower arrow).

- *Ventilation/perfusion (V/Q) lung scan*: macroaggregated particles or microspheres of human albumin, labelled with a gamma-emitting radioisotope, technetium-99m, are injected intravenously. These particles impact in the pulmonary capillaries and the radioactivity emitted from the lung fields is detected by a gamma camera, thus outlining the distribution of pulmonary perfusion. The distribution of ventilation in the lungs is similarly outlined after the patient has inhaled radiolabelled xenon. A completely normal pattern of pulmonary perfusion is strong evidence against pulmonary embolism. 'Cold areas' are evident on the scan where there is defective blood flow and these may occur in association with localised abnormalities apparent on a chest X-ray (e.g. pleural effusion, carcinoma, bulla). In these circumstances ventilation is usually decreased in the same areas resulting in 'matched defects' in ventilation and perfusion scans. The classic pattern seen in pulmonary embolism consists of multiple areas of perfusion defects that are not matched with defects in ventilation. A *V/Q* scan may therefore show: normal perfusion, in which case pulmonary embolism is unlikely ('low probability'); areas of perfusion defects not matched with ventilation defects in the presence of a normal chest X-ray that indicates a 'high probability' of pulmonary embolism; or it may show matched ventilation and perfusion defects in which case interpretation is difficult and the scan is regarded as 'indeterminate'. Patients with a suspected pulmonary embolism but an indeterminate scan require further imaging, such as CTPA.

- *Imaging of peripheral veins*: demonstration of thrombus in the peripheral veins by venography, Doppler ultrasound or ^{125}I-fibrinogen isotope scan provides support for the decision to anti-coagulate a patient who has clinical features of pulmonary embolism but an 'indeterminate' *V/Q* scan.

Diagnosing pulmonary embolism

The British Thoracic Society recommends a step-wise approach and use of a probability scoring system in diagnosing pulmonary embolism.

- **Assess the probability of pulmonary embolism.** The main clinical features are breathlessness, increased respiratory rate (>20/min), pleuritic pain, haemoptysis or sudden collapse.
- **Are other diagnoses unlikely?** (e.g. pneumothorax, COPD, pneumonia etc): if Yes, score +1
- **Is a major risk factor for venous thrombosis present?** (e.g. surgery, pregnancy, previous venous thrombosis, immobility, major medical illness): if Yes, score +1
- Patients scoring 2 have a high probability of pulmonary embolism. Heparin should be started immediately and CTPA should be organised to confirm the diagnosis. Patients scoring 1 have an intermediate probability of pulmonary embolism. Measurement of D-dimer is then useful as a negative D-dimer in this situation makes pulmonary embolism unlikely. If D-dimer is positive then heparin should be started and CTPA should be arranged. Patients scoring 0 may have an alternative diagnosis accounting for their symptoms. A negative D-dimer in these circumstances would make pulmonary embolism unlikely. However if D-dimer is positive then further investigations by CTPA may be needed. **D-dimer assays can be used to exclude but not to confirm venous thromboembolism** and can reduce the need for CTPA in some circumstances.

Pregnancy

The diagnosis of pulmonary embolism in a woman who is pregnant requires particular consideration. Pulmonary embolism is a leading cause of maternal death and accurate diagnosis is essential. CTPA exposes the foetus to less radiation than an isotope perfusion scan but exposes the mother's breasts to

a significant dose of radiation at a time when they are particularly vulnerable, increasing the risk of future breast cancer. **Ultrasound of the legs for DVT** is a useful initial investigation. If this is negative and chest x-ray is normal a **half-dose perfusion scan** is recommended, and **CTPA** is reserved for patients with indeterminate initial investigations.

Treatment

Anti-coagulant therapy

When a clinical diagnosis of suspected pulmonary embolism or DVT has been made, anti-coagulants should be started at once unless there is a strong contraindication (e.g. active haemorrhage). The decision as to whether anti-coagulants should be continued in the long term is made later based upon the results of subsequent investigations. **Low-molecular weight heparin** (e.g. **tinzaparin 175units/kg subcutaneously once daily**) is now the standard initial treatment for patients with pulmonary embolism. The dose is determined by the patient's weight and anti-coagulant monitoring is not needed. An alternative is unfractionated heparin (e.g. heparin given as an initial intravenous bolus followed by an infusion), and this requires monitoring of the activated partial thromboplastin time (APTT) with adjustment of the dose to maintain the APTT at 1.5–2.5 times the control value. Intravenous heparin may be preferred to subcutaneous heparin in patients with a massive pulmonary embolism or where rapid reversal of anti-coagulation may be needed (e.g. in patients at risk of haemorrhage). Adverse effects of heparin include haemorrhage, bruising and thrombocytopenia. Once the clinical suspicion of pulmonary embolism or DVT has been supported by subsequent investigations **oral anti-coagulation** is commenced using **warfarin**. Usually 10 mg is given on the first day as a loading dose, and then the international normalised ratio (INR) is measured and the dosage adjusted to maintain a ratio of about 2–3. Since warfarin takes at least 48–72 hours to establish its anti-coagulant effect heparin needs to be continued for this period. The optimal duration of warfarin treatment is uncertain but it is usually continued for 3–6 months after a first episode of idiopathic venous thromboembolism. Patients with recurrent or unexplained thromboembolic disease should have investigations for hypercoagulable states (e.g. anti-thrombin III, protein S or C deficiencies; anti-cardiolipin antibody disease) and may require long-term anti-coagulation.

The patient should be given an **anti-coagulant information booklet** that explains the nature and side-effects of treatment, states the indication for and proposed duration of treatment, provides contact numbers for obtaining advice and instructions on avoiding medications that interfere with therapy. Many drugs enhance the effect of warfarin (e.g. non-steroidal anti-inflammatory drugs, aspirin, ciprofloxacin, erythromycin, etc.) and others reduce the effect (e.g. carbamazepine, barbiturates, rifampicin, etc.). Warfarin is teratogenic and women of child-bearing age should be warned of this danger, and may require specialist contraceptive advice. Precise details of INR, warfarin dosage and clinic appointments are included in the booklet and this provides a useful method of communication with the patient and with all involved in the care of the patient (e.g. general practitioner, dentist, nurses etc.).

Thrombolytic therapy

The aim of thrombolytic therapy is to actively dissolve clots, but its use is reserved for those patients with acute massive pulmonary embolism who remain in severe haemodynamic collapse (e.g. hypotensive, poorly perfused, hypoxaemic). These patients have survived the immediate impact of the pulmonary embolism but remain critically ill. If all the clinical features and bedside tests (e.g. ECG, chest X-ray) suggest a massive pulmonary embolism and exclude alternative diagnoses (pneumothorax, post-operative haemorrhage, myocardial infarction, aortic dissection etc.), a decision may have to be taken that the circumstances justify the use of thrombolytic therapy. Contraindications to thrombolytic therapy include active haemorrhage, recent major surgery or trauma. Typically **alteplase 50 mg** is given as a bolus via a peripheral vein. Thereafter heparin anti-coagulation is commenced.

Patients with acute pulmonary embolism require **high-flow oxygen** to correct hypoxaemia, and **analgesia** (e.g. diamorphine) to relieve pain and distress. In patients with active haemorrhage contraindicating the use of anti-coagulant, or recurrent pulmonary emboli despite adequate anti-coagulation, **a venous filter** procedure may be useful. This involves the passing of a specially designed filter into the inferior vena cava to prevent further emboli from reaching the lungs from DVT in the pelvis or lower limbs (Fig. 15.3).

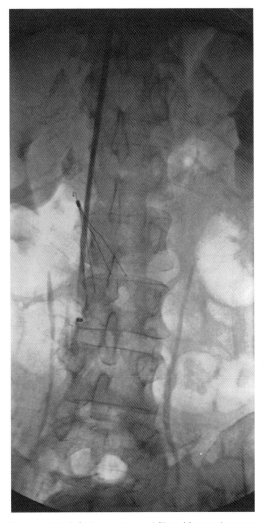

Figure 15.3 Inferior vena caval filter. Most pulmonary emboli arise from thrombi in the deep veins of the leg. An inferior vena caval filter can be used to prevent emboli from reaching the lungs. They are used in patients who have suffered recurrent pulmonary emboli despite adequate anti-coagulation and in those in whom anti-coagulant therapy is contraindicated. This 64-year-old woman had had major pulmonary emboli from a deep vein thrombosis in her right femoral vein. She then suffered major haemorrhage from a gastric ulcer while on heparin therapy, which was discontinued. A filter device was passed through the venous system from the internal jugular vein to be placed in the inferior vena cava.

DVT Prophylaxis

A variety of measures are directed against Virchow's triad of factors predisposing to DVT. Early **ambulation**, use of graded elastic **compression stockings** and leg **exercises** reduce venous stasis. Prophylactic **low-dose heparin** is now widely used to reduce the risk for patients on surgical, obstetric and medical wards. Typically, **tinzaparin 3500 units/day** is given subcutaneously. For patients undergoing surgery with a higher risk of DVT (e.g. hip replacement) the dosage may be increased to 4500 units given 12 hours before surgery and then daily until the patient is mobile again.

Other materials that may occasionally embolise to the lungs include **fat** (after fracture of long bones), **amniotic fluid** (post-partum), **air** (e.g. from disconnected central venous lines), **tumour** (from tumour invasion of venous system), **infected vegetations** (from tricuspid endocarditis) and **foreign materials** (from contamination of drugs injected by drug misusers).

Pulmonary hypertension

In normal lungs the pulmonary arterial pressure is about 20/8 mmHg (compared with typical systemic artery systolic/diastolic pressures of 120/80 mmHg) and the mean pulmonary artery pressure is 12–15 mmHg. Pulmonary hypertension is defined as a mean pulmonary artery pressure >25 mmHg at rest. It may occur as a result of hypoxaemia and chronic lung disease, when it is often referred to as **cor pulmonale**, but in some cases there is no demonstrable cause and this is termed **idiopathic pulmonary hypertension**.

Cor pulmonale

Some confusion arises from the differing ways in which this term is used but it essentially refers to the development of pulmonary hypertension and right ventricular hypertrophy secondary to disease of the lungs. **Hypoxaemia** is a powerful stimulus for pulmonary vasoconstriction and this is the most common mechanism giving rise to cor pulmonale (e.g. chronic hypercapnic respiratory failure in COPD). Other mechanisms giving rise to pulmonary hypertension include **vascular obstruction** (e.g. chronic pulmonary emboli, pulmonary artery stenosis), **increased blood flow** (e.g.

left-to-right intracardiac shunts – atrial and ventricular septal defects) and **loss of pulmonary vascular bed** (e.g. fibrotic lung disease, emphysema).

The clinical features of cor pulmonale are **elevation of jugular venous pressure**, **hepatomegaly** (as a result of congestion), peripheral **oedema**, a prominent left **parasternal heave**, a **loud pulmonary secondary sound** and a systolic murmur of **tricuspid regurgitation**. A chest X-ray may show large pulmonary arteries with pruning of the vessels in the lung fields. ECG typically shows p pulmonale (tall p wave in leads II III AVF) with a tall R wave in V_1 and ST segment depression with T-wave inversion in V_1–V_3. Echocardiography can assess the structure and dimension of the right heart chambers and the pulmonary artery pressure can be estimated from the velocity of the tricuspid regurgitation jet.

Idiopathic pulmonary hypertension

This is a rare disease, affecting about two per million of the population per annum, in which pulmonary hypertension occurs **without a demonstrable cause**. It particularly affects young women. Some cases of familial pulmonary hypertension are inherited as an autosomal dominant trait due to mutations in the bone morphogenetic protein receptor 2 gene. Some cases are associated with human immunodeficiency virus (**HIV**) infection or with use of **appetite-suppressant drugs** (e.g. aminorex, fenfluramine) but in most cases no cause is apparent. Pulmonary hypertension also occurs as a complication of **collagen vascular diseases** such as systemic sclerosis (scleroderma), mixed connective tissue disease and systemic lupus erythematosus (SLE). Some patients with generalised systemic sclerosis develop severe pulmonary fibrosis (see Chapter 13) but there is also a limited cutaneous variant of systemic sclerosis characterised by subcutaneous calcinosis, Raynaud's phenomenon, oesophageal involvement, sclerodactyly and telangiectasia (CREST syndrome). Patients with the CREST syndrome usually have anti-centromere antibodies and may develop pulmonary hypertension as a primary vascular phenomenon, often in the absence of significant pulmonary fibrosis. Patients present with dyspnoea, fatigue, angina and syncope on exertion. Investigations (e.g. echocardiography, V/Q scans, pulmonary artery catheterisation) are particularly directed towards excluding other causes of pulmonary hypertension such as left-to-right cardiac shunts and chronic thromboembolic disease. The pathophysiology of the disease involves pulmonary artery vasoconstriction, vascular wall remodelling and thrombosis *in situ*. Treatment of patients with pulmonary hypertension is complex and is delivered from specialist centres. Supportive treatments include warfarin, diuretics and oxygen therapy. Pulmonary endarterectomy is a surgical procedure in which organised thrombi are removed from the proximal pulmonary arteries in appropriate patients with chronic thromboembolic disease. Calcium-channel blocker drugs (e.g. nifedipine) produce useful vasodilatation in a small number of these patients. Prostacycline drugs produce vascular smooth muscle relaxation and inhibit vascular smooth muscle growth, and include: epoprostenol given as a continuous intravenous infusion via an indwelling central venous catheter; iloprost that is given by inhalation; and treprostinil given as a subcutaneous infusion. Endothelial receptor antagonists (e.g. bosentan) reduce vascular tone and proliferation in pulmonary hypertension. Selective phosphodiesterase-5-inhibitors (e.g. sildenafil) also reduce pulmonary artery pressure. Atrial septostomy involves the creation of a right-to-left interatrial shunt and can be used to decompress the failing right heart. Heart–lung or lung transplantation also needs to be considered as the disease is usually progressive.

Pulmonary vasculitis

When pulmonary vasculitis occurs it is usually as part of a more widespread systemic vasculitis such as Wegener's granulomatosis, polyarteritis nodosa, Churg–Strauss syndrome, Goodpasture's disease or collagen vascular diseases (e.g. scleroderma, SLE; see also Chapter 13).

Wegener's granulomatosis

This is characterised by necrotising granulomatous inflammation and vasculitis affecting in particular the **upper airways** (rhinitis, sinusitis, bloodstained nasal discharge), the **lungs** (cavitating nodules, endobronchial disease) and **kidneys** (glomerulonephritis). **Anti-neutrophil cytoplasmic antibodies** (ANCA) are usually present in the serum. It is treated with a combination of corticosteroids and cyclophosphamide.

Churg–Strauss syndrome

This is an unusual disease consisting of allergic granulomatosis and angiitis. It consists of an initial phase of **asthma** followed by marked peripheral blood **eosinophilia** and **eosinophilic vasculitis** giving rise to pulmonary infiltrates, myocarditis, myositis, neuritis, rashes and glomerulonephritis. It usually responds rapidly to corticosteroids.

Polyarteritis nodosa

This consists of a vasculitis of medium and small arteries resulting in **aneurysm** formation, **glomerulonephritis** and **vasculitic lesions** in various organs. Pulmonary involvement is unusual but may result in haemoptysis, pulmonary haemorrhage, fibrosis and pleurisy. There is often considerable overlap in the clinical features of the various vasculitic syndromes.

Goodpasture's syndrome

This consists of a combination of **glomerulonephritis** and **alveolar haemorrhage** in association with circulating **anti-basement membrane antibody** that binds to lung and renal tissue. Pulmonary involvement is more common in smokers and may cause severe pulmonary haemorrhage resulting in haemoptysis, infiltrates on chest X-ray, hypoxaemia and anaemia. Transfer factor may be elevated because of binding of the inhaled carbon monoxide to haemoglobin in the alveoli. Treatment consists of corticosteroids and cyclophosphamide, with plasmapheresis to remove circulating antibodies.

 Respiratory emergencies **Pulmonary embolism**

- Consider the **diagnosis** of pulmonary embolism in all patients with unexplained breathlessness, pleuritic pain, haemoptysis or sudden collapse.
- Chest X-ray, electrocardiogram, arterial gases are the key initial tests.
- Assess the probability of pulmonary embolism
  - are other diagnoses unlikely?
  - is a major risk factor present?

- **D-dimer** is useful in excluding the diagnosis but not in confirming it as it is often elevated in patients with infection, systemic illness and after surgery.
- **CT pulmonary angiography** is the definitive test to confirm or exclude pulmonary embolism.
- **Tinzaparin 175 units/kg subcutaneously once daily** should be started immediately when pulmonary embolism is suspected.
- **Warfarin** should be started when the diagnosis is confirmed, and continued for 3–6 months after a first episode.
- **High-flow oxygen** and **analgesia** (e.g. diamorphine) are given as needed.
- **Thrombolysis (e.g. alteplase 50 mg)** intravenous bolus should be considered for patients with acute massive pulmonary embolism who have severe haemodynamic compromise.

 KEY POINTS

- Most pulmonary emboli arise from thrombosis in the deep veins of the legs, which is common in immobilised patients in the community and in hospital on medical, surgical and obstetric wards.
- Assessing patients with suspected pulmonary emboli involves an appraisal of compatible clinical features and risk factors, exclusion of alternative diagnoses and measurement of D-dimer levels.
- CTPA is increasingly being used as the main imaging modality to confirm or exclude the diagnosis of pulmonary embolism.
- Heparin is used to achieve rapid anti-coagulation, followed by warfarin. Thrombolytic therapy is only given to patients with circulatory compromise from a massive pulmonary embolism.
- Pulmonary hypertension (mean pressure >25 mmHg) may arise from chronic thromboembolic disease, as a result of chronic hypoxic lung disease, or in the form of idiopathic pulmonary hypertension.

 FURTHER READING

Blann AD, Lip GYH. Venous thromboembolism. *BMJ* 2006; **332**: 215–19.

British Thoracic Society Standards of Care Committee Pulmonary Embolism Guideline Development Group. British Thoracic Society guidelines for the management of suspected acute pulmonary embolism. *Thorax* 2003; **58**: 470–84 (www.brit-thoracic.org.uk).

Ghuysen A, Ghaye B, Willems V. Computed tomographic pulmonary angiography and prognostic significance in patients with acute pulmonary embolism. *Thorax* 2005; **60**: 956–61.

National Pulmonary Hypertension Centres of the UK and Ireland. Consensus statement on the management of pulmonary hypertension in clinical practice. *Thorax* 2008; **63** (suppl II): 1–41.

Pulmonary Hypertension Asociation: www.phassociation.uk.com/.

Rubin LJ. Pulmonary arterial hypertension. *Proc Am Thorac Soc* 2006; **3**: 111–15.

Sanchez O, Planquette B, Meyer G. Update on acute pulmonary embolism. *Eur Respir Rev* 2009; **18**: 137–47.

Pneumothorax and pleural effusion

Pneumothorax

Pneumothorax is the presence of air in the pleural space. Usually the air enters the pleural space as the result of a leak from a hole in the underlying lung, but rarely it enters from outside as a result of a penetrating chest injury. Pneumothoraces may be classified as **spontaneous** or **traumatic**, and spontaneous pneumothoraces may be **primary**, without evidence of other lung disease, or occur **secondary** to underlying lung disease (e.g. chronic obstructive pulmonary disease (COPD), cystic fibrosis).

Pathogenesis

Spontaneous primary pneumothorax typically occurs in a previously healthy young adult and is most common in tall thin men. Most seem to arise from the rupture of **subpleural blebs or bullae** at the apex of an otherwise normal lung. The aetiology of these blebs is uncertain but they may represent congenital lesions aggravated by the more negative pleural space pressure at the apex of the lung. Smoking is associated with a greatly increased risk of pneumothorax. The intrapleural pressure is normally negative because of the retractive force of lung elastic recoil so that when a communication is established between the atmosphere and the pleural space air is sucked in and the lung deflates. A small hole in the lung often closes off as the lung deflates. Sometimes the hole remains open and the air leak will then continue until the pressure equalises. Occasionally, the opening from the lung to the pleural space functions as a valve allowing air to leak into the pleural space during inspiration but not to re-enter the lung on expiration. This is a potentially lethal situation as the air accumulates in the pleural space under increasing pressure giving a **tension pneumothorax** in which the lung is pushed down, the mediastinum is shifted to the opposite side and the venous return to the heart and cardiac output are impaired.

There is an increased risk of pneumothorax in association with virtually all lung diseases. These spontaneous secondary pneumothoraces are particularly common in patients with COPD and bullous emphysema. A pneumothorax resulting from rupture of a bulla may render an already disabled patient critically ill. Pneumothorax is a well-recognised complication of positive pressure endotracheal ventilation in patients on intensive therapy units (ITUs) with underlying lung disease. Traumatic pneumothorax usually arises from puncture of the lung by a fractured rib but air may enter the pleural space from outside via a penetrating injury

Respiratory Medicine Lecture Notes, Eighth Edition. Stephen J. Bourke and Graham P. Burns.
© 2011 John Wiley & Sons, Ltd. Published 2011 by John Wiley & Sons, Ltd.

or from rupture of alveoli, oesophagus, trachea or bronchi. **Iatrogenic** ('doctor-induced') pneumothorax may arise as a complication of invasive chest procedures such as the insertion of a catheter into the subclavian vein, percutaneous needle aspiration of a lung lesion or transbronchial lung biopsy.

Clinical features

Pneumothorax typically presents with acute **pleuritic pain** and **breathlessness**. An otherwise healthy young adult may tolerate a pneumothorax quite well but older patients with underlying lung disease often develop severe respiratory distress with cyanosis. The clinical signs of pneumothorax are **reduced breath sounds** and **hyper-resonance** on the side of the pneumothorax, but these may be difficult to detect. Sometimes a left-sided pneumothorax is associated with a clicking noise if the cardiac beat produces friction on movement of the layers of the pleura. Signs of **mediastinal shift** such as displacement of the trachea and apex beat to the opposite side may be detectable in a tension pneumothorax.

The **chest X-ray** shows a black gas space, containing no lung markings, between the margin of the collapsed lung and the chest wall (Fig. 16.1). Typically the visceral pleural of the margin of the lung is visible as a laterally convex 'pleural line' that runs parallel to the chest wall and the pulmonary vascular markings are absent lateral to this line. Identification of a convex pleural line helps to differentiate a pneumothorax from a large bulla (see Chapter 11, Fig. 11.5). A chest X-ray taken after expiration may accentuate the radiological features and may help to detect a small pneumothorax but expiratory X-rays are not needed routinely. It is often difficult to detect a pneumothorax if the chest X-ray is performed with the patient lying supine (e.g. on ventilation in the ITU) because the air in the pleural space, in this position, rises anteriorly giving an appearance of hyperlucency of the lower chest, such that the mediastinal contours and costophrenic angle are outlined with increased clarity (Fig. 16.2). If the patient cannot be imaged in an upright position, a lateral decubitus film should be performed. The size of a pneumothorax can be quantified arbitrarily as being 'small' if the rim of air between the margin of the collapsed lung and chest wall is, <2 cm, or 'large' if it is >2 cm. The volume of a 2-cm rim of air is approximately a 50% pneumothorax.

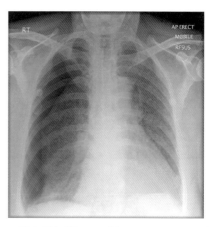

Figure 16.1 This 75-year-old woman presented with sudden onset of breathlessness and right pleuritic pain. Examination showed diminished breath sounds and hyper-resonance over the right lung. Chest X-ray shows a right pneumothorax with a large gas-filled pleural space without lung markings in the right hemithorax, deflation of the right lung and a clear 'pleural line' running parallel to the chest wall at the margin of the collapsed lung. She was given oxygen and analgesia, and an intercostal chest tube was inserted into the right pleural space, with successful re-expansion of the lung (see Fig. 16.3a).

Treatment

- *No intervention:* a small (rim of air <2 cm) pneumothorax that is not causing respiratory distress may not require any intervention because it will **resolve spontaneously at a rate of about 1–2% per day**. Such patients may be allowed home with advice to return to hospital immediately if symptoms deteriorate. They should not undertake an airplane flight until 1 week after the chest X-ray shows complete resolution of the pneumothorax because the reduced barometric pressure at altitude causes expansion of enclosed thoracic air pockets. A follow-up appointment should be arranged for clinical assessment and chest X-ray to ensure resolution of the pneumothorax and to exclude underlying lung disease. If a patient with a pneumothorax is admitted to hospital for observation **high-flow oxygen** (e.g. 10 L/min) should be administered, with appropriate caution in patients with COPD who may be sensitive to higher concentrations of oxygen. Inhalation of oxygen reduces the total pressure of gases in the pleural capillaries by reducing the partial pressure of

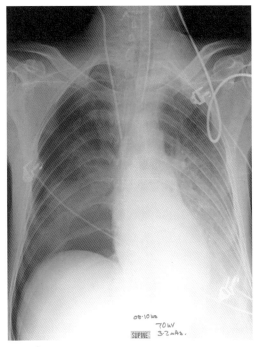

Figure 16.2 Chest X-ray of a pneumothorax in a patient lying flat. This patient was in the intensive care unit receiving endotracheal ventilation. His condition deteriorated with hypoxia, tachycardia and hypotension. The chest X-ray shows an endotracheal tube in satisfactory position, a cannula in the right internal jugular vein, left lower lobe consolidation and evidence of a right pneumothorax. When a patient with a pneumothorax is lying flat the air in the pleural space tends to collect anteriorly and inferiorly giving the appearance of hyperlucency with unusual clarity of the mediastinal contour and the costophrenic angle, and the typical 'pleural line' at the margin of the lung, which is characteristic of a pneumothorax in an upright patient, is often not present.

nitrogen. This increases the pressure gradient between the pleural capillaries and the pleural cavity and increases absorption of air from the pneumothorax.

- *Aspiration:* air may be aspirated from the pleural space by inserting a French gauge 16 cannula (such as an intravenous cannula) through the second intercostal space in the mid-clavicular line after injection of local anaesthetic. Once the pleural cavity is entered, the needle is removed and the cannula is connected via a three-way tap to a syringe, and air is aspirated. Aspiration should be abandoned if 2.5 L of air have been aspirated as this indicates a persistent air leak from the lung. A chest X-ray is performed to

assess the success of the procedure. This technique is simple, less distressing to the patient than insertion of a chest tube, and very effective for primary pneumothoraces. Even large primary pneumothoraces can be aspirated but chest tube insertion is needed if aspiration is unsuccessful.

- *Intercostal tube drainage* (Fig. 16.3): intercostal tube drainage is needed for most secondary pneumothoraces (i.e. in patients with underlying

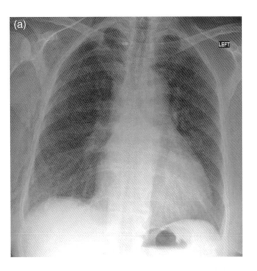

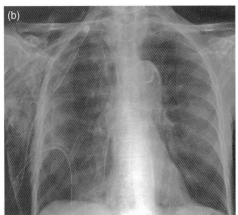

Figure 16.3 (a) Chest X-ray showing a small calibre tube that was inserted using a Seldinger technique (tube passed over a guide wire) into the pleural space of a 75-year-old woman who had presented with a pneumothorax (see Fig. 16.1). (b) Chest X-ray showing two large calibre tubes that were inserted by blunt dissection, in a patient with COPD who had suffered a secondary pneumothorax with a large air leak. Air has tracked into the tissues of the right chest wall causing 'subcutaneous emphysema'.

lung disease e.g. COPD) or where simple aspiration has failed.

- **Small calibre (e.g. size 8–14F) tubes** (Fig. 16.3a) can be passed into the pleural space to drain air or fluid using a **Seldinger technique** whereby, after injection of local anaesthetic (e.g. 10 mls of 1% lidocaine (lignocaine)), a guide wire is inserted via a specially designed cannula and then the tube is passed over the guide wire into the pleural space. The tube is sutured in place and attached to an underwater seal. These small calibre tubes are very effective at draining air and fluid from the pleural space and they cause less pain and discomfort to the patient than large calibre tubes. Whenever possible chest tubes should be inserted in the **'triangle of safety'**, which is bordered anteriorly by the lateral edge of pectoralis major, laterally by the lateral edge of latissimus dorsi, inferiorly by the line of the fifth intercostal space (level of nipple) and by the base of the axilla. This position minimises the risk of damage to underlying structures (e.g. internal mammary artery) and avoids damage to muscle and breast tissue resulting in unsightly scarring.
- **Large calibre (e.g. size 24–32F) tubes** (Fig. 16.3b) are needed if there is a very large air leak from the lung that exceeds the capacity of the smaller tubes. The insertion of a large calibre chest tube is a frightening procedure for the patient, who needs adequate **explanation and reassurance**. Pre-medication with atropine (300–600 mg intravenously) prevents vasovagal reactions, and a small dose of a sedative (e.g. midazolam 1–2 mg intravenously) may be considered for anxious patients. Chest tubes should be inserted in a clean environment using full aseptic technique including sterile gloves, gowns, drapes and skin cleansing. The skin, subcutaneous tissues, intercostal muscles and parietal pleura are anaesthetised by injection of 10–20 ml of 1% **lidocaine (lignocaine)**. Aspiration of air into the syringe confirms that the pleural space has been entered. The skin is incised and **blunt dissection** with a forceps is used to make a track through the intercostal muscles into the pleural space, taking care to avoid the neurovascular bundle, usually situated in the groove on the lower surface of each rib. The chest tube may then be inserted through the track, and directed towards the apex. The track made by blunt dissection should be sufficiently wide **to allow the drain to slide in easily without force**, and care must be taken to avoid causing damage to the underlying lung or other structures. The tube is securely **anchored in place** with a suture and connected to an underwater seal. The end of the tube should be 2–3 cm below the level of the water in the bottle. **Oscillation** of the meniscus of the water in the tube indicates that the tube is patent and in the pleural space. **Bubbling** on respiration or coughing indicates continued drainage of air. Breathing with a chest tube in place is painful and **adequate analgesia** should be prescribed. The position of the tube and the degree of re-expansion of the lung should be checked by chest X-ray. Low-pressure (-10 to $-20\,\text{cmH}_2\text{O}$) suction applied to the tube may expedite the removal of air.

- *Surgical intervention:* surgical treatment is required for persistent or recurrent pneumothoraces. Failure of re-expansion of the lung with profuse bubbling of air through the underwater drain suggests a bronchopleural fistula (i.e. a persistent communication between the lung and pleural space). **Surgical closure of the hole** with pleurodesis is usually necessary and may be performed via a thoracotomy or via thoracoscopy. The hole is oversewn and blebs on the surface of the lung are excised. **Pleurodesis** involves the obliteration of the pleural space and can be achieved by instilling tetracycline or talc, which provokes adhesions between the visceral and parietal pleura. **Pleurectomy** involves the removal of the parietal pleura. Usually, an apicolateral pleurectomy (leaving the posterobasal pleura intact) prevents recurrence without compromising lung function. There is quite a high risk of recurrence after a first spontaneous primary pneumothorax, with about 50% of patients suffering a second pneumothorax within 4 years. Surgical intervention is usually recommended after a second pneumothorax. This is also the case if the patient has suffered a pneumothorax on both sides, because of the risk of catastrophic simultaneous bilateral pneumothoraces. Particular thought must be given to the best procedure for patients with complicated pneumothoraces secondary to diseases such as cystic fibrosis so as not to compromise potential future lung transplantation. A limited apicolateral surgical abrasion pleurodesis may be the best option in these circumstances.

Pleural effusion

A pleural effusion is a collection of fluid in the pleural space.

Pleural fluid dynamics

The parietal and visceral pleural surfaces are normally in close contact and the potential space between them contains only a very thin layer of fluid. Pleural fluid dynamics are complex and incompletely understood but Fig. 16.4 shows, in a simplified form, some of the main factors governing fluid filtration and absorption. The parietal pleura is perfused by the systemic circulation, and the high systemic capillary pressure, negative intrapleural pressure and pleural oncotic pressure overcome the plasma oncotic pressure resulting in fluid filtration into the pleural space. The visceral pleura is mainly perfused by the pulmonary circulation with its low pulmonary capillary pressure so that the balance of forces results in movement of fluid outward from the pleural space to the veins and lymphatics. The balance between **fluid filtration** by the parietal pleura and **fluid absorption** by the visceral pleura is such that fluid does not normally collect in the pleural space. Pleural effusions may develop from **increased capillary pressure** (e.g. left ventricular failure), **reduced plasma oncotic pressure** (e.g. hypoalbuminaemia), increased capillary permeability (e.g. disease of pleura) or **obstruction of lymphatic drainage** (e.g. carcinoma of lymphatics).

Clinical features

Patients with pleural effusions typically present with **dyspnoea**, sometimes with pleuritic pain, and often with features of associated diseases (e.g. cardiac failure, carcinoma etc.). The signs of pleural effusion are **decreased expansion** on the side of the effusion, **stony dullness, diminished breath sounds** and **reduced tactile vocal fremitus**. Sometimes **bronchial breathing** is heard at the upper level of the fluid. In taking the patient's history it is important to enquire about clues to possible causes of pleural effusion such as asbestos exposure, contact with tuberculosis, smoking, drugs (e.g. dantrolene, bromocriptine) or systemic disease. A full careful physical examination is essential to detect signs of underlying disease (e.g. cardiac failure, breast lump, lymphadenopathy etc.).

Investigations (Fig. 16.5)

- *Radiology*: **chest X-ray** characteristically shows a dense white shadow with a concave upper edge (Fig. 16.6). Small effusions cause no more than blunting of a costophrenic angle whereas very large effusions cause 'white out' of an entire hemithorax with shift of the mediastinum to the

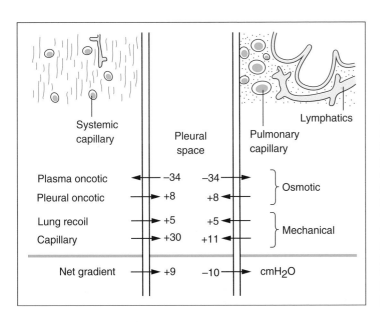

Figure 16.4 **Pleural fluid dynamics**. In the normal pleural space the mechanical and oncotic pressures are in equilibrium such that net filtration of fluid by the parietal pleura is balanced by net absorption of fluid by the visceral pleura. Pleural effusion may arise from changes in the mechanical and oncotic pressures (transudates) or from increased capillary permeability brought about by disease of the pleura (exudates).

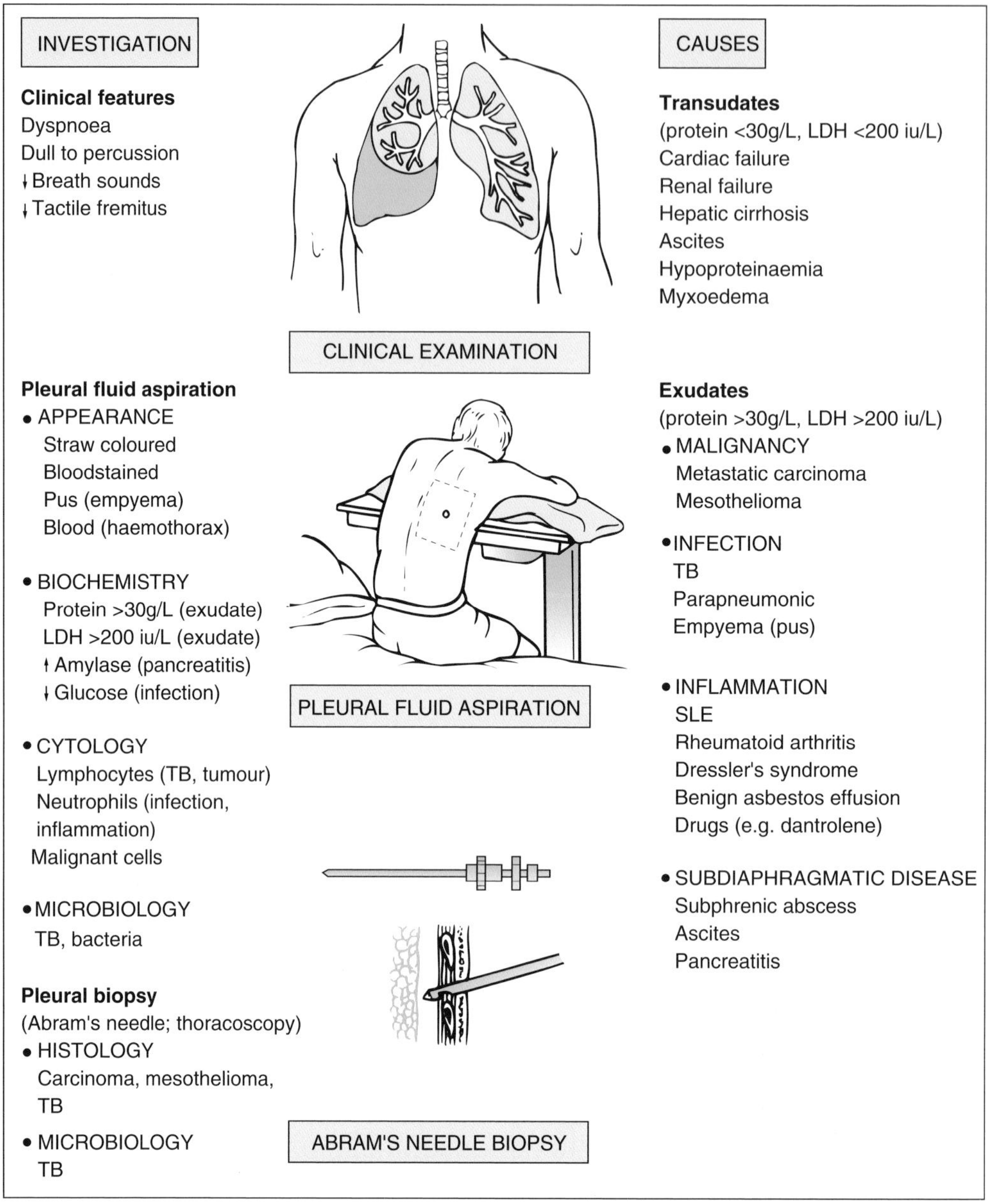

INVESTIGATION

Clinical features
Dyspnoea
Dull to percussion
↓Breath sounds
↓Tactile fremitus

CLINICAL EXAMINATION

Pleural fluid aspiration
- APPEARANCE
  Straw coloured
  Bloodstained
  Pus (empyema)
  Blood (haemothorax)

- BIOCHEMISTRY
  Protein >30g/L (exudate)
  LDH >200 iu/L (exudate)
  ↑Amylase (pancreatitis)
  ↓Glucose (infection)

PLEURAL FLUID ASPIRATION

- CYTOLOGY
  Lymphocytes (TB, tumour)
  Neutrophils (infection, inflammation)
  Malignant cells

- MICROBIOLOGY
  TB, bacteria

Pleural biopsy
(Abram's needle; thoracoscopy)
- HISTOLOGY
  Carcinoma, mesothelioma, TB

- MICROBIOLOGY
  TB

ABRAM'S NEEDLE BIOPSY

CAUSES

Transudates
(protein <30g/L, LDH <200 iu/L)
Cardiac failure
Renal failure
Hepatic cirrhosis
Ascites
Hypoproteinaemia
Myxoedema

Exudates
(protein >30g/L, LDH >200 iu/L)
- MALIGNANCY
  Metastatic carcinoma
  Mesothelioma

- INFECTION
  TB
  Parapneumonic
  Empyema (pus)

- INFLAMMATION
  SLE
  Rheumatoid arthritis
  Dressler's syndrome
  Benign asbestos effusion
  Drugs (e.g. dantrolene)

- SUBDIAPHRAGMATIC DISEASE
  Subphrenic abscess
  Ascites
  Pancreatitis

Figure 16.5 Summary of the causes and investigation of pleural effusions. LDH, lactate dehydrogenase; SLE, systemic lupus erythematosus; TB, tuberculosis.

opposite side. Pleural fluid can be difficult to detect if the chest X-ray is performed with the patient lying supine, and may only be suspected by haziness on the affected side. A **lateral decubitus** film may be useful in demonstrating mobility of the fluid, distinguishing the features from pleural thickening. **Ultrasound** imaging is helpful in localising loculated effusions and in positioning chest tubes (Fig. 16.7). **Computed tomography(CT)** may be helpful in detecting pleural tumours (e.g. mesothelioma) and in assessing the underlying lung and mediastinum.

- *Pleural fluid aspiration (thoracocentesis)* is the key initial investigation. A **protein** level >30 g/L

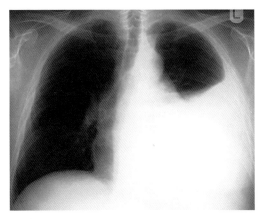

Figure 16.6 This 68-year-old man presented with a 6-week history of progressive breathlessness and left pleuritic pain. On examination there was stony dullness and diminished breath sounds over the left hemithorax. The chest X-ray shows features of a large pleural effusion with a dense white shadow with a concave upper border over the left side of the chest. The pleural fluid was bloodstained and showed metastatic adenocarcinoma on cytology. Bronchoscopy showed the primary tumour partly occluding the left lower lobe bronchus. An intercostal drain was inserted to evacuate the fluid and tetracycline was instilled to achieve pleurodesis.

and **lactate dehydrogenase(LDH)** level>200 units/L indicate that the effusion is an exudate and that further investigations for pleural disease are indicated. Both transudates and exudates are

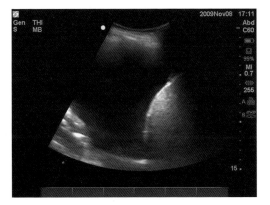

Figure 16.7 Ultrasound is useful in assessing pleural effusions and in guiding the insertion of chest drains. This 40-year-old man had an exudative pleural effusion secondary to a pneumonia. The pleural fluid appears black on ultrasound with no loculations within the fluid. The curvilinear white line to the right of the image is the diaphragm above the liver.

typically a yellow, straw colour. **Bloodstained** fluid points towards malignancy, pulmonary infarction or severe inflammation. **Pus** indicates an empyema, **milky** white fluid suggests a chylothorax and frank **blood** suggests a haemothorax (e.g. as a result of trauma). A low **glucose** content points towards infection or a connective tissue disease as a cause of the effusion. A high **amylase** content is characteristic of pleural effusion associated with pancreatitis but also sometimes occurs with adenocarcinoma. **Neutrophils** are the predominant cells in acute inflammation or infection and **lymphocytes** in chronic effusions particularly caused by tuberculosis or malignancy. **Cytology** may show malignant cells (e.g. mesothelioma or metastatic carcinoma).**Microbiology** examination of the fluid may identify tuberculosis or bacterial infection, for example.

- *Pleural biopsy* may be performed using a specially designed needle such as the **Abram's needle**. After injection of local anaesthetic, incision of the skin and blunt dissection of the intercostal muscles, the needle is passed into the pleural space. The Abram's needle is in two parts which can be rotated on each other; pleural fluid can be aspirated when the window of the needle is rotated to the open position. The needle is then pulled back until some parietal pleural tissue is caught in the notch of the needle. The inner cylinder of the needle has a sharp cutting edge that when rotated cuts off pleural tissue caught in the notch (Fig. 16.5). This 'blind' biopsy technique has a low diagnostic yield such that CT-guided biopsy or biopsy under direct thracoscopic vision is often preferred. **Radiologically guided biopsy** is particularly useful in diagnosing malignant disease of the pleura when CT has shown a focal area of pleural thickening. Histology of pleural biopsy samples is particularly useful in diagnosing malignant effusions or tuberculosis(e.g. caseating granuloma). A sample of the biopsy should also be sent for culture for *Mycobacterium tuberculosis*. **Video-assisted thoracoscopy** allows direct inspection of the pleural surfaces with direct biopsy of abnormal tissue.

Further investigations (e.g. bronchoscopy for suspected lung carcinoma or ultrasound of abdomen for suspected subphrenic disease) may be required depending on the clues to diagnosis elicited on initial assessment.

Causes

Pleural effusions are classified as transudates or exudates. Transudates are characterised by a low protein content ($< 30\,g/L$) and a low LDH level ($< 200\,units/L$). They arise as a result of changes in hydrostatic or osmotic pressures across the pleural membrane rather than from disease of the pleura. Exudates are characterised by a high protein (>30 g/L) and LDH ($>200\,units/L$) content, and result from increased permeability associated with disease of the pleura. Sometimes, in patients with borderline protein and LDH levels, there is difficulty in distinguishing between transudates and exudates, and comparison of pleural to serum ratios may be helpful: exudates have a pleural fluid/serum protein ratio >0.5 and an LDH ratio >0.6.

Transudates

The main causes of transudative pleural effusions are **cardiac failure**, **renal failure**, **hepatic cirrhosis** and **hypoproteinaemia** caused by malnutrition or nephrotic syndrome, for example. In most cases transudative effusions are bilateral, although they may be asymmetrical and initially unilateral. **Ascitic fluid** may pass through pleuroperitoneal communications, which are more common in the right hemidiaphragm. Similarly, **peritoneal dialysis fluid** may give rise to a right pleural effusion. Rare causes of transudates are **myxoedema** and Meigs' syndrome (benign ovarian fibroma, ascites and pleural effusion, which may be a transudate or exudate). Sometimes, treatment of cardiac failure with diuretics results in an increase in fluid protein content so that the effusion appears to be an exudate. Treatment of transudates involves correction of the underlying hydrostatic or osmotic mechanisms (e.g. treatment of cardiac failure or hypoproteinaemia), and further investigation of the pleura is not usually necessary.

Exudates

A variety of diseases that affect the pleura are associated with increased capillary permeability or reduced lymphatic drainage. Exudates are often unilateral and investigations are directed towards identifying the cause because this determines treatment.

- *Malignancy:* **metastases** to the pleura most commonly arise from **lung**, **breast**, **ovarian** or **gastrointestinal** cancers and from **lymphoma**. **Mesothelioma** is a primary tumour of the pleura related to asbestos exposure (see Chapter 14). In malignant effusions the fluid is often blood-stained with a high lymphocyte count, and cytology often shows malignant cells. If cytology of a pleural aspirate is negative, pleural biopsy may be diagnostic. Sometimes, confirmation of the diagnosis is difficult and thoracoscopy with biopsy of lesions under direct vision may be necessary. Malignancy may give rise to pleural effusions by means other than direct involvement of the pleura. **Lymphatic involvement** by tumours may obstruct drainage and cause pleural effusions with negative cytology. **Chylous effusions**, caused by malignancy in the thoracic duct, are characterised by a milky cloudy appearance of the pleural fluid. **Superior vena caval obstruction** may give rise to pleural effusions as a result of elevation of systemic venous pressure. Treatment of a pleural effusion associated with malignancy is directed against the underlying tumour (e.g. chemotherapy). **Drainage of the fluid** by needle aspiration or intercostal chest tube relieves dyspnoea. It is usually advisable to remove the fluid slowly at no more than 1–1.5 L at a time as too rapid removal may provoke re-expansion pulmonary oedema, although the risk is small. The risk of recurrence of the effusion may be reduced by the instillation of a sclerosing agent (e.g. tetracycline 1–1.5 g, doxycycline 500 mg or sterile talc 2–5 g in 50 mL saline) into the pleural space to provoke chemical **pleurodesis**. Lidocaine (lignocaine) 3 mg/kg, maximum 250 mg may be instilled intrapleurally before the sclerosing agent to provide local anaesthesia. It is important that the effusion has been drained to dryness before insertion of the sclerosing agent so that the two pleural surfaces can be apposed so as to promote adhesions. If chemical pleurodesis is not successful, surgical pleurodesis or **pleurectomy via thoracoscopy** may be helpful.
- *Infection:* pneumonia may be complicated by an inflammatory reaction in the pleura resulting in a **parapneumonic effusion**. Secondary infection of this effusion with multiplication of bacteria in the pleural space produces an **empyema,** which is the presence of pus in the pleural cavity. If a parapneumonic effusion has a low pH (< 7.2) there is a high risk of an empyema developing and early tube drainage is indicated. Various organisms may give rise to an empyema including *Streptococcus pneumoniae, Staphylococcus*

aureus, Streptococcus milleri and anaerobic organisms (e.g. *Bacteroides*). Empyema is particularly associated with aspiration pneumonia (e.g. related to unconsciousness, alcohol, vomiting, dysphagia etc.). **Actinomycosis** is an unusual infection that spreads from the lung to the pleura and chest wall with a tendency to form sinus tracts. **Tuberculosis** must always be borne in mind as a cause of pleural effusion or empyema (see Chapter 7). Initial **antibiotic treatment** is often with co-amoxiclav and metronidazole, adjusted in accordance with results of microbiology tests. The key treatment of empyema, however, is **drainage of the pus**. Placement of the drainage tube is best guided by ultrasound imaging as the effusion is often loculated as a result of fibrin deposition and adhesions. Instillation of a **fibrinolytic agent** (e.g. streptokinase 250000 units or urokinase 100000 units in 20 mL of saline, left in situ for 2 hours, daily for 3–5 days) through the chest tube into the pleural space has been used in an attempt to improve drainage by promoting lysis of fibrin adhesions. It may be effective in selected patients with empyema but clinical trials have not confirmed overall benefit and it is not recommended routinely. More recently combinations of fibrinolytics and deoxyribonuclease (DNAse) are being studied in trials. **Surgical intervention** is necessary if these measures fail and a variety of approaches may be used including rib resection with open drainage, or thoracotomy with removal of infected debris and decortication (stripping of the pleura and empyematous sac).

- *Inflammatory diseases*: various inflammatory diseases may involve the pleura. Effusions associated with **connective tissue diseases** (e.g. rheumatoid arthritis, systemic lupus erythematosus) characteristically have a low glucose content. **Drug reactions** involving the pleura have been described with dantrolene, bromocriptine, nitrofurantoin and methysergide, for example. **Asbestos** may give rise to **benign asbestos-related pleural effusions** that may recur producing diffuse pleural thickening (see Chapter 14). Small pleural effusions may complicate **pulmonary embolism** and infarction (see Chapter 15). **Dressler's syndrome** consists of inflammatory pericarditis and pleurisy of uncertain aetiology following a myocardial infarction or cardiac surgery.
- *Subdiaphragmatic disease*: **pancreatitis** may be associated with pleural effusions probably as a result of diaphragmatic inflammation. Such effusions are usually left sided and characterised by a high amylase content. **Ascites** may traverse the diaphragm through pleuroperitoneal communications causing a pleural effusion. Spread of infection or inflammation from a **subphrenic abscess** or **intrahepatic abscess** may also cause a pleural effusion.

Oesophageal rupture

Oesophageal rupture may give rise to a pyopneumothorax (air and pus in the pleural cavity). This may result from external **trauma** or be **iatrogenic** (e.g. perforation during endoscopy). **Spontaneous rupture of the oesophagus** (Boerhaave's syndrome) is a rare but catastrophic condition that typically occurs when the patient attempts to suppress vomiting by closure of the pharyngeal sphincter. Intraoesophageal pressure rises steeply and rupture typically occurs in the lowest third of the oesophagus. It is a more severe form of the Mallory–Weiss syndrome of haematemesis caused by mucosal tears from protracted vomiting. Characteristically, vomiting is followed by chest pain and subcutaneous emphysema (palpable air in skin) as air and gastric contents leak into the mediastinum. A few hours later the pleural membrane gives way and air and food debris pass into the pleural cavity producing pleuritic pain, pleural effusion and empyema. Chest X-ray typically shows an initial pneumomediastinum (a rim of air around mediastinal structures) followed by a hydropneumothorax. The diagnosis is notoriously difficult to make and a radiocontrast oesophagogram is the key investigation. Thoracotomy with repair of the oesophagus is usually the best treatment.

 Respiratory emergencies
Pneumothorax

- Acute **pleuritic pain** and **breathlessness** with diminished breath sounds are the typical features of a pneumothorax. Severe distress with cardiorespiratory compromise suggests a **tension pneumothorax**.

- **Chest X-ray** shows a convex **'pleural line'** at the margin of the collapsed lung with a black gas space containing **no lung markings** between the collapsed lung and chest wall. If a distinct pleural line in not visible the appearances may be as a result of a **bulla** and CT scan may be needed to clarify. A 2 cm rim of air approximately equates to a 50% pneumothorax.
- **Conservative management**: a small pneumo-thorax not causing distress may not require intervention. It is likely to resolve spontaneously at a rate of 1–2% per day.
- **Aspiration** is recommended for a spontaneous primary pneumothorax (no underlying lung dis-ease) using a 16 G cannula inserted via the second intercostal space anteriorly.
- **A chest tube** is needed for a symptomatic secondary pneumothorax (underlying lung dis-ease e.g. COPD) and for primary pneu-mothoraces where aspiration has failed. A small calibre (8–14F) tube is inserted using a Seldinger technique over a guide wire in the **'triangle of safety'** and connected to an un-derwater seal.
- **Care of a chest drain**: check the tube position on X-ray. Examine the drain frequently to ensure that it is securely anchored in place and not kinked or blocked. **Oscillation** of the meniscus of water in the tube indicates that the tube is patent. **Bubbling** indicates on-going drainage of air. Ensure adequate pain control (e.g. ibuprofen and morphine). The drain is removed when bubbling has stopped and X-ray confirms re-expansion of the lung.
- Persistent bubbling indicates an on-going air leak. **Low pressure suction** (-10 to -20 cmH$_2$O) may be applied. If the air leak persists **thoracic surgical assessment** is needed for thoracoscopic closure of the hole and pleurod-esis or pleurectomy.
- At discharge advise the patient **not to smoke** and to avoid air travel for at least 7 days.

 KEY POINTS

- Pneumothorax is the presence of air in the pleural space and this usually occurs from rupture of subpleural cysts in the underlying lung.
- A small pneumothorax (<2 cm rim of air) may not require intervention. A larger pneumothorax (>2 cm rim of air) is treated by simple aspiration or insertion of an intercostal tube.
- A pleural effusion is a collection of fluid in the pleural space.
- Transudative effusions result from changes in hydrostatic pressure (e.g. cardiac failure). Exudative effusions result from diseases of the pleura (e.g. malignancy, infection, inflammation).
- Investigation of an exudative effusion involves clinical assessment, imaging (e.g. CT), pleural fluid aspiration (for biochemistry, cytology and microbiology) and pleural biopsy.

 FURTHER READING

Bouros D, Antoniou KM, Light RW. Intrapleural streptokinase for pleural infection. *BMJ* 2006; **332**: 133–4.

British Thoracic Society Pleural Disease Guideline Group. British Thoracic Society pleural disease guideline. *Thorax* 2010; **65**: (suppl II): 1–76 (www.brit-thoracic.org.uk/).

Curtis HJ, Bourke SJ, Dark JH, et al. Lung trans-plantation outcome in cystic fibrosis patients with previous pneumothorax. *J Heart Lung Transplant* 2005; **24**: 865–9.

Henry MT. Simple sequential treatment for prima-ry spontaneous pneumothorax: one step closer. *Eur Resp J* 2006; **27**: 448–50.

Light RW. Parapneumonic effusions and empy-ema. *Proc Am Thorac Soc* 2005; **3**: 75–80.

Maskell NA, Davies CW, Nunn AJ, et al. UK con-trolled trial of intrapleural streptokinase for pleural infection. *N Engl J Med* 2005; **352**: 865–74.

Acute respiratory distress syndrome

Introduction

The acute respiratory distress syndrome (ARDS) is a form of **acute respiratory failure** caused by **permeability pulmonary oedema** resulting from **endothelial damage** due to a cascade of **inflammatory events** developing in response to an **initiating injury or illness**.

It had long been recognised that soldiers wounded in battle often died of respiratory failure some days later. During World Wars I and II it was thought that this was because of lung infection or excessive fluid administration. Further experience of the condition during the Vietnam War showed that despite successful surgical management of wounds and optimal fluid replacement, soldiers were still dying of pulmonary dysfunction some days later and that the lungs showed features such as oedema, atelectasis, haemorrhage and hyaline membrane formation. It was not until 1967 that this condition was recognised as a specific clinical entity separate from the precipitating injury, and that it could also arise from civilian injuries and illnesses. The term adult respiratory distress syndrome was sometimes used because of the superficial similarity of the pathology of the disease, showing hyaline membranes, to the infant respiratory distress syndrome (caused by surfactant deficiency in premature babies), although the term acute respiratory distress syndrome is more appropriate.

Pathogenesis

In most situations pulmonary oedema arises as a result of increased pulmonary capillary **pressure** (e.g. left ventricular failure) but in ARDS it arises because of increased alveolar capillary **permeability**.

Pressure pulmonary oedema (Fig. 17.1)

In the normal situation the hydrostatic pressure and the osmotic pressure exerted by the plasma proteins are in a state of equilibrium between the pulmonary capillaries and lung alveoli. An **increase in hydrostatic pressure** is the most common cause of pulmonary oedema and this typically occurs secondary to elevated left atrial pressure from left ventricular failure (e.g. after myocardial infarction) or from mitral valve disease (e.g. mitral stenosis). **Volume overload** may also increase pulmonary capillary pressure and this may arise from excessive intravenous fluid administration or fluid

Respiratory Medicine Lecture Notes, Eighth Edition. Stephen J. Bourke and Graham P. Burns.
© 2011 John Wiley & Sons, Ltd. Published 2011 by John Wiley & Sons, Ltd.

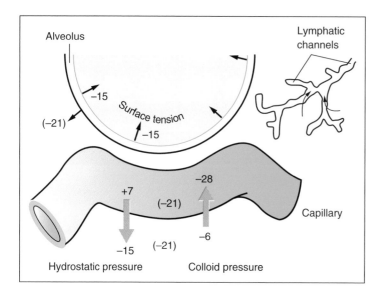

Figure 17.1 Diagram illustrating approximate values for hydrostatic and colloid pressures in millimetres of mercury (mmHg) between the pulmonary capillary and alveolus. Pulmonary oedema may arise from increased hydrostatic pressure (e.g. cardiogenic pulmonary oedema), from reduced colloid pressure (e.g. hypoalbuminaemia) or from increased capillary permeability (e.g. acute respiratory distress syndrome).

retention (e.g. renal failure). **Reduced osmotic pressure** may contribute to pulmonary oedema and this occurs in hypoproteinaemic states (e.g. severely ill, malnourished patients; nephrotic syndrome with renal protein loss). In the early stages of pulmonary oedema there is an increase in the fluid content of the interstitial space between the capillaries and alveoli but as the condition deteriorates flooding of the alveoli occurs.

Permeability pulmonary oedema

In ARDS a cascade of inflammatory events arises over a period of hours from a focus of tissue damage. In particular, activated neutrophils aggregate and adhere to endothelial cells, releasing various toxins, oxygen radicals and mediators (e.g. arachidonic acid, histamine, kinins). This **systemic inflammatory response** may be initiated by a variety of injuries or illnesses and gives rise to **acute lung injury** as one of its earliest manifestations, with the development of **endothelial damage** and **increased alveolar capillary permeability**. The alveoli become filled with a protein-rich exudate containing abundant neutrophils and other inflammatory cells and the airspaces show a rim of proteinaceous material – the hyaline membrane. The characteristic feature of permeability pulmonary oedema in ARDS is that the pulmonary capillary wedge pressure is not elevated. This may be measured by passing a special balloon-tipped pulmonary artery catheter (e.g. Swan–Ganz catheter) via a central vein through the right side of the heart

to the pulmonary artery. The balloon of the catheter is then inflated and is carried forward in the blood flow until it wedges in a pulmonary capillary. The measurement of pulmonary capillary wedge pressure reflects left atrial pressure and in ARDS it is typically ≤ 18 mHg, whereas in cardiogenic pulmonary oedema it is elevated.

Clinical features

ARDS develops in response to a variety of injuries or illnesses that affect the lungs either **directly** (e.g. aspiration of gastric contents, severe pneumonia, lung contusion) or **indirectly** (e.g. systemic sepsis, major trauma, pancreatitis). About 12–48 hours after an initiating event the patient develops respiratory distress with increasing dyspnoea and tachypnoea. Arterial blood gases show deteriorating hypoxaemia that responds poorly to oxygen therapy. Diffuse bilateral infiltrates develop on chest X-ray in the absence of evidence of cardiogenic pulmonary oedema. ARDS is the most severe end of the spectrum of acute lung injury and is characterised by the following features:

- a history of an **initiating injury or illness** (Table 17.1);
- **hypoxaemia** refractory to oxygen therapy (e.g. Po_2, 8.0 kPa (60 mmHg) on 40% oxygen). The degree of hypoxaemia may be expressed as the ratio of arterial oxygen tension (Po_2) to the

Table 17.1 Acute respiratory distress syndrome: initiating injuries and illnesses

Direct	Indirect
Aspiration of gastric contents	Sepsis
Severe pneumonia	Major trauma
Smoke inhalation	Multiple blood transfusions
Lung contusion	Pancreatitis
Fat embolism	Extensive burns
Amniotic fluid embolism	Anaphylaxis
Chemical inhalation (e.g. silo filler's lung)	Hypotensive shock
Oxygen toxicity/ ventilator lung	Disseminated intravascular coagulation

Various illnesses and injuries, which affect the lungs directly or indirectly, initiate a cascade of inflammatory responses resulting in endothelial damage and the characteristic permeability pulmonary oedema of ARDS.

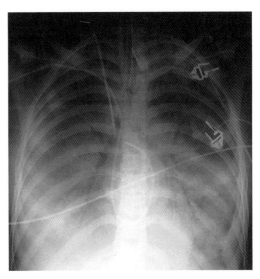

Figure 17.2 This 21-year-old diabetic patient was admitted to the intensive therapy unit (ITU) having vomited and inhaled gastric contents while unconscious with severe ketoacidosis. Despite antibiotics and treatment of ketoacidosis she developed acute respiratory distress syndrome (ARDS) with progressive respiratory distress and severe hypoxaemia refractory to oxygen therapy. The chest X-ray shows diffuse bilateral shadowing with air bronchograms (black tubes of air against the white background of consolidated lung). An endotracheal tube is in place and the patient is being mechanically ventilated, with a positive end-expiratory pressure (PEEP) of 7.5 cmH$_2$O. Electrocardiogram monitor leads are visible and a central venous line has been inserted via the right internal jugular vein. A Swan–Ganz catheter has been passed from the right subclavian vein and can be seen, looped around through the right side of the heart into the pulmonary artery. Pulmonary capillary wedge pressure was low at 8 mmHg indicating that the lung shadowing was not caused by cardiogenic pulmonary oedema, but by increased capillary permeability of ARDS. Despite requiring prolonged ventilation and support on ITU the patient made a full recovery.

fractional inspired oxygen concentration (F_io$_2$/ 100% oxygen = F_io$_2$ of 1). In ARDS Po$_2$/F_io$_2$ is < 26 kPa (200 mmHg);

- bilateral **diffuse infiltrates on chest X-ray** (Fig. 17.2);
- no evidence of cardiogenic pulmonary oedema (e.g. **pulmonary capillary wedge pressure** < 18 mmHg).

Recognition of critically ill patients

Patients who subsequently develop ARDS may appear deceptively well in the initial stages of their illness. Early recognition and careful observation of at-risk patients is of crucial importance in detecting the signs of deterioration and in identifying the need for intensive therapy unit (ITU) care. Certain warning signs are applicable in a wide variety of clinical circumstances because there is often a common physiological pathway of deterioration in the severely ill that can be detected by simple observations of the **pulse rate, respiratory rate, blood pressure, temperature, urine output** and **level of consciousness** (Table 17.2). Arterial blood gas measurements provide useful additional information about gas exchange and the metabolic state of the patient.

Treatment

The treatment of ARDS consists of optimal management of the initiating illness or injury combined with supportive care directed at preserving

Table 17.2 Features indicating a critically ill patient. A patient demonstrating any of these warning signs needs urgent attention and consideration for intensive therapy unit care

Respiratory rate	<8 or >30/min
Pulse rate	<40 or >130/min
Blood pressure	<90 mmHg
Temperature	Hyperthermia (>38 °C, 100.4 °F)
	Hypothermia (<36 °C, 96.8 °F)
Urine output	<30 mL/hour for 3 hours
Level of consciousness	Not responding to commands
Oxygenation	O_2 saturation <90% or
	$P_aO_2 < 8$ kPa (60 mmHg)
	despite 60% inspired oxygen
Acidosis	pH <7.2; bicarbonate
	<20 mmol/L

adequate oxygenation, maintaining optimal haemodynamic function and compensating for multiorgan failure; which often supervenes.

Treatment of initiating illness

Prompt and complete treatment of the initiating injury or illness is essential. This includes rapid resuscitation with correction of hypotension in patients with multiple trauma for example, and eradication of any source of sepsis (e.g. intra-abdominal abscess or ischaemic bowel post-surgery).

Respiratory support

Characteristically, the hypoxaemia of ARDS is refractory to **oxygen therapy** because of shunting of blood through areas of lung that are not being ventilated as a result of the alveoli being filled with a proteinaceous exudate and undergoing atelectasis. **Continuous positive airway pressure(CPAP)** can be applied via a tight-fitting nasal mask to prevent alveolar atelectasis and thereby reduce ventilation/perfusion mismatch and the work of breathing. However, **endotracheal intubation and mechanical ventilation** rapidly become necessary and the patient may need to be transferred to a **specialist ITU** with expertise and facilities for treating ARDS. Intermittent positive pressure ventilation mechanically inflates the lungs, delivering oxygen-enriched air at a set tidal volume and rate. Adjustments in the volume, inflation pressure, rate and percentage oxygen are made to achieve

adequate ventilation. A **positive end-expiratory pressure(PEEP)** of 5–15 cmH$_2$O is usually applied at the end of the expiratory cycle to prevent collapse of the alveoli. High airway pressures may be generated in ventilating the non-compliant stiff lungs in ARDS and this can reduce cardiac output and carries the risk of barotrauma (e.g. pneumothorax). High ventilation pressures combined with high oxygen concentrations may themselves result in microvascular damage that perpetuates the problem of permeability pulmonary oedema ('ventilator lung/oxygen toxicity'). A variety of lung-protective ventilatory techniques have been developed to overcome these problems. **Permissive hypercapnia** is a technique that allows the patient to have a high $P_a$co$_2$ level (e.g. 10 kPa; 75 mmHg) in order to reduce the alveolar ventilation and to avoid excessive airway pressure. **Inverse ratio ventilation** prolongs the inspiratory phase of ventilation such that it is longer than the expiratory phase allowing the tidal volume to be delivered over a longer time at a lower pressure. However, this may cause progressive air trapping. **High-frequency jet ventilation** is a technique whereby small volumes are delivered as an injected jet of gas at high frequencies (e.g. 100–300/min). Ventilation of the patient in the **prone posture** may be beneficial as it reduces gravity-dependent fluid deposition and atelectasis. **Extra corporeal membrane oxygenation** (ECMO) involves the diversion of the patient's circulation through an artificial external membrane to provide oxygen and remove carbon dioxide. None of these ventilatory strategies has yet achieved a major improvement in the overall prognosis of ARDS but each may be useful in individual circumstances. Nursing patients in a semi-recumbent position at 45 degrees reduces the incidence of ventilator-associated pneumonia.

Optimising haemodynamic function

Reducing the pulmonary artery pressure may help to reduce the degree of pulmonary capillary leak. This is achieved by avoiding excessive fluid administration, by judicious use of **diuretics** and by use of drugs that act as **vasodilators** of the pulmonary arteries. Treatment is sometimes guided by use of a balloon-tipped pulmonary artery catheter (Swan–Ganz) that measures pulmonary artery pressures, pulmonary capillary wedge pressure (reflecting left atrial pressure) and cardiac output (using a thermal dilution technique).

Haemodynamic management essentially consists of achieving an **optimal balance** between a **low pulmonary artery pressure** to reduce fluid leak to the alveoli, an **adequate systemic blood pressure** to maintain perfusion of tissues and organs (e.g. kidneys) with a satisfactory **cardiac output** and optimal **oxygen delivery** to tissues (oxygen delivery is a function of the haemoglobin level, oxygen saturation of blood and cardiac output). Most drugs used to vasodilate the pulmonary arteries, such as nitrates or calcium antagonists, also cause systemic vasodilatation with hypotension and impaired organ perfusion. Inotropes and vasopressor agents, such as **dobutamine** or **norepinephrine** (noradrenaline) may be needed to maintain systemic blood pressure and cardiac output particularly in patients with the sepsis syndrome (caused by septicaemia or peritonitis, for example) in which sepsis is associated with systemic vasodilatation. Inhaled **nitric oxide** (NO) may be used as a selective pulmonary artery vasodilator. Because it is given by inhalation it is selectively distributed to ventilated regions of the lung where it produces vasodilatation. This vasodilatation to ventilated alveoli may significantly improve ventilation/perfusion matching with improved gas exchange. NO is rapidly inactivated by haemoglobin preventing a systemic action. It is necessary to monitor the level of inspired gas, nitrogen dioxide (NO_2) and methaemoglobin to avoid toxicity. Nebulised **prostacyclin** is a vasodilator with similar effects to NO but less risk of toxicity. Unfortunately these selective pulmonary vasodilator agents have not been shown to reduce mortality.

General management

Correction of anaemia by **blood transfusions** improves oxygen carriage in the blood and oxygen delivery to the tissues. **Nutritional support** (e.g. by enteral feeding via a jejunostomy) is crucial in maintaining the patient's overall fitness in the face of critical illness, and correction of hypoalbuminaemia improves the osmotic pressure of the plasma reducing fluid leak from the circulation. The ventilated patient with ARDS is particularly vulnerable to **hospital-acquired pneumonia** and bronchoalveolar lavage may be helpful in identifying pathogens. **Multiorgan failure** often complicates ARDS requiring further specific interventions (e.g. dialysis for renal failure).

Anti-inflammatory therapies

A key target for potential treatment is the cascade of inflammatory events arising from the tissue damage resulting from the initiating illness. Unfortunately, these events are poorly understood and no anti-inflammatory drug has yet achieved an established role in treating ARDS. Corticosteroids have not been beneficial. Ibuprofen has been used in an attempt to reduce neutrophil activation and pentoxifylline has been used because of its action in reducing the production of interleukin-1. Haemofiltration is a procedure primarily used to control fluid balance but it may have an additional beneficial effect in patients with sepsis by removal of endotoxins. Recently it has been recognised that there is a link between the coagulation system and the immune response to sepsis with activation of cytokines, neutrophils, monocytes, complement, coagulation and fibrinolytic systems as part of the systemic inflammatory response to infection. Recombinant human activated protein C has an anti-inflammatory effect by blocking the production of cytokines and cell adhesion and by inhibiting thrombin production. This drug has been shown to reduce mortality when used early in the treatment of patients with severe sepsis and multiple organ failure.

Prognosis

Despite intensive research into the inflammatory mechanisms giving rise to ARDS and major advances in ventilatory techniques and haemodynamic control, the mortality of patients with ARDS remains very high at >50%. Patients who survive may be left with lung fibrosis and impaired gas diffusion but some patients make a remarkably full recovery despite having been critically ill with gross lung injury requiring prolonged treatment in ITU.

KEY POINTS

- ARDS is a form of acute pulmonary oedema due to increased endothelial permeability caused by an inflammatory response to illness or injury.
- Precipitating factors include systemic sepsis, trauma, burns, pancreatitis and aspiration of gastric contents.
- Patients are severely hypoxic with diffuse infiltrates on chest X-ray with no evidence of cardiac failure.
- Treatment involves correction of the initiating illness and supportive care using lung-protective ventilation with PEEP.

 FURTHER READING

Adhikari NK, Burns KE, Friedrich JO, et al. Effect of nitric oxide on oxygenation and mortality in acute lung injury: systematic review and meta-analysis. *BMJ* 2007; **334**: 779–82.

Ashbaugh DG, Bigelow DB, Petty TL, Levine BE. Acute respiratory distress in adults. *Lancet* 1967; **ii**: 319–23.

Baudouin SV. Manipulation of inflammation in ARDS: achievable goal or distant Target? *Thorax* 2006; **61**: 464–5.

Baudouin S, Evans T. Improving outcomes for severely ill medical patients. *Clin Med* 2002; **2**: 92–4.

Bernard GR. Acute respiratory distress syndrome: a historical perspective. *Am J Resp Crit Care Med* 2005; **172**: 798–806.

Bernard GR, Artigas A, Brigham KL, et al. Report of the American–European Consensus Conference on ARDS. *Intens Care Med* 1994; **20**: 225–32.

MacIntyre NR. Current issues in mechanical ventilation for respiratory failure. *Chest* 2005; **128** (suppl): 561–7.

Matthay MA, Zimmerman GA. Acute lung injury and acute respiratory distress syndrome. *Am J Resp Cell Mol Biol* 2005; **33**: 319–27.

Peter JV, John P, Graham PL, et al. Corticosteroids in the prevention and treatment of acute respiratory distress syndrome in adults: meta-analysis. *BMJ* 2008; **336**: 1006–9.

Sleep-related breathing disorders

Introduction

People spend almost one-third of their lives asleep but it is only relatively recently that we have become aware of the important effects of sleep on respiratory physiology, and of specific breathing disorders occurring during sleep, such as the obstructive sleep apnoea syndrome (OSAS). The sleep disruption that results from OSAS has important consequences for the patient's quality of life in terms of daytime sleepiness, poor concentration and decreased cognitive function. It is now becoming clear that the diagnosis and treatment of OSAS also has major public health implications as OSAS is being increasingly recognised as a risk factor for cardiovascular disease, stroke and hypertension and a significant cause of accidents at home, at work and on the road.

Sleep physiology

Although familiar to everyone as a state in which the eyes are closed, postural muscles relaxed and consciousness suspended, sleep is an enigmatic condition that has essential refreshing and restorative effects on the mind and body. Electroencephalogram (EEG) studies show that sleep may be divided into five stages and two major categories. Stages 1–4 are characterised by loss of alpha wave activity and progressive slowing in the frequency with increase in the amplitude of the EEG wave form, and during these stages rapid eye movements are absent: **non-REM sleep**. Stage 5 is characterised by rapid eye movement: **REM sleep**. Typically, a person drifts from an awake relaxed state into sleep, progressing serially through EEG stages 1–4, becoming less responsive to stimuli and less rousable. After about 70 minutes of non-REM sleep the person usually enters a period of deep sleep associated with rapid eye movements. This usually lasts about 30 minutes and is often followed by a brief awakening and a return to stage 1 sleep. Cycles of REM and non-REM sleep continue throughout the night with the period spent in REM sleep becoming longer, such that it occupies about 25% of total sleep time. During REM sleep the person is difficult to rouse and has reduced muscle tone. This stage of sleep is associated with dreaming and a variety of autonomic changes including penile erection and changes in respiration, blood pressure, pulse rate and pupil diameter. Irregularity of respiration and heart rate are common in this stage of sleep and apnoeic episodes lasting 15–20 seconds are common in normal individuals. The exact sleep

Respiratory Medicine Lecture Notes, Eighth Edition. Stephen J. Bourke and Graham P. Burns.
© 2011 John Wiley & Sons, Ltd. Published 2011 by John Wiley & Sons, Ltd.

'architecture' (depth, character and changes) varies with age and circumstances (e.g. unfamiliar environment, disruption of regular routine), so that it can be difficult to define precisely normal and abnormal patterns by arbitrary cut-off points. Although sleep has major beneficial effects on the mind and body, the physiological changes during sleep may aggravate pre-existing respiratory disease, and specific breathing disorders may arise during sleep.

Oxygen desaturation during sleep in respiratory disease

During sleep the respiratory centre in the medulla receives less stimulation from higher cortical centres and becomes less responsive to chemical (e.g. hypercapnia) and mechanical (e.g. from chest wall and airway receptors) stimuli. Minute ventilation (tidal volume and respiratory rate), falls, Pco_2 rises, functional residual capacity decreases and there is diminished activity of the intercostal and accessory respiratory muscles. These changes are most marked during REM sleep. Although they are not associated with any adverse effects in normal individuals they may produce profound nocturnal hypoxaemia and hypercapnia in patients with underlying respiratory disease, who are dependent on accessory respiratory muscle activity and who are already hypoxic when awake and on the steep part of the oxyhaemoglobin dissociation curve. Sleep-related oxygen desaturation is most important in diseases associated with hypercapnic (type 2) respiratory failure such as **chronic obstructive pulmonary disease(COPD)**, **neuromuscular disease** (e.g. muscular dystrophy, motor neurone disease) and **thoracic cage disorders** (e.g. kyphoscoliosis). The nocturnal oxygen desaturation in these disorders results from the deleterious effect of sleep physiology on pre-existing respiratory insufficiency and is quite distinct from OSAS (see below).

Treatment

Optimising the management of the **underlying respiratory disease** is the first priority (e.g. bronchodilators in COPD). Avoidance of **aggravating factors**, such as use of alcohol or sedative medication is important. Supplemental **oxygen** may alleviate oxygen desaturation but may provoke further hypoventilation and carbon dioxide retention because in many of these patients respiratory drive is partly dependent on the stimulant effect of hypoxaemia. Some non-sedative tricyclic and serotonin-reuptake inhibitor antidepressants reduce the time spent in REM sleep, but they are not an effective treatment for nocturnal oxygen desaturation.

There are very few drugs that have **respiratory stimulant** effects but an intravenous infusion of doxapram may occasionally be useful for a short period during a crisis. **Ventilatory support** can be delivered in the short term by endotracheal ventilation in an intensive therapy unit (ITU) to tide the patient over a crisis. However, long-term ventilatory support is often required and this is nowadays usually given as domiciliary nocturnal **non-invasive positive pressure ventilation** (NIPPV). A tight-fitting mask is strapped in place over the nose and connected to a specifically designed ventilating machine. The spontaneous respiratory efforts of the patient trigger the ventilator to deliver additional tidal volume under positive pressure. Despite the cumbersome nature of this form of ventilatory support it is very well tolerated by patients who usually can manage to sleep while receiving nasal ventilation after a few nights of acclimatisation. Control of nocturnal desaturation by NIPPV not only improves the quality of their sleep and nocturnal symptoms but also improves daytime symptoms and gas exchange. It seems that improvement of arterial blood gas levels during ventilation, resting fatigued respiratory muscles, recruiting atelectatic alveoli, relief of sleep deprivation and control of nocturnal hypoventilation by NIPPV all result in some recalibration of ventilatory responses with sustained improvement that ameliorates daytime arterial blood gas levels also. NIPPV represents an important advance in the treatment of patients with ventilatory failure caused by kyphoscoliosis, for example (Fig. 18.1).

Obstructive sleep apnoea syndrome (Fig. 18.2)

OSAS is a condition of sleep-related pharyngeal collapse, in which recurrent episodes of **upper airway occlusion** occur **during sleep** causing diminution (hypopnoea) or cessation of airflow

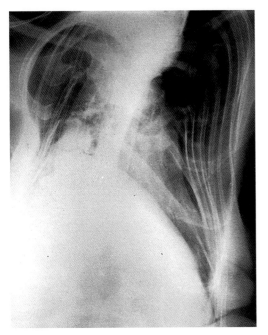

Figure 18.1 This 39-year-old woman with severe ky-phoscoliosis developed sleep disturbance, tiredness, headaches and oedema. She was erroneously treated with sedatives for insomnia. Spirometry showed a severe restrictive defect with forced expiratory volume in 1 second (FEV$_1$) of 0.4 L and forced vital capacity (FVC) of 0.5 L. Po_2 was 5.6 kPa (42 mmHg) and Pco_2 10.2 kPa (76 mmHg). Her sleep was fragmented with multiple arousals and profound oxygen desaturation. She was unable to tolerate oxygen because of deteriorating hypercapnia. Nocturnal ventilatory support was commenced using NIPPV delivered via a tight nasal mask. She has now been using NIPPV for about 8 hours at night at home for 2 years. She works as a secretary and can do housework but is breathless on walking 150 metres. NIPPV is an effective form of ventilatory support for patients with hypercapnic respiratory failure caused by thoracic cage disorders or neuromuscular disease.

(apnoea) in the pharynx provoking arousals and **sleep fragmentation**, resulting in daytime **sleepiness**.

Pathogenesis

The oropharyngeal dilator muscles play an important part in maintaining patency of the upper airway. During deep sleep there is reduced muscle tone so that the pharyngeal airway is most vulnerable to collapse during REM sleep. Use of sedatives or alcohol may cause a further loss of muscle tone. Narrowing of the upper airway predisposes to occlusion and this is usually a result of fat deposition in the neck from obesity, but other factors such as bone morphology (e.g. micrognathia), soft tissue deposition (e.g. hypothyroidism, acromegaly) or enlargement of tonsils or adenoids in children may be important. Contraction of the diaphragm and intercostal muscles during inspiration creates a negative pressure in the airways drawing air into the lungs. The negative pressure in the airway, however, also acts as a force sucking in or collapsing the upper airway. An increase in upper airway resistance such as occurs in nasal obstruction (e.g. deviated nasal septum, polyps) or in enlargement of tonsils and adenoids, requires a greater inspiratory effort to overcome it, and thus increases the forces sucking in the pharyngeal airway. Although upper airway reflexes and neuromuscular control of respiration may also be important, the main factors involved in upper airway patency are the **calibre of the pharyngeal airway**, the action of **oropharyngeal dilator muscles** and the **inspiratory effort** needed to overcome **upper airway resistance**.

OSAS is characterised by recurrent episodes of pharyngeal airway obstruction during sleep with apnoea, arousal and sleep fragmentation. As the patient with a compromised pharyngeal airway (e.g. narrowed by obesity) enters deep sleep the reduction in oropharyngeal dilator muscle tone results in collapse of the airway causing apnoea (cessation of airflow) or hypopnoea (reduction of airflow) with a fall in oxygen saturation. Inspiratory effort increases as the diaphragm and intercostal muscles try to overcome the closed upper airway. The apnoea is terminated by a brief arousal from sleep and this is associated with a burst of sympathetic nerve activity, release of catecholamines and fluctuations in pulse rate and blood pressure. Resumption of pharyngeal airflow is accompanied by loud snoring, which is an inspiratory noise arising from vibration of the soft tissues of the oropharynx. Arousals are often associated with generalised body movement. Hundreds of episodes of apnoea and arousal throughout the night disrupt sleep, resulting in daytime sleepiness.

Clinical features

Patients with OSAS may have no detectable respiratory abnormality when awake but *daytime*

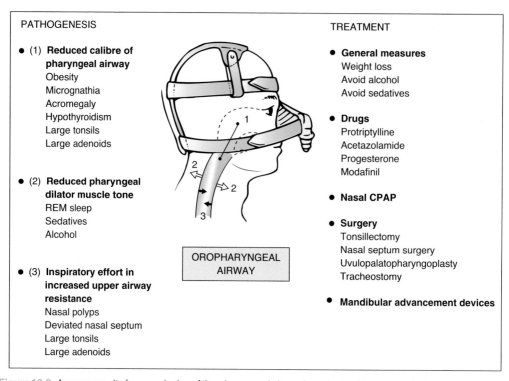

PATHOGENESIS

- (1) **Reduced calibre of pharyngeal airway**
  Obesity
  Micrognathia
  Acromegaly
  Hypothyroidism
  Large tonsils
  Large adenoids

- (2) **Reduced pharyngeal dilator muscle tone**
  REM sleep
  Sedatives
  Alcohol

OROPHARYNGEAL AIRWAY

- (3) **Inspiratory effort in increased upper airway resistance**
  Nasal polyps
  Deviated nasal septum
  Large tonsils
  Large adenoids

TREATMENT

- **General measures**
  Weight loss
  Avoid alcohol
  Avoid sedatives

- **Drugs**
  Protriptylline
  Acetazolamide
  Progesterone
  Modafinil

- **Nasal CPAP**

- **Surgery**
  Tonsillectomy
  Nasal septum surgery
  Uvulopalatopharyngoplasty
  Tracheostomy

- **Mandibular advancement devices**

Figure 18.2 Apnoea results from occlusion of the pharyngeal airway in patients with narrowed airways when there is loss of pharyngeal dilator muscle tone in sleep. Increased inspiratory effort, when there is increased upper airway resistance, 'sucks in' the pharyngeal airway. Nasal continuous positive airway pressure (CPAP) acts as a splint preventing collapse of the airway and is the main treatment used for sleep apnoea.

symptoms include excessive **sleepiness, poor concentration, irritability, morning headaches** and **loss of libido**. Sleepiness is usually a prominent feature and may result in the patient falling asleep inappropriately when reading, watching television, listening to a lecture, travelling on a bus or driving a car, for example. It is important to recognise the importance of such symptoms and their relationship to sleep-disordered breathing as such symptoms may be erroneously dismissed as laziness. **The Epworth sleepiness scale** is a useful method of assessing the likelihood of falling asleep in various situations and a score of ten or more suggests the need for evaluation for an underlying sleep disorder (Table 18.1). Patients with OSAS have a high rate of accidents at home, at work and when driving. It is estimated that about 5% of commercial drivers have OSAS and that sleep-related **road traffic accidents** comprise 15–20% of all crashes, resulting in many serious injuries and deaths. Patients with OSAS should be advised to notify their driving licence authority of their condition and to avoid driving until their sleepiness has been controlled by treatment. The patient may be unaware of *night-time symptoms* but the bed partner may report loud **snoring**, witnessed **apnoeas** and **restless sleep**. It is important to enquire about use of sedatives or alcohol that may aggravate OSAS. *Examination* focuses on risk factors for OSAS such as **obesity, increased neck circumference**, anatomical abnormalities reducing **pharyngeal calibre** (e.g. micrognathia, enlarged tonsils), and **nasal obstruction** (e.g. polyps, deviated septum).

Cardiovascular complications associated with OSAS include hypertension, myocardial infarction, stroke, cardiac arrhythmias, structural cardiac changes and cardiac failure. Although some of these associations may be explained by confounding variables such as obesity, evidence is accumulating of an independent direct relationship between OSAS and hypertension, stroke and cardiovascular disease that may be caused by a combination of factors such as hypoxaemia, changes in

Table 18.1 The Epworth sleepiness score is useful in screening patients for excessive sleepiness. How likely are you to doze off or fall asleep in these situations?

Situation	Score (0–3)
1 Sitting and reading	
2 Watching television	
3 Sitting inactive in a public place (e.g. theatre)	
4 As a passenger in a car for an hour without a break	
5 Lying down to rest in the afternoon	
6 Sitting and talking to someone	
7 Sitting quietly after lunch (when you've had no alcohol)	
8 In a car, while stopped in traffic	

Patients rate their sleepiness using the following scale: 0, would never doze; 1, slight chance of dozing; 2, moderate chance of dozing; 3, high chance of dozing. A total score of 10 or more suggests the need for further evaluation for an underlying sleep disorder.

blood pressure and sympathetic nervous system activation during apnoeas and arousals. There is an association between OSAS and the metabolic syndrome (visceral obesity, insulin resistance, hypertension, dyslipidaemia). Recurrent apnoeas and arousals with deoxygenation and reoxygenation increase the formation of reactive oxygen species that are damaging to the vasculature. Reactive oxygen species also provoke inflammatory responses with activation of cytokines, adhesion molecules, endothelial cells, circulating leucocytes and platelets. It is important to reduce cardiovascular risk factors in these patients by checking smoking history, blood pressure, and lipid and glucose levels, and intervening as appropriate. In addition to catecholamine release, OSAS is associated with other **hormonal changes** including reduced testosterone and growth hormone levels. Although hypoxaemia, hypercapnia and elevation of pulmonary artery pressure occur during apnoeas, cor pulmonale is unusual unless there is concomitant lung disease (e.g. COPD). The long-term prognosis of OSAS is not fully understood but some studies have shown a significantly higher mortality in patients who refused treatment than in those whose sleep apnoea was controlled by continuous positive airway pressure (CPAP).

Polysomnography

Although OSAS may be diagnosed on the basis of clinical features and a limited sleep study with overnight oximetry, definitive assessment requires polysomnography. This involves the recording of signals relating to oxygenation, airflow, chest wall movement and stage of sleep. An **EEG** records the stage of sleep. An **electrooculogram (EOG)** detects rapid eye movement. A thermistor detects **airflow** at the nose and mouth, and **ribcage** and **abdominal movements** are measured using magnetometers or impedance plethysmography. **Oximetry** detects oxygen desaturation and an **electrocardiogram (ECG)** records heart rate. These tracings are often combined with a video recording of the patient during sleep that permits observation of the patient's position and movement in relation to apnoeas and arousals.

The number of apnoeas increases with age and there is a continuum from normality to full-blown OSAS, so that it is difficult to define precise diagnostic criteria. However, OSAS is usually diagnosed when there are more than 15 apnoeas or hypopnoeas per hour, each lasting 10 seconds: **apnoea/hypopnoea index >15**. These are usually associated with **oxygen desaturation of >4%**. For OSAS to be regarded as clinically significant, requiring treatment, the patient should have typical symptoms (e.g. daytime sleepiness) combined with an apnoea/hypopnoea index>15. Using these criteria about 4% of middle-aged men and 2% of women have OSAS.

Treatment

• *General measures*: **weight loss** is an important treatment for patients who are overweight, although it is difficult to achieve. Even a small loss in weight can result in a significant improvement with a 10% reduction in weight typically resulting in an improvement in the apnoea/hypopnoea index. Dietary advice, increased exercise and behavioural modification are crucial in achieving and maintaining weight reduction. Aggravating factors should be removed by **avoidance of alcohol and sedatives** before sleep. Snoring and OSAS are more common when the patient sleeps lying on his or her back so that sometimes measures such as sewing a tennis ball onto the back of the pyjamas **discourages sleeping on the back**. Tonsillectomy, excision of nasal polyps or correction of a deviated nasal septum may be appropriate in some cases. Attention should also be directed towards eliminating any concomitant risk factors for cardiovascular disease. Any underlying lung disease (e.g. COPD) should be treated appropriately. One unusual study showed that training of the upper airway muscles by **didgeridoo playing** reduced the collapsibility of the upper airways and improved sleepiness and the apnoea/hypopnoea index.

- *Nasal CPAP* (e.g. 5–15 cmH$_2$O) applied via a tight-fitting **nasal mask** has become the standard first choice treatment for OSAS. It is very effective and acts by splinting the pharyngeal airway open, counteracting the tendency to airway collapse. However, it is a cumbersome treatment and some patients have difficulty in adhering to this treatment in the long term. The attention of a trained CPAP nurse or technician is helpful in overcoming any practical difficulties and in adjusting the level of CPAP required.
- *Pharmacological treatments*: a number of drugs have been tried in the treatment of OSAS but their effectiveness is disappointing and none has an established role in clinical practice. **Modafinil**, a stimulant alerting drug, may improve alertness in some patients who remain sleepy despite CPAP. **Protriptylline** is a non-sedative antidepressant that reduces the time spent in REM sleep. **Progesterone** has some effect in stimulating respiratory drive. **Acetazolamide** enhances ventilatory drive by producing a metabolic acidosis through inhibition of renal tubular secretion of hydrogen ion.
- *Surgery*: **uvulopalatopharyngoplasty** (UPPP) involves the surgical excision of redundant tissue of the soft palate, uvula and pharyngeal walls in order to increase the calibre of the pharyngeal airway. It is effective in stopping snoring but its effect on sleep apnoea is unpredictable and where beneficial the effect is often short lived. Side-effects include post-operative pain, changes in the quality of the voice and sometimes nasal regurgitation during swallowing. **Tracheostomy** is effective but is a treatment of last resort. Surgical correction of bone abnormalities, such as **mandibular advancement** for micrognathia, can be effective in appropriate cases. The lower jaw may be held in an open, slightly advanced position by the use of specifically designed **mandibular advancement devices** that are worn over the teeth. The forward movement of the mandible increases the cross-sectional area of the oropharynx.

Patients with obstructive sleep apnoea are at high risk for developing complications when having any surgery under general anaesthesia and require careful assessment and monitoring in the perioperative period.

Central sleep apnoea

Central sleep apnoea is a relatively uncommon condition in which cessation of airflow at the nose and mouth is associated with a lack of respiratory muscle activity. It is associated with an **unstable ventilatory control system** that may arise in a variety of different circumstances. For example **Cheyne–Stokes respiration** is a pattern of irregular breathing with periods of apnoea followed by hyperventilation, seen in patients with cardiac failure when the carotid body is slow in responding to changes in ventilation because of a prolonged circulation time. Periodic breathing develops in most people at high altitude, when hypoxia results in hyperventilation, hypocapnia and ventilatory instability. Sometimes obstructive sleep apnoea seems to provoke reflex inhibition of inspiratory drive so that central apnoeas follow classic obstructive apnoeas. Patients with this reflex central apnoea respond to nasal CPAP. Primary central sleep apnoea is rare but may result from instability of respiratory drive because of damage to the respiratory centres by brain stem infarcts or syringobulbia, for example. Most of these patients also have hypercapnic respiratory failure when awake, and NIPPV is the main form of treatment used.

 KEY POINTS

- Obstructive sleep apnoea is due to pharyngeal collapse during sleep, resulting in apnoea, arousal, sleep fragmentation and daytime sleepiness.
- It is a serious condition causing daytime sleepiness, poor quality of life and road accidents.
- It is associated with an increased risk of hypertension, strokes and myocardial infarctions.
- CPAP is the main treatment and acts by splinting the pharyngeal airway open during sleep.

FURTHER READING

American Sleep Apnoea Association: http://www .sleepapnea.org/.

Johansson K, Neovius M, Lagerros YT, et al. Effect of a very low energy diet on moderate and severe obstructive sleep apnoea in obese men: a randomised controlled trial. *BMJ* 2009; **339**: 1365.

John MW. A new method for measuring daytime sleepiness: the Epworth sleepiness scale. *Sleep* 1991; **14**: 540–5.

McNicholas WT. Diagnosis of obstructive sleep apnoea in adults. *Proc Am Thorac Soc* 2008; **5**: 154–60.

Ozsancak A, D'Ambrosio C, Hill NS. Nocturnal non-invasive ventilation. *Chest* 2008; **133**: 1275–86.

Peters RW. Obstructive sleep apnoea and cardiovascular disease. *Chest* 2005; **127**: 1–3.

Puhan MA, Suarez A, Cascio CL, Zahn A, Heitz M, Braendli O. Didgeridoo playing as alternative treatment for obstructive sleep apnoea syndrome: a randomised controlled trial. *BMJ* 2006; **332**: 266–8.

Scottish Intercollegiate Guidelines Network. *Management of Obstructive Sleep Apnoea/Hypopnoea Syndrome in Adults*. Edinburgh: Scottish Intercollegiate Guidelines Network, 2003 (www.sign .ac.uk).

Sleep Apnoea Trust: www.sleep-apnoea-trust.org.

Suratt PM, Findley LJ. Serious motor vehicle crashes: the cost of untreated sleep apnoea. *Thorax* 2001; **56**: 505.

Tasali E, IpMS. Obstructive sleep apnoea and metabolic syndrome: alterations in glucose metabolism and inflammation. *Proc Am Thorac Soc* 2008; **5**: 207–17.

West SD, McBeath HA, Stradling JR. Obstructive sleep apnoea in adults. *BMJ* 2009; **338**: 1165–7.

19

Lung transplantation

Introduction

Lung transplantation is now an established treatment option for selected patients with end-stage lung disease who have failed to respond to maximum medical treatment. However, lung transplantation is a major surgical procedure with a substantial mortality and a limited long-term prognosis. The critical shortage of donor organs severely restricts the application of the procedure. The first heart transplantation was performed in 1967 in Groote Schuur hospital, South Africa, when a man in end-stage cardiac failure received the heart of a young woman killed in a road traffic accident. Initial attempts at lung transplantation were unsuccessful but surgical advances, better selection of suitable patients and the introduction of ciclosporin immunosuppression introduced a new era, with the first successful heart–lung transplantation performed in 1981 in Stanford, USA, for a patient with primary pulmonary hypertension.

Types of operation

Surgical techniques have been developed to transplant a single lung, both lungs or the heart and lungs. Approximately 2700 procedures are now performed every year worldwide.

Heart–lung transplant

The recipient's diseased lungs and heart are removed through a median sternotomy and the donor lungs and heart are implanted as a block. If the recipient's heart is normal it may be donated to another patient (domino procedure).

Single-lung transplant

A diseased lung is removed through a thoracotomy incision, leaving the heart and contralateral lung intact. The donor lung is then implanted using a bronchial anastomosis. The residual native lung must be free of infection or it will be a source of sepsis in the post-operative period when the patient is immunosuppressed, so that this procedure is not suitable for patients with cystic fibrosis, for example. The donor's heart and other lung are available to transplant to other patients.

Bilateral-lung transplant

- *Double-lung transplant*: the diseased lungs are removed through a median sternotomy, leaving the heart intact. The donor lungs are implanted as a block using a tracheal anastomosis.
- *Bilateral sequential single-lung transplant*: a transverse bilateral thoracotomy is performed dividing the sternum horizontally (clamshell incision). The diseased lungs are removed and two separated lungs are implanted with separate bronchial anastomoses.

Respiratory Medicine Lecture Notes, Eighth Edition. Stephen J. Bourke and Graham P. Burns.
© 2011 John Wiley & Sons, Ltd. Published 2011 by John Wiley & Sons, Ltd.

Donor organs are most commonly procured from patients who are less than 55 years of age who have suffered a catastrophic spontaneous intracranial haemorrhage or a major head injury who have been ventilated on an intensive therapy unit (ITU) and who are then diagnosed as having suffered brain stem death. There are strict criteria for the diagnosis of brain stem death and the process of organ donation. Because of the vulnerability of the lungs to injury and infection only about 20% of suitable heart donors will also be potential lung donors. Ideally there should be no history of significant respiratory disease and no major chest trauma. The chest X-ray should be clear and gas exchange adequate (Po_2 >12 kPa (90 mmHg) on <35% inspired oxygen). The shortage of donor organs has led to some relaxation of these criteria without any detrimental effects on outcomes. Techniques have been developed to preserve the donor lungs for up to 6–8 hours allowing emergency transport (e.g. by plane) of donor organs to the recipient. The donor and recipient are matched for ABO blood group, cytomegalovirus status and chest size.

Living lobar transplantation

This is a less common procedure whereby a child or small young adult receives two lower lobes from two living donors, but this technique involves significant risks to the living donors, and the technique is not suitable for the majority of patients on a lung transplant waiting list.

Indications for transplantation

Although in theory many types of end-stage lung disease would be amenable to transplantation, in practice the lack of donor organs severely restricts the procedure. The median waiting time to transplantation is about 18 months and unfortunately up to 40–50% of patients identified as suitable candidates to undergo lung transplantation die of their underlying lung disease before an organ becomes available. Lung transplantation has proved a successful treatment for patients with cystic fibrosis, idiopathic pulmonary hypertension, emphysema caused by α_1-anti-trypsin deficiency, idiopathic pulmonary fibrosis and a variety of rare diseases such as lymphangioleiomyomatosis. There is a window of opportunity in which the patient is **ill enough to need a lung transplant** but **not so ill as to be unable to withstand** the surgery. Furthermore, the patient must be aware of the limitations, risks and benefits of transplantation and must actively **want to undergo** the operation. In patients with cystic fibrosis, for example, a forced expiratory volume in 1 second (FEV$_1$), 30% predicted, a Po_2 <7.5 kPa (55 mmHg) and a Pco_2 >6.5 kPa (50 mmHg) are associated with a 50% mortality within 2 years, and it is at this stage that lung transplantation may be the best treatment option. (Fig. 19.1). The patient needs time to understand the severity of the disease, the predicted prognosis and what is involved in lung transplantation. Addressing these issues is traumatic for the patient and his or her family. Some patients with advanced lung disease want to try all available treatment options, whereas other patients fear high-intensity unpleasant interventions and would prefer to take a palliative approach to the terminal stages of their disease. **Contraindications** to lung transplantation include the presence of other major organ dysfunction such as **hepatic** or **renal disease**, **uncontrolled infection**, **malignancy**, **inability to adhere** to a complex treatment regimen, the presence of an **aspergilloma** and **poor nutritional** status. In patients with cystic fibrosis poor outcomes have been reported in patients with *Burkholderia cenocepacia* such that infection with this organism is now considered a contraindication to transplantation. The success of lung transplantation programmes is based upon careful selection of the small number of patients who can benefit from the procedure and who can be supported long enough to have a realistic chance of getting a donor organ.

Post-transplantation complications and treatment

In the first few days post-transplantation **re-implantation injury** may occur with infiltrates developing in the donor lung because of increased capillary permeability as a result of surgical trauma, ischaemia, denervation and lymphatic interruption. Early post-operative

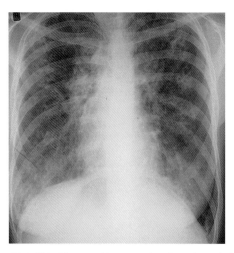 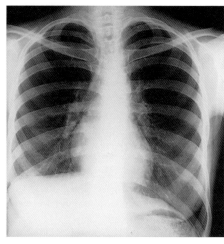

Figure 19.1 This 29-year-old woman developed respiratory failure (P_{O_2} 6 kPa (45 mmHg), P_{CO_2} 8 kPa (60 mmHg)) as a result of advanced cystic fibrosis lung disease (FEV_1 0.5 L). (a) Her chest X-ray shows hyperinflated lungs with diffuse bronchiectasis and peribronchial fibrosis. She was accepted onto a lung transplantation waiting list and supported by oxygen therapy, antibiotics, physiotherapy and nutritional supplements while awaiting donor lungs. Her hypercapnic respiratory failure deteriorated and she was 'bridged' to transplantation by domiciliary intermittent positive pressure ventilation delivered via a tight-fitting nasal mask. (b) Bilateral sequential single-lung transplantations were performed 14 months after being accepted onto the waiting list. She subsequently died 5 years post-transplantation of obliterative bronchiolitis.

surgical complications include haemorrhage and dehiscence of the anastomosis. Prophylactic antibiotics are given to counter **'donor-acquired' infection** because the donor lungs are often contaminated by bacteria. Lavage of the donor organ is performed before implantation to identify infection. Intense **immunosuppression**, using a combination of ciclosporin, azathioprine and corticosteroids, is needed to prevent rejection of the donor lungs. Anti-thymocyte globulin may be given for the first few days to suppress T-cell function. Patients remain on ciclosporin, prednisolone and azathioprine indefinitely and are at ongoing risk from two particular hazards: **rejection** and **infection**. Both may present with similar clinical features of malaise, pyrexia, infiltrates on chest X-ray, impaired oxygenation and reduced lung function. Bronchoscopy, with bronchoalveolar lavage and transbronchial biopsy are the key investigations in identifying rejection of the donor lung and infection. Episodes of **acute rejection** are treated by intensification of immunosuppression (e.g. intravenous methylprednisolone). The treatment of infection is crucially dependent upon identification of the causative organism because the patient is at risk from both bacterial and **opportunistic infections** (e.g. *Pneumocystis*

pneumonia, cytomegalovirus or fungi (see Chapter 6)). *Pneumocystis* pneumonia prophylaxis (e.g. co-trimoxazole) is given routinely. **Lymphoproliferative disorders** such as Epstein–Barr-virus-related B-cell lymphoma may develop as a result of immunosuppression. Treatment consists of aciclovir with a reduction in immunosuppression. **Bronchiolitis obliterans syndrome** is the most important complication threatening the long-term survival of patients after lung transplantation. It results from chronic rejection of the donor lungs and is characterised by progressive airways obstruction as a result of obliteration of the bronchioles by organising fibrosis. It may be treated by intensifying or changing the immunosuppressive regimen (e.g. use of tacrolimus, sirolimus, mycophenolate mofetil), and azithromycin has a beneficial effect in stabilising lung function. Lung transplant patients are also vulnerable to **gastroesophageal reflux** and gastric aspiration; which is damaging to the lungs. **Drug toxicity** is important and levels of drugs such as ciclosporin must be monitored to ensure adequate immunosuppression and to avoid toxicity such as hypertension, neurotoxicity and renal failure. Care must be taken when prescribing other drugs that may interfere with ciclosporin levels. **Recurrence of the primary disease** in the donor lungs has been documented in recipients with sarcoidosis but the outcome has not been affected by this in most cases.

Prognosis

Overall survival rates post-lung transplantation are approximately 80% at 1 year, and 55% at 5 years and 30% at 10 years. The quality of life of patients is dramatically improved by a successful lung transplantation but the long-term prognosis is limited particularly by the occurrence of bronchiolitis obliterans syndrome.

Future prospects

The shortage of donor organs and the occurrence of obliterative bronchiolitis are the two main problems to be overcome in lung transplantation. The general public are encouraged to carry **donor cards** in order to raise the general awareness of organ donation issues. However, less than 20% of cadaveric donors have lungs suitable for donation because the lungs of a ventilated brain-dead patient are very vulnerable to infection, aspiration and lung injury. Management aimed at **optimising donor lung function** prior to retrieval and better identification of the criteria that make a lung unsuitable for donation might increase the number of useable organs. **Xenotransplantation** (the use of animal organs for transplantation in humans) has not been successful because of hyperacute rejection, and there are also concerns about the potential for the spread of animal viruses to humans. There are attempts to increase the number of donor organs that can be used by a process of 're-conditioning', whereby explanted donor lungs are placed in a chamber connected to a heart bypass machine, and then treated with nutrient-rich solution to allow damaged cells to repair. This allows some donor organs that initially appear unsuitable, to be used. It is hoped that developments in **immunosuppressive**

therapies will reduce the occurrence of obliterative bronchiolitis. These include total lymphoid irradiation and drugs such as tacrolimus, sirolimus, mycophenolate mofetil and ciclosporin microemulsion formulations.

 KEY POINTS

- Lung transplantation is now an established option for some patients with end-stage lung disease.
- There is a critical shortage of donor organs.
- The transplanted lungs are very vulnerable to infection and rejection.
- Bronchiolitis obliterans syndrome is a form of chronic rejection that limits long-term survival.
- Survival rates post-lung transplantation are 80% at 1 year and 55% at 5 years.

 FURTHER READING

Fisher AJ, Donnelly SC, Pritchard G, Dark JH, Corris PA. Objective assessment of criteria for selection of donor lungs suitable for transplantation. *Thorax* 2004; **59**: 434–7.

Iversen M, Corris PA. Lung transplantation: immunosuppression. *Eur Respir Monog* 2009; **45**: 147–68.

Meachery G, DeSoyza A, Nicholson A, et al. Outcome of lung transplantation for cystic fibrosis in a large UK cohort. *Thorax* 2008; **63**: 725–31.

National Institute for Health and Clinical Excellence. *Living-Donor Lung Transplantation for End-Stage Lung Disease. Interventional Procedure Guidance 170.* London: NICE, 2006 (www.nice.org.uk).

Verleden GM, Fisher AJ. Indication, patient selection and timing of referral for lung transplantation. *Eur Respir Mon* 2009; **45**: 1–5.

Yates B, Murphy DM, Forrest IA, et al. Azithromycin reverses airflow obstruction in established bronchiolitis obliterans syndrome. *Am J Respir Crit Care Med* 2005; **172**: 772–5.

Multiple choice questions

Chapter 1: Anatomy and physiology of the lungs

1.1 The principal muscle(s) involved in forced expirations is (are):
  A the diaphragm
  B rectus abdominus
  C the scalene muscles
  D sternocleidomastoids
  E the intercostals

1.2 Lung compliance:
  A increases as lung volume increases
  B is reduced in emphysema
  C is reduced in lung fibrosis
  D is the change in pleural pressure per unit change in lung volume
  E is the principal factor determining forced expiratory flow

1.3 In relation to airways resistance:
  A overall airways resistance increases as lung volume increases
  B in health the greater part of airways resistance is situated in the small airways at high lung volume.
  C airways resistance is reduced in emphysema due to diminished retractive force on the airway
  D is proportional to the cubed power of the radius of the airway (r^3)
  E in asthma the greater part of airways resistance is situated in the small airways

1.4 In relation to ventilation (V) and perfusion (Q):
  A the upper zones of the lungs are ventilated more than the lower zones
  B the upper zones of the lungs receive more perfusion than the lower zones
  C V/Q is greater in the lower zones
  D poor VQ matching leads to a rise in P_{CO_2}
  E reduced overall ventilation leads to a fall in P_{O_2}

1.5 In a patient breathing room air at sea level the arterial blood gases were: pH 7.36, P_{CO_2} 4.0, P_{O_2} 10.5, $aHCO_3$– 19 base excess – 5. What is the alveolar–arterial gradient?

Chapter 2: History taking and examination

2.1 A 72-year-old man presents with breathlessness, clubbing and prominent bibasal crackles on auscultation of his chest. The most likely diagnosis is:
  A pulmonary oedema
  B idiopathic pulmonary fibrosis
  C bronchiectasis
  D emphysema
  E lung cancer

2.2 A 76-year-old man presents with breathlessness. On examination there is diminished expansion of the left hemithorax, dullness to percussion and decreased breath sounds with reduced tactile vocal fremitus at the left base posteriorly. These features suggest:
  A a pleural effusion
  B pneumonic consolidation
  C a pneumothorax
  D atelectasis
  E bronchiectasis

2.3 A 45-year-old woman is admitted to hospital with a 3-day history of cough, breathlessness and right pleuritic pain. She has smoked 20 cigarettes/day for 25 years. On examination chest expansion is equal on both sides. There is dullness over the right lung base with increased tactile vocal fremitus, bronchial breathing and crackles. These features suggest:
  A atelectasis due to a bronchial carcinoma
  B pneumonic consolidation

Respiratory Medicine Lecture Notes, Eighth Edition. Stephen J. Bourke and Graham P. Burns.
© 2011 John Wiley & Sons, Ltd. Published 2011 by John Wiley & Sons, Ltd.

C pneumothorax
D emphysema
E a pleural effusion

2.4 A 25-year-old man presents with a sudden onset of right pleuritic pain while playing rugby. He has smoked 10 cigarettes/day for 8 years. On examination there are decreased breath sounds over the right hemithorax with hyper-resonance on percussion. The trachea is central, jugular venous pressure is normal, heart sounds are normal and there is no tenderness on palpation of the chest. These features suggest:

A a pulmonary embolism
B pleurisy with a pleural effusion
C a traumatic rib fracture
D pneumonic consolidation with pleurisy
E a pneumothorax

2.5 An 80-year-old man presents with progressive breathlessness. He stopped smoking 10 years ago having previously smoked 20 cigarettes/day for 50 years. He had worked as a coalminer for 30 years. On examination he was not clubbed. Respiratory rate was 22/min. He was cyanosed. His chest was hyperinflated with decreased cricosternal distance. The costal margins moved inwards during inspiration. The chest was hyper-resonant to percussion on both sides. There was bilateral wheeze but no crackles. These features suggest a diagnosis of:

A chronic obstructive pulmonary disease
B asthma
C coalminer's pneumoconiosis
D pneumothorax
E pulmonary oedema

Chapter 3: Pulmonary function tests

3.1 The volume of gas in the lungs after a normal tidal inspiration is:

A residual volume
B total lung capacity minus residual volume
C functional residual capacity
D tidal volume plus functional residual capacity
E vital capacity minus residual volume

3.2 The lung function test results: FEV_1 reduced, FEV_1/VC normal, $T_{L}CO$ normal, KCO increased would be most in keeping with:

A kyphoscoliosis
B idiopathic pulmonary fibrosis
C pulmonary hypertension
D asthma
E COPD

3.3 The arterial blood gases: pH 7.33, P_{CO_2} 8.4 kPa, P_{O_2} 12.6 kPa, $sHCO_3$ 28 mmol/L, O_2 saturation 97% is most in keeping with:

A a chronic metabolic acidosis
B an acute on chronic metabolic acidosis.
C an overcompensated metabolic alkalosis
D an acute on chronic respiratory acidosis
E a chronic respiratory acidosis

3.4 Given the arterial blood gases: pH 7.33, P_{CO_2} 8.4, kPa P_{O_2} 12.6 kPa, $sHCO_3$ 28 mmol/L, O_2 saturation 97%, one could confidently conclude that:

A the patient is breathing supplemental oxygen
B the patient has COPD
C the patient needs to be transferred to ITU
D the condition is chronic and stable
E the lungs are normal

3.5 A 24-year-old woman presents to hospital as an emergency with breathlessness. Her arterial blood gases while breathing room air were: pH 7.49, P_{CO_2} 3.3 kPa, P_{O_2} 11.9 kPa, $sHCO_3$ 24 mmol/L, O_2 saturation 97%. This presentation is most in keeping with:

A pulmonary embolism
B anxiety
C opiate overdose
D excess vomiting
E pneumonia

Chapter 4: Radiology of the chest

4.1 Cavitation is a characteristic feature of:

A a hamartoma
B fibrotic lung disease
C *Haemophilus influenzae* pneumonia
D dermoid cysts
E squamous carcinoma

4.2 An air bronchogram in an area of consolidation suggests:

A bronchial obstruction due to carcinoma
B infarction secondary to a pulmonary embolism
C an arteriovenous malformation
D pneumonia
E sarcoidosis

4.3 A 1-cm peripheral lung nodule with avid uptake of FDG on PET–CT scan is most likely to be a:

A tuberculous granuloma
B hamartoma
C carcinoma
D neurofibroma
E rheumatoid nodule

4.4 A 65-year-old smoker presents with cough, purulent sputum and left chest pain. Chest X-ray shows features of left lower lobe collapse. The most likely diagnosis is:

A pneumonia
B pneumonia with a parapneumonic effusion
C mucus plugging of the left lower lobe bronchus
D bronchial carcinoma
E an inhaled foreign body in the left lower lobe bronchus

4.5 A 60-year-old woman is found to have an anterior mediastinal mass on chest X-ray and CT. The most likely cause is a:

A hiatus hernia
B thymoma
C oesophageal cyst
D pericardial cyst
E neurofibroma

Chapter 5: Upper respiratory tract infections and influenza

5.1 Acute epiglottitis is usually caused by:

A *Streptococcus pneumoniae*
B *Mycoplasma pneumoniae*
C infectious mononucleosis
D *Haemophilus influenzae* type B
E *Staphylococcus aureus*

5.2 Contact with birds is a risk factor for infection with:

A *Chlamydophila pneumoniae*
B *Mycoplasma pneumoniae*
C *Coxiella burnetti*
D *Legionella pneumophila*
E *Chlamydophila psittaci*

5.3 Severe seasonal influenza is usually caused by:

A influenza virus type A
B *Haemophilus influenzae*
C influenza virus type B
D influenza virus type C
E *Staphylococcus aureus*

5.4 Recurrent sinusitis is a characteristic feature of:

A cystic fibrosis
B chronic obstructive pulmonary disease
C atopic asthma
D chronic bronchitis
E obstructive sleep apnoea syndrome

5.5 Influenza pandemics occur because of:

A emergence of new coronaviruses
B antigenic shift in influenza viral antigens
C overuse of antibiotics
D lack of uptake of influenza vaccination
E antigenic drift in influenza viral antigens

Chapter 6: Pneumonia

6.1 The commonest cause of community-acquired pneumonia is:

A *Mycoplasma pneumoniae*
B *Haemophilus influenzae*
C *Pseudomonas aeruginosa*
D *Streptococcus pneumoniae*
E *Staphylococcus aureus*

6.2 *Chlamydophila psittaci*:

A is associated with contaminated water
B is associated with foreign travel
C is a zoonosis
D is associated with recent influenza infection
E is a common cause of hospital-acquired pneumonia

6.3 A 40-year-old man presents with cough, fever and purulent sputum. Chest X-ray shows consolidation in the right lower lobe. He is alert with respiratory rate of 22/min, blood pressure of 122/78 mmHg, urea of 5.6 mmol/L, white cell count 18.4×10^9/L. His CURB-65 score is:

A 0
B 1
C 2
D 4
E 5

6.4 Severe acute respiratory syndrome (SARS) is caused by:

A *Legionella pneumophila*
B a coronavirus
C methicillin-resistant *staphylococcus aureus* (MRSA)
D a retrovirus
E *Chlamydophila pneumoniae*

6.5 A 28-year-old man is admitted to hospital with severe respiratory failure (Po_2 7.5 kPa), and diffuse bilateral consolidation in the peirhilar areas on chest X-ray. HIV test is positive and CD4 count is 100/mm³. The most likely cause of his lung consolidation is:

A pneumocystis pneumonia
B Kaposi's sarcoma
C *Mycobacterium avium intracellulare* infection
D HIV pneumonitis
E *Streptococcus pneumoniae*

Chapter 7: Tuberculosis

7.1 A 70-year-old man who lives in a hostel for homeless men and who has a history of alcohol excess presents with a chronic cough. Chest X-ray shows diffuse consolidation in the left upper lobe with cavitation. Tuberculosis is suspected but initial sputum AAFB stains are negative. The next definitive investigation to confirm the diagnosis is:
A interferon gamma release assay
B Mantoux test
C Heaf test
D bronchoscopy and bronchoalveolar lavage
E gastric washings

7.2 The main usefulness of interferon gamma release assays for tuberculosis is in:
A detecting active tuberculosis
B detecting latent tuberculosis
C confirming immunity after BCG vaccination
D detecting non-tuberculosis mycobaterial infection
E monitoring a response to drug treatment

7.3 The lifetime risk of latent tuberculosis becoming active is approximately:
A 1%
B 10%
C 40%
D 60%
E 90%

7.4 The most important adverse effect of ethambutol is:
A renal toxicity
B hepatitis
C rashes

D peripheral neuropathy
E optic neuritis

7.5 A 65-year-old woman who has recently arrived in the UK from India presents with cough. Chest X-ray shows bilateral upper zone consolidation. Sputum AAFB stains are positive. Standard treatment consists of:

A isoniazid, rifampicin, ethambutol and pyrazinamide for 6 months
B isoniazid for 6 months
C isoniazid and rifampicin for 3 months
D isoniazid and rifampicin for 6 months with ethambutol and pyrazinamide for the initial 2 months
E isoniazid and rifampicin for 9 months with ethambutol and pyrazinamide for the initial 2 months

Chapter 8: Bronchiectasis and lung abscess

8.1 A 32-year-old man has diffuse bronchiectasis, *Pseudomonas aeruginosa* infection, nasal polyps and infertility due to obstructive azospermia. The main diagnosis to consider is:
A HIV infection
B cystic fibrosis
C allergic bronchopulmonary aspergillosis
D hypogammaglobulinaemia
E Kartagener's syndrome

8.2 Allergic bronchopulmonary aspergillosis is characterised by:
A the halo sign on chest X-ray
B low IgG levels
C non-tuberculous mycobaterial infection
D reduced specific antibodies to polysaccahride antigens
E proximal bronchiectasis on CT scans

8.3 Definitive diagnosis of bronchiectasis is made by:
A high-resolution CT scanning
B sputum microbiology
C bronchoscopy
D clinical history
E lung function tests

8.4 In bronchiectasis, due to previous pneumonia, sputum clearance is facilitated by:
A nebulised colistin
B oral ciprofloxacin
C nebulised hypertonic saline

D   nebulised DNAse

E   azithromycin

8.5 **A 55-year-old woman has bilateral basal bronchiectasis that is thought to have arisen from childhood pneumonia. She has chronic lung infection with *Pseudomonas aeruginosa*. Her symptoms are troublesome despite intermittent courses of antibiotics and regular chest clearance physiotherapy. The most appropriate additional treatment to recommend is:**

A   long-term oral doxycycline

B   nebulised colistin or tobramycin

C   intravenous immunoglobulin therapy

D   long-term prednisolone

E   surgery with resection of areas of bronchiectasis

Chapter 9: Cystic fibrosis

9.1 **A newborn baby is diagnosed as having cystic fibrosis. His parents ask about the risk of future children of theirs having cystic fibrosis. The risk of a further child of these parents having cystic fibrosis is approximately:**

A   10%

B   25%

C   50%

D   75%

E   90%

9.2 **The most common bacterium causing lung infection in an adult with cystic fibrosis is:**

A   *Burkholderia cepacia* complex

B   Methicillin resistant *Staphylococcus aureus*

C   *Pseudomonas aeruginosa*

D   *Achromobacter xylosoxidans*

E   *Mycobacterium abscessus*

9.3 **A 16-year-old boy with cystic fibrosis and chronic *Pseudomonas aeruginosa* infection attends the clinic because of an increase in his cough and sputum. There is a mild reduction in his FEV_1. He is undertaking exams and it is decided that he should have a course of tablet antibiotics at home. The most appropriate choice of antibiotic is:**

A   co-amoxiclav

B   colistin

C   ciprofloxacin

D   tobramycin

E   amoxicillin

9.4 **Men with cystic fibrosis usually:**

A   have normal fertility

B   are infertile due to absence of the vas deferens

C   are infertile because of failure to produce sperm in the testes

D   have reduced fertility due to ciliary dysfunction

E   have reduced fertility because of testosterone deficiency

9.5 **In a child with cystic fibrosis diarrhoea and failure to thrive typically occurs because of:**

A   diabetes

B   antibiotic-associated diarrhoea

C   liver disease

D   pancreatic dysfunction

E   deficiency of Vitamins A, D and E

Chapter 10: Asthma

10.1 **Most patients with asthma:**

A   are overoptimistic in their expectations of what can be achieved with treatment

B   are fastidious about treatment compliance

C   can manage simple inhalers well

D   need more that just the basics (inhaled corticosteroids and short-acting bronchodilators) to maintain good control

E   are capable of managing the disease themselves

10.2 **In a patient presenting with breathlessness which of the following most strongly supports a diagnosis of asthma:**

A   breathlessness on exertion

B   a family history of hay fever

C $FEV_1/VC < 0.7$ at the time of clinic visit

D   nocturnal wakening due to cough

E   asymmetry of chest expansion on examination

10.3 **Which of the following are features of a life threatening attack of asthma:**

A   PEF 33–50% of best or predicted

B   respiratory rate ≥ 25 /min

C O_2 saturation $< 92\%$

D   respiratory rate ≥ 25 /min

E   heart rate ≥ 110 bpm

10.4 **In chronic asthma management which of the following most accurately reflects current protocols and treatment:**

A   use of reliever medication only once per day suggests good control

B inhaled corticosteroids do not improve symptoms

C long-acting bronchodilators should never be used without inhaled corticosteroids

D omalizumab is a new effective oral medication for severe disease.

E leukotriene receptor antagonists are effective in most patients

10.5 Which of the following is NOT a common trigger for asthma:

A cigarette smoke

B influenza vaccine

C beta-blockers

D aspirin

E cold air

Chapter 11: Chronic obstructive pulmonary disease

11.1 Which of the following statements best describes the physiological changes typically seen in COPD:

A FEV_1 reduced, T_Lco normal, Kco reduced

B FEV_1/FVC reduced, FEV_1 normal, FVC normal

C FVC reduced, total lung capacity increased, residual volume increased.

D FEV_1/FVC reduced, total lung capacity reduced, residual volume reduced

E FEV_1/FVC reduced, FEV_1 reduced, T_Lco normal

11.2 Which statement best describes the pathological changes typically seen in COPD:

A chronic bronchitis principally affects the distal airways

B emphysema results in increased elastic recoil of the lung

C airway inflammation causes airway obstruction

D emphysema can show some recovery with smoking cessation

E emphysema is independent of airways obstruction

11.3 In relation to oxygen therapy in COPD

A long-term oxygen therapy can extend life

B long-term oxygen therapy can slow the progression of COPD

C most patients experiencing limiting dyspnoea will benefit from ambulatory oxygen

D short-burst oxygen therapy is only used in the terminal stages of the disease

E in an acute exacerbation oxygen should be delivered to achieve a saturation >94%

11.4 In the management of COPD, which one of the following CANNOT be achieved by some intervention:

A improved spirometry (FEV_1/VC ratio)

B improved mortality (extension of life)

C disease modification (slowing of the decline in FEV_1)

D reduced frequency of exacerbations

E improved exercise tolerance

11.5 In relation to epidemiology which of the following best reflects current evidence:

A COPD was a disease of the twentieth century and as smoking patterns change the global prevalence is now falling

B COPD affects all socioeconomic groups equally

C most COPD in the industrial world is caused by occupational exposures and air pollution

D in the UK, COPD affects urban more than rural populations

E most smokers develop COPD

Chapter 12: Carcinoma of the lung

12.1 The most common type of bronchial carcinoma is:

A squamous cell carcinoma

B small-cell carcinoma

C carcinoid tumour

D adenocarcinoma

E large-cell undifferentiated carcinoma

12.2 A 71-year-old man, who is usually fit and well, is coincidentally found to have a 2-cm mass in the periphery of the right upper lobe on a chest X-ray that was performed when he underwent cholecystectomy. He is a smoker. PET/CT scan confirms avid uptake of FDG in a 2-cm mass in the right upper lobe with no other abnormality. The features suggest a bronchial carcinoma. Confirmation of the cell type is best sought by:

A bronchoscopy

B endobronchial ultrasound guided needle aspiration

C   video-assisted thoracoscopic biopsy

D   percutaneous CT-guided needle aspirate

E   mediastinoscopy

12.3 A 60-year-old woman who has smoked and has mild COPD presents with swelling of her face and arms, with dilated veins over her chest wall. Chest X-ray shows a widened bulky mediastinal shadow with a 2-cm opacity in the left upper lobe. The clinical features suggest:

A   dissection of the thoracic aorta

B   nephrotic syndrome

C   central venous thrombosis

D   superior vena caval obstruction

E   thymoma

12.4 A 72-year-old man is diagnosed as having a $T_1N_0M_0$ adenocarcinoma of the left upper lobe of lung. PET/CT confirms avid uptake of FDG within the tumour, without any other abnormality. He is otherwise fit and well with an FEV_1 of 3.2 L (98% predicted) and a WHO performance status of zero. The best treatment option is:

A   left pneumonectomy

B   radical radiotherapy

C   chemotherapy

D   left upper lobectomy

E   monitoring of the tumour by serial CT scans until symptoms arise

12.5 A 65-year-old woman is diagnosed as having an extensive stage small-cell carcinoma of lung with bone metastases. After discussion she decides to have chemotherapy as the initial treatment option. In advising her about her prognosis, her 5-year survival is likely to be approximately:

A   80%

B   60%

C   40%

D   20%

E   0%

Chapter 13: Interstitial lung disease

13.1 Bilateal hilar lymphadenopathy and erythema nodosum suggest a diagnosis of:

A   extrinsic allergic alveolitis

B   sarcoidosis

C   lymphoid interstitial pneumonia

D   systemic sclerosis

E   systemic lupus erythematosis

13.2 A 70-year-old man, who has smoked heavily, presents with progressive breathlessness, clubbing, bibasal crackles and reticular shadowing on chest X-ray. The most likely diagnosis is:

A   cryptogenic organising pneumonia

B   lympoid interstitial pneumonia

C   desquamative interstitial pneumonia

D   idiopathic pulmonary fibrosis

E   respiratory bronchiolitis-interstitial lung disease

13.3 In sarcoidosis bronchoalveolar lavage typically shows a high count of:

A   lymphocytes

B   eosinophils

C   neutrophils

D   macrophages

E   histiocytes

13.4 Ground-glass shadowing with areas of decreased attenuation and air trapping on high-resolution CT scanning are characteristic features of:

A   sarcoidosis

B   lymphocytic interstitial pneumonia

C   non-specific interstitial pneumonia

D   extrinsic allergic alveolitis

E   idiopathic pulmonary fibrosis

13.5 The worst prognosis is associated with a diagnosis of:

A   non-specific interstitial pneumonia

B   cryptogenic organising pneumonia

C   idiopathic pulmonary fibrosis

D   sarcoidosis

E   extrinsic allergic alveolitis

Chapter 14: Occupational lung disease

14.1 The most common work-related lung disease in the UK is:

A   coalminer's pneumoconiosis

B   asbestosis

C   extrinsic allergic alveolitis

D   asthma

E   silicosis

14.2 Isocyanate induced occupational asthma is a substantial hazard for:

A   healthcare workers

B   cleaners

C   paint sprayers

D   hairdressers

E   coalminers

14.3 A 70-year-old man who has smoked 20 cigarettes daily for 50 years and who has worked for 10 years as a pipe lagger in shipyards presents with right chest pain and breathlessness. Chest X-ray shows a right pleural effusion. CT shows nodular pleural thickening extending onto the mediastinal pleura. The most likely diagnosis is:

A mesothelioma
B benign asbestos pleurisy
C lung carcinoma
D diffuse pleural thickening
E pleural plaques

14.4 Eggshell calcification of mediastinal nodes on chest X-ray is a characteristic feature of:

A simple coalworker's pneumoconiosis
B coalworker's progressive massive fibrosis
C silicosis
D asbestos pleural plaques
E Caplan's syndrome

14.5 There is an increased risk of tuberculosis in patients with:

A asbestosis
B coalminer's pneumoconiosis
C siderosis
D byssinosis
E silicosis

Chapter 15: Pulmonary vascular disease

15.1 A 24-year-old woman using a combined oestrogen progesterone contraceptive pill complains of pleuritic pain. Her pulse is 90/min, blood pressure 120/70 mmHg, respiratory rate 16/min. Chest X-ray is normal. D-dimer level is normal. The next most appropriate course of action is:

A proceed to CT pulmonary angiography
B reassure her that no further tests are needed
C proceed to ultrasound of legs
D commence heparin
E commence warfarin

15.2 A 26-year-old woman who is 32-weeks' pregnant presents with pleuritic pain and breathlessness. Pulmonary embolism is suspected. Chest X-ray is normal. The best next investigation is:

A ultrasound of legs
B D-dimer
C isotope perfusion scan
D CT pulmonary angiography
E pulmonary angiography

15.3 A 60-year-old man presents with a 6-month history of bloodstained nasal discharge, arthralgia and general malaise. He is admitted to hospital with renal failure. Chest X-ray shows cavitating nodules. Anti-neutrophil cytoplasmic antibodies are present in the serum. The most likely diagnosis is:

A pulmonary embolism with infarction
B Wegener's granulomatosis
C Churg–Strauss syndrome
D metastataic lung cancer
E systemic lupus erythematosis

15.4 A 70-year-old man has confirmed deep vein thrombosis with pulmonary emboli and he has been started on warfarin. Seven days later he develops haemetemesis with haemoglobin falling to 5 g/dl. Endoscopy confirms a bleeding duodenal ulcer. His thromboembolic disease is best managed by:

A subcutaneous tinzaparin
B intravenous heparin
C aspirin
D insertion of an inferior vena caval filter
E warfarin

15.5 A 50-year-old woman presents with breathlessness. Investigations confirm pulmonary arterial hypertension. She has Raynaud's phenomenon, facial telangiectasia and scerodactyly, with positive anti-centromere antibodies. The most likely cause of her pulmonary hypertension is:

A mitral stenosis
B chronic thromboembolic disease
C CREST syndrome
D Wegener's granulomatosis
E HIV infection

Chapter 16: Pneumothorax and pleural effusion

16.1 The characteristic features of a pneumothorax are:

A dullness to percussion
B bronchial breathing
C tenderness on palpation of the chest wall

D   decreased breath sounds

E   crackles

16.2 An 18-year-old man who is usually fit and well presented with left pleuritic pain. A chest X-ray showed a small left apical pneumothorax. He is now asymptomatic. The most appropriate management of his pneumothorax is:

A   no intervention

B   aspiration

C   chest drain insertion

D   thoracoscopy with pleurodesis

E   limited apicolateral surgical pleurectomy

16.3 A 50-year-old man is admitted to hospital with a left lower lobe pneumonia. Chest X-ray shows a small left pleural effusion. Pleural aspiration under ultrasound guidance yields straw-coloured fluid with a protein of 40 g/L, LDH of 300 units/L, ph of 7.5. These features indicate:

A   an empyema requiring insertion of a chest drain

B   an exudative parapneumonic effusion not requiring insertion of a chest drain

C   a transudative effusion not requiring intervention

D   an exudative parapneumonic effusion requiring insertion of a chest drain

E   probable tuberculosis

16.4 A transudative pleural effusion in a 70-year-old man is most likely to be because of:

A   lung carcinoma

B   mesothelioma

C   left ventricular failure

D   pneumonia

E   rheumatoid arthritis

16.5 A 75-year-old man presented acutely unwell with a 16-hour history of left chest pain, breathlessness and fever, following an episode of vomiting the previous night. There was dullness on percussion of the left side of the chest with diminished breath sounds. Subcutaneous emphysema was palpable in the neck. Chest X-ray showed a left hydropneumothorax. The most likely diagnosis is:

A   oesophageal rupture

B   perforated duodenal ulcer

C   aspiration pneumonia and empyema

D   pneumothorax with bronchopleural fistula

E   aspiration pneumonia and parapneumonic effusion

Chapter 17: Acute respiratory distress syndrome

17.1 Pulmonary oedema in the acute respiratory distress syndrome is characterised by:

A   an elevated pulmonary artery pressure

B   volume overload

C   increased hydrostatic pressure

D   decreased colloid pressure

E   increased alveolar capillary permeability

17.2 A 40-year-old man is admitted to hospital with severe pancreatitis. Three days later he develops progressive breathlessness, severe hypoxia and diffuse bilateral shadowing on chest X-ray. The most likely diagnosis is:

A   pulmonary embolism

B   left ventricular failure

C   acute respiratory distress syndrome

D   hospital acquired pneumonia

E   fat embolism

17.3 The mortality rate of patients requiring endotracheal ventilation for acute respiratory distress syndrome is approximately:

A   10%

B   20%

C   30%

D   50%

E   80%

17.4 With regard to the acute respiratory distress syndrome:

A   the pulmonary capillary wedge pressure is typically less than 18 mmHg

B   pulmonary oedema usually results from excessive fluid administration

C   left ventricular failure is usually a major factor in the development of pulmonary oedema

D   lung infiltrates on chest X-ray usually indicate pneumonia

E   lymphatic obstruction gives rise to pulmonary congestion

17.5 The most common precipitating factor for the acute respiratory distress syndrome is:

A   acute pulmonary embolism

B myocardial infarction with cardiogenic shock

C systemic sepsis

D an acute exacerbation of chronic obstructive pulmonary disease

E multiple blood transfusions

Chapter 18: Sleep-related breathing disorders

18.1 The most effective treatment of obstructive sleep apnoea is:

A oxygen

B nitrazepam night sedation

C continuous positive airway pressure

D uvulopalatopharyngoplasty

E mandibular advancement devices

18.2 The prevalence of obstructive sleep apnoea in middle-aged men is approximately:

A 4%

B 10%

C 20%

D 30%

E 40%

18.3 The main treatment for oxygen desaturation during sleep in patients with neuromuscular disease is:

A oxygen

B continuous positive airway pressure

C weight reduction

D mandibular advancement devices

E non-invasive positive pressure ventilation

18.4 Obstructive sleep apnoea:

A particularly occurs during non-REM sleep

B is less common in men than women

C does not occur in children

D is more common when lying supine

E only occurs in overweight people

18.5 Obstructive sleep apnoea results from:

A weakness of the respiratory muscles

B episodes of upper airways obstruction

C loss of ventilatory drive from the respiratory centre in the brain stem

D nocturnal bronchospasm

E pulmonary oedema and paroxysmal nocturnal dyspnoea

Chapter 19: Lung transplantation

19.1 Patients with cystic fibrosis are not suitable for:

A single-lung transplantation

B bilateral lung transplantation

C living lobar transplantation

D heart–lung transplantation

E double-lung transplantation

19.2 Patients with cystic fibrosis are not suitable for lung transplantation if they have:

A *Pseudomonas aeruginosa* infection

B respiratory failure

C *Burkholderia cenocepacia* infection

D diabetes

E previous pneumothorax

19.3 The 5-year survival post lung transplantation is approximately:

A 80%

B 70%

C 50%

D 30%

E 10%

19.4 A major late complication, occurring 5–10 years post transplantation is:

A reimplantation injury

B lung cancer

C donor-acquired infection

D dehiscence of the anastomosis

E bronchiolitis obliterans syndrome

19.5 Lung transplantation is not a suitable option for patients with:

A idiopathic pulmonary fibrosis

B lung cancer

C idiopathic pulmonary hypertension

D emphysema

E cystic fibrosis

Answers to multiple choice questions

Chapter 1: Anatomy and physiology of the lungs

1.1 B

The diaphragm is the main muscle of inspiration; quiet expiration is a rather passive process. Forced expiration requires positive pressure to be generated in the thorax quickly, to achieve this, the abdominal musculature contracts quickly, which increases the intra-abdominal pressure, forcing the diaphragm up into the thorax.

1.2 C

Lung compliance is the change in lung volume brought about by a unit change in transpulmonary (intrapleural) pressure. The fibrotic lung is less compliant.

1.3 E

Airway resistance in health resides principally in the central (large) airways at high lung volume. As lung volume decreases it moves peripherally to the smaller airways. It is increased in emphysema and is proportional to r^4.

1.4 E

Most of the ventilation goes to the bases, but an even greater proportion of the perfusion goes to the bases. Poor V/Q leads to a fall in Po_2 but does not affect Pco_2. Reduced overall ventilation causes a rise in Pco_2 and a fall in Po_2.

1.5 5.5 kPa

$$P_AO_2 = P_IO_2 - \frac{P_aco_2}{0.8}$$

$$P_AO_2 = 21 - \frac{4.0}{0.8} = 16$$

$$P_AO_2 - P_aO_2 = 16 - 10.5 = 5.5\text{kPa}$$

This is elevated, implying a problem with VQ matching within the lung.

Chapter 2: History taking and examination

2.1 B

Bilateral crackles and clubbing are characteristic features of pulmonary fibrosis.

2.2 A

Dullness to percussion suggests a pleural effusion, pleural thickening or pneumonic consolidation. In consolidation tactile vocal fremitus is often increased whereas in a pleural effusion it is characteristically reduced.

2.3 B

Pneumonic consolidation is characterised by dullness to percussion, increased tactile vocal fremitus, bronchial breathing and crackles. Pneumonia is sometimes associated with inflammation of the overlying pleura causing pleuritic pain.

2.4 E

Pneumothorax typically causes acute pleuritic pain and is characterised by reduced breath sounds and hyper-resonance on the side of the pneumothorax.

2.5 A

He has been a smoker and shows features of airways obstruction with paradoxical inward movement of the costal margins on inspiration (in a normal person they move outwards) with a hyperinflated chest (reduced cricosternal distance) and wheeze. The presence of cyanosis indicates hypoxia and respiratory failure.

Chapter 3: Pulmonary function tests

3.1 D

See Figure 3.1.

3.2 A

The normal FEV/VC and reduced FEV_1 implies restriction. The elevated Kco suggests the cause is extrapulmonary.

3.3 D

The pH is low so this is an acidosis; the Pco$_2$ is high so this is a respiratory acidosis. The bicarbonate is high suggesting there has been time to attempt to compensate (chronic). However, the pH would be in the normal range had this been a chronic stable state; there must be an acute component. Remember too that physiological compensatory mechanisms do not over compensate.

3.4 A

If you assume the patient is breathing room air (P_Io$_2 = 21$ kPa), then the alveolar–arterial gradient would be negative, suggesting that the patient was a net contributor of oxygen to the environment! This seems unlikely. The inspired Po$_2$ therefore must be greater than 21 kPa. The condition is clearly not stable as the pH is outside the normal range. As we are not given the P_Io$_2$ we cannot conclude the lungs are normal. The A–a gradient may be very high.

3.5 A

This is a primary respiratory alkalosis so the answer must be either anxiety-driven hyperventilation or pulmonary embolism. The alveolar arterial gradient is increased implying a problem within the lungs (affecting V/Q matching), which anxiety cannot explain.

Chapter 4: Radiology of the chest

4.1 E

Cavitation is the presence of an area of radiolucency within a mass lesion. It is a feature of bronchial carcinoma (particularly squamous carcinoma), tuberculosis, lung abscess, pulmonary infarcts, Wegener's granulomatosis and some pneumonias (e.g. *Staphylococcus aureus*, *Klebsiella pneumoniae*).

4.2 D

An air bronchogram is visible as a black tube of air against the white background of consolidated lung. It indicates that the bronchus is patent, and not occluded. It is a feature of pneumonic consolidation.

4.3 C

Avid uptake of FDG on PET scanning is a feature of bronchial carcinoma, but can also occur in inflammatory conditions such as tuberculosis, sarcoidosis, histoplasmosis and coccidioidomycosis.

4.4 D

Collapse of a lobe is a sinister feature suggesting occlusion of the bronchus by a mass lesion such as a carcinoma.

4.5 B

Thymic tumours, thyroid masses and dermoid cysts are most commonly situated in the anterior mediastinum, whereas neurofibromas and oesophageal cysts are often situated posteriorly.

Chapter 5: Upper respiratory tract infections and influenza

5.1 D

Acute epiglottitis is a serious illness that is usually caused by virulent strains of *H. influenzae* type B. It typically affects young children, may cause occlusion of the airway and is often accompanied by septicaemia.

5.2 E

Chlamydophila psittaci is primarily a disease of birds that is transmitted to humans as a zoonosis. *Chlamydophila pneumoniae* typically causes mild upper respiratory tract infections, and is spread from person to person.

5.3 A

Influenza A is the main cause of seasonal influenza, which is characterised by systemic symptoms of headache, malaise, myalgia and prostration in addition to upper respiratory tract symptoms.

5.4 A

Recurrent sinusitis is a feature of cystic fibrosis, hypogammaglobulinaemia and ciliary dyskinesia, all of which also cause bronchiectasis.

5.5 B

Influenza A undergoes frequent changes in its surface antigens. Minor changes referred to as 'antigenic drift' result in outbreaks of seasonal influenza, but major changes, referred to as 'antigenic shift' result in epidemics and pandemics.

Chapter 6: Pneumonia

6.1 D

Streptococcus pneumoniae is the most common cause of community-acquired pneumonia.

6.2 C

Chlamydophila psittaci is primarily an infection of birds that can be transmitted to humans as a zoonosis.

6.3 A

This patient's CURB-65 score is zero. He is not **C**onfused, his **U**rea is normal at 5.6 mmol/L, his **R**espiratory rate is not elevated above 30/min, his **B**lood pressure is normal, and he is not over **65** years of age. This indicates a low risk for developing complications and he is likely to be suitable for treatment at home rather than in hospital.

6.4 B

SARS was a very severe pneumonic illness caused by a newly identified coronavirus, that caused a global pandemic in 2003. The pandemic was brought to an end by public health measures including rapid case detection, case isolation, contact tracing and strict infection control procedures.

6.5 A

Pneumocystis pneumonia is likely to occur in patients with HIV infection whose CD4 count is <200/mm^3. The diagnosis may be confirmed by detecting *Pneumocystis jirovecii* in induced sputum or in bronchoalveolar lavage fluid. He requires treatment with high-dose intravenous co-trimoxazole, prednisolone and oxygen.

Chapter 7: Tuberculosis

7.1 D

Obtaining bronchoalveolar lavage fluid will allow rapid diagnosis of active tuberculosis by AAFB staining, and culture will allow tests of sensitivity to drugs.

7.2 B

Interferon gamma release assays are useful in diagnosing latent tuberculosis but are not recommended as a routine test for active tuberculosis.

7.3 B

The term 'latent tuberculosis' refers to the situation where a person has been infected with TB at some time but does not currently have active disease. There is an approximately 10% risk of the TB becoming active at some stage. This risk may be reduced by prophylactic treatment with isoniazid and rifampicin for 3 months.

7.4 E

Because of the risk of optic neuritis visual acuity should be tested before starting treatment and patients should be advised to report visual changes. The dose should be reduced in renal impairment (creatinine clearance <30 mls/minute).

7.5 D

Standard treatment consists of isoniazid and rifampicin for 6 months with ethambutol and pyrazinamide for the initial 2 months.

Chapter 8: Bronchiectasis and lung abscess

8.1 B

Bronchiectasis, pseudomonas infection, nasal polyps and infertility due to obstructive azospermia (no sperm in ejaculate) are all characteristic features of cystic fibrosis. It is recommended that all children and adults up to the age of 40 years with bronchiectasis should have sweat tests and DNA analysis for cystic fibrosis. About 6–10% of patients with cystic fibrosis are diagnosed in adulthood.

8.2 E

Allergic bronchopulmonary aspergillosis is characterised by severe bronchial inflammation with mucus plugging and bronchiectasis that is typically proximal in location. The halo sign is a feature of an aspergilloma (a fungal ball within a cavity) rather than allergic bronchopulmonary aspergillosis.

8.3 A

High-resolution CT scanning is the key investigation in diagnosing bronchiectasis. Chest X-ray is not sufficiently sensitive.

8.4 C

Nebulised hypertonic saline improves sputum clearance in patients with bronchiectasis. Nebulised DNase is a treatment for patients with cystic fibrosis but is not effective in other forms of bronchiectasis.

8.5 B

This patient has chronic *Pseudomonas aeruginosa* lung infection and is therefore likely to benefit from nebulised anti-pseudomonas antibiotics e.g. colistin or tobramycin. Doxy-cycline is not effective against *Pseudomonas aeruginosa.*

Chapter 9: Cystic fibrosis

9.1 B

Cystic fibrosis is an autosomal recessive disease. The child with cystic fibrosis has two mutations of the cystic fibrosis gene, having inherited one abnormal gene from each of his parents. Each of his parents is a carrier of cystic fibrosis. The risk of a child of carrier parents having the disease is 1:4 (25%).

9.2 C

Patients with cystic fibrosis are particularly vulnerable to *Pseudomonas aeruginosa* infection, and this is the most common infection in adults.

9.3 C

The only oral antibiotic with activity against *Pseudomonas aeruginosa* is ciprofloxacin. Co-amoxiclav and amoxicillin are not active against *Pseudomonas aeruginosa.* Colistin and tobramycin can be given intravenously or by nebulisation, but are not available in an oral formulation.

9.4 B

Nearly all men with cystic fibrosis are infertile because of congenital bilateral absence of the vas deferens resulting in azospermia (no sperm in the ejaculate). However, normal sperm are usually produced by the testes such that these men can achieve biological fatherhood by assisted reproduction techniques involving aspiration of sperm from the testes and in vitro fertilisation. Women with cystic fibrosis have essentially normal fertility.

9.5 D

Approximately 85% of children with cystic fibrosis have pancreatic insufficiency such that there is a lack of pancreatic enzymes resulting in malabsorption of fat; which causes diarrhoea and failure to thrive.

Chapter 10: Asthma

10.1 E

Patients often have inappropriately low expectations of what can be achieved with treatment. Adherence to treatment is a major issue in any chronic disease, the additional complexity of inhaled medication (as opposed to oral) only adds to this. Inhaler technique is generally very poor. This is usually the prescribing clinician's fault, not the patient's. Most people can be managed perfectly well at step two of the BTS guidelines provided attention is paid to the detail. Self-monitoring and management is key to good control in this variable condition. Education is crucial.

10.2 D

Any cause of breathlessness tends to be worse on exertion. Although hay fever may be linked with asthma, the associating of a family history and a personal diagnosis of asthma is a little weak. $FEV_1/VC <0.7$ confirms airway obstruction, variability is required for a diagnosis of asthma. Nocturnal symptoms of cough or breathlessness suggest diurnal variability consistent with asthma. Asymmetry of chest expansion on examination suggests the diagnosis is something else.

10.3 C

All are features of acute severe asthma, only (C) is a feature of a life-threatening attack.

10.4 C

The need for reliever medication more than three times per week implies inadequate control. Of course corticosteroids improve symptoms; they just do not do it instantly. Omalizumab is given by injection. Leukotriene receptor antagonists can be very effective in a minority of patients.

10.5 B

Influenza is a common trigger of asthma, such that influenza vaccine is recommended.

Chapter 11: Chronic obstructive pulmonary disease

11.1 C

$T_{L}CO$ is reduced, FEV_1 is reduced, FVC is usually also reduced (although not as much as FEV_1).

11.2 C

Chronic bronchitis principally affects the larger airways. Emphysema results in reduced elastic recoil. Airway inflammation, in conjunction with emphysema and chronic bronchitis all contribute to airway obstruction. Emphysema is permanent.

11.3 A

Long-term oxygen therapy can extend life in severe disease associated with hypoxia by slowing the progression of cor pulmonale, it has no effect on the progression of COPD (FEV$_1$ decline). Many breathless patients are not hypoxic, supplemental oxygen is of no benefit to them. Short-burst oxygen is often used as a 'palliative' measure but is not confined to the terminal stages of the disease. Emergency oxygen should be delivered to achieve a saturation of 88–92% pending arterial blood gas assessment.

11.4 They are all achievable!

Bronchodilators work in COPD (just not as dramatically as in asthma). Long-term oxygen therapy extends life. The rate of decline of FEV$_1$ will be slowed by smoking cessation. Combination inhalers and tiotropium reduce exacerbation frequency. Many interventions including pulmonary rehabilitation improve exercise tolerance.

11.5 D

Global prevalence of COPD is increasing, COPD affects lower socioeconomic groups more – largely because of smoking prevalence. Smoking is the main cause of COPD in the developed world, although only about 15% of smokers will develop the condition.

Chapter 12: Carcinoma of the lung

12.1 A

Squamous carcinoma is the most common form of lung cancer. Small-cell carcinoma accounts for approximately 20%, and non-small-carcinoma 80%, comprising squamous carcinoma 45%, adenocarcinoma 20% and undifferentiated carcinoma 15%.

12.2 D

The nodule is peripherally located such that it is not likely to be amenable to biopsy at bronchoscopy or by endobronchial ultrasound. Percutaneous fine needle aspirate of the nodule under CT scan guidance provides the best method of seeking cytological diagnosis and is less invasive than video-assisted thoracoscopic biopsy. Mediastinoscopy gives access to the mediastinal nodes but not to nodules in the lung.

12.3 D

Obstruction of the superior vena cava causes oedema of the face, neck and arms, with dilatation of collateral veins, often visible on the chest wall.

12.4 D

This patient has a stage I adenocarcinoma that is best treated by surgical resection in the form of a left upper lobectomy. He has adequate lung function and general fitness for lobectomy. Pneumonectomy is not required to resect the tumour. Radiotherapy or chemotherapy are not appropriate as they offer a much lower chance of cure for stage I carcinoma.

12.5 E

Small-cell carcinoma is a highly malignant cancer. She has extensive stage disease at presentation. Average survival without treatment is approximately 6 weeks, improving to 8 months with chemotherapy, but long-term survival is extremely unlikely.

Chapter 13: Interstitial lung disease

13.1 B

Bilateral hilar lymphadenopathy (BHL) on chest X-ray is a characteristic feature of sarcoidosis. It may also be caused by lymphoma, metastatic carcinoma, tuberculosis, and fungal infections such as histoplasmosis. Erythema nodosum consists of round, red raised nodules, often on the shins. It is a feature of hypersensitivity and is also found in streptococcal infections, tuberculosis, ulcerative colitis, Crohn's disease and with drugs (e.g. contraceptive pill). The combination of BHL and erythema nodosum is highly suggestive of sarcoidosis, and this form of the disease has an excellent prognosis, often resolving spontaneously.

13.2 D

Idiopathic pulmonary fibrosis is the most common form of interstitial lung disease. The fibrosis is predominantly basal and subpleural, giving rise to crackles on auscultation and reticular shadowing on X-ray. Approximately 60–70% have clubbing.

13.3 A

Both sarcoidosis and extrinsic allergic alveolitis are characterised by high lymphocyte counts in bronchoalveolar lavage fluid. Bronchoalveolar lavage is also useful in excluding infection in patients presenting with diffuse shadowing on chest X-ray.

13.4 D

High-resolution CT is a key investigation in interstitial lung disease. Diagnosis is based upon the integration of clinical, radiological and histopathology features in a multidisciplinary meeting. Extrinsic allergic alveolitis has a characteristic CT pattern of ground-glass shadowing with areas of decreased attenuation and air trapping, best seen on expiratory views.

13.5 C

Idiopathic pulmonary fibrosis is a serious disease that usually progresses relentlessly and responds poorly to treatment. In contrast diseases such as cryptogenic organising pneumonia and non-specific interstitial pneumonia have a greater inflammatory component that usually responds to prednisolone.

Chapter 14: Occupational lung disease

14.1 D

Occupational asthma is now the most common type of occupational lung disease. In the UK about 3000 new cases are diagnosed each year.

14.2 C

Isocyanates are a potent cause of occupational asthma. They are used in spray paints, varnishes, adhesives and polyurethane foams.

14.3 A

The CT scan features of nodular pleural thickening extending onto the mediastinal pleura is a characteristic feature of mesothelioma. He has had heavy exposure to asbestos that was used for pipe lagging in shipyards.

14.4 C

Eggshell calcification of mediastinal nodes is a characteristic feature of silicosis. It may also occur in long-standing sarcoidosis. Asbestos causes calcified pleural plaques (but not calcification of mediastinal nodes).

14.5 E

Silica interferes with the ability of macrophages to kill tubercle bacilli. There is a significantly increased risk of tuberculosis in patients with silicosis.

Chapter 15: Pulmonary vascular disease

15.1 B

The combined low-dose oestrogen contraceptive pill is associated with only a mildly increased risk of venous thrombosis. This patient does not have breathlessness and has a normal respiratory rate. The negative D-dimer provides strong evidence in excluding pulmonary embolism in these circumstances. She should be reassured and does not need further imaging or anti-coagulation.

15.2 A

There is a high probability of pulmonary embolism here as the patient has a major risk factor (pregnancy) and has typical symptoms. CTPA exposes the mother's breasts to radiation with an increased risk of future breast cancer. Isotope perfusion scan exposes the foetus and mother to a small radiation dose. Ultrasound of legs may be useful if it confirms DVT, thereby avoiding the need for CTPA or perfusion scanning.

15.3 B

Wegener's granulomatosis characteristically involves the nose, lungs and kidneys and is an ANCA-associated vasculitis.

15.4 D

This patient has conflicting problems of haemorrhage and thrombosis. Anti-coagulation poses a major risk of provoking further bleeding from his duodenal ulcer. Insertion of an inferior vena caval filter prevents major emboli from reaching the lungs, and is indicated in these circumstances.

15.5 C

This patient has some clinical features of CREST syndrome (calcinosis, Raynaud's phenomenon, oesophageal dysmotility and telangiectasia), which is a particular, limited form of systemic sclerosis. It is a recognised cause of pulmonary hypertension and is often associated with anti-centromere antibodies.

Chapter 16: Pneumothorax and pleural effusion

16.1 D

The typical signs of a pneumothorax are diminished breath sounds, decreased expansion and hyper-resonance on the side of the pneumothorax, although these signs are often difficult to detect. Shift of the trachea and apex beat to the opposite side with severe distress and cardiorespiratory compromise indicates a tension pneumothorax.

16.2 A

Conservative management of small, asymptomatic primary spontaneous pneumothoraces has been shown to be safe. This man is fit and well with no known pre-existing lung disease (primary pneumothorax) and is asymptomatic. No intervention is needed. He may be allowed to go home with a follow-up appointment arranged. He should be advised to return to the accident and emergency department in the unlikely event that he deteriorates.

16.3 B

The elevated protein and LDH indicate an exudate. The fluid is straw-coloured with a normal pH so that the small pleural effusion is likely to resolve with antibiotics and does not need drainage. A pH of <7.2 indicates that a parapneumonic effusion requires drainage.

16.4 C

Transudative pleural effusions have a protein content of <30 g/L and an LDH <200 units/L. They arise as a result of changes in hydrostatic or osmotic pressures across the pleural membrane rather than by disease of the pleura. The main causes of transudative effusions are cardiac failure, renal failure, hepatic cirrhosis and hypoproteinaemia.

16.5 A

Spontaneous rupture of the oesophagus (Boerhaave's syndrome) occurs when the patient attempts to suppress vomiting by closure of the pharyngeal sphincter. Air and fluid leak from the ruptured oesophagus into the pleural space causing a hydropneumothorax. Air can leak into the tissues giving palpable subcutaneous emphysema.

Chapter 17: Acute respiratory distress syndrome

17.1 E

ARDS is characterised by permeability pulmonary oedema. The systemic inflammatory response results in endothelial damage with leakage of a protein-rich exudate into the alveoli.

17.2 C

Severe pancreatitis is a typical initiating illness that gives rise to the inflammatory processes and endothelial damage resulting in ARDS.

17.3 D

ARDS is a very serious disease with a high mortality of approximately 50%.

17.4 A

In cardiogenic pulmonary oedema (e.g. caused by left ventricular failure) pulmonary artery pressure is typically elevated whereas in ARDS the pulmonary oedema results from an increase permeability of the endothelium rather than 'pressure pulmonary oedema' and the pulmonary artery pressure is typically <18 mmHg.

17.5 C

Severe systemic sepsis is the most common cause of ARDS in most circumstances.

Chapter 18: Sleep-related breathing disorders

18.1 C

CPAP is very effective and has become the standard treatment of obstructive sleep apnoea. Uvulopalatopharyngoplasty is primarily used to reduce snoring but its effect on sleep apnoea is unpredictable.

18.2 A

About 4% of middle-aged men and 2% of women have obstructive sleep apnoea.

18.3 E

Patients with neuromuscular weakness who hypoventilate during sleep require non-invasive ventilation rather than CPAP.

18.4 D

Apnoeas are more common when patients are supine, lying on their backs. Sleep apnoea is more common during REM sleep. It is not confined to people who are overweight. It also occurs in children when it may be related to enlarged tonsils and adenoids.

18.5 B

Obstructive sleep apnoea results from recurrent episodes of upper airways occlusion during sleep. Sleep disturbance from nocturnal wheeze in patients with asthma and from pulmonary oedema in patients with

paroxysmal nocturnal dyspnoea due to cardiac failure, is not due to obstructive sleep
apnoea.

Chapter 19: Lung transplantation

19.1 A

Patients with cystic fibrosis are not suitable
for single lung transplantation as the residual
native lung contains infection which would
act as a source of sepsis in the post-operative
period.

19.2 C

Unfortunately the results of transplanting
patients with cystic fibrosis who had *Burkho-
deria cenocepacia* infection were so poor
that transplant centres now regard this
infection as a major contraindication to

transplantation. Previous pneumothorax is
not a contraindication to transplantation.

19.3 C

Survival rates post-lung transplantation
are approximately 80% at 1 year, 50–55% at
5 years and 30% at 10 years.

19.4 E

Re-implantation injury, dehiscence of the
anastomosis and donor-acquired infection
are risks early after transplantation. The
bronchiolitis obliterans syndrome is the
most important complication threatening
the long-term survival of patients with transplanted lungs.

19.5 B

Lung transplantation is a potential treatment
for many forms of advanced lung disease,
but is not suitable for patients with lung
cancer.

Index

Page numbers in *italics* denote figures, those in **bold** denote tables.

abdominal paradox 18
Abram's needle 175
abscess
  lung 39, 84–5, *84*
accessory muscles of respiration 16
acetazolamide, obstructive sleep
    apnoea 190
acid-base balance 32, *33*
  disturbances of 33–4, *33, 34*
acquired immunodeficiency
    syndrome *see* HIV/AIDS
actinomycosis 177
acute respiratory distress syndrome
    see ARDS
adenovirus, HIV/AIDS 65
aegophony 20
aeroallergens 99
air bronchogram 38
air pollution 117
air travel, COPD 125–6
airway inflammation 98
  treatment 108
airway obstruction 116, *116, 117*
  reversibility 103
  variability 103
airway remodelling 101
airway resistance 5–7, *5, 6*
  disease effects 6–7
  flow-limiting mechanism 6
  and lung volume 7
  maximal, site of 5–6, *5, 6*
    lung volume 7
airway responsiveness 103
alteplase 165
alveolar cell carcinoma 140
alveolar gas equation 11–12
alveolar-arterial gradient 11
alveoli 1–2, *2, 3*
aminoglycosides, pneumonia 58
aminophylline 123
amiodarone, lung fibrosis 142
amoxicillin
  bronchiectasis 84
  COPD 126
  cystic fibrosis 94
  pneumonia 58, 59

amylase, pleural effusion 175
amyloidosis, cystic fibrosis 92
anaemia 16
anti-cardiolipin antibody
    disease 160
anti-neutrophil cytoplasmic
    antibodies (ANCA) 167
anti-thrombin III 160
anti-thymocyte globulin 194
antibiotics
  bronchiectasis 83–4
  COPD 126
  cystic fibrosis 94
  lung abscess 85
  pneumonia 58
  see also individual drugs
anticoagulants, pulmonary
    embolism 164–5
antigens
  environmental 142
  extrinsic allergic alveolitis 146–7,
    147
apex beat 18
ARDS 179–84
  clinical features 180–1, *181*, **181**
  diagnosis 181, **182**
  initiating injuries **181**
  pathogenesis 179–80, *180*
    permeability pulmonary
      oedema 180
    pressure pulmonary
      oedema 179–80, *180*
  prognosis 183
  treatment 181–3
arterial blood gases 32–6, **32**
  acid-base balance 32, *33*
  acid-base disturbances 33–4, *33,
    34*
  arterial oxygenation 35–6
  bicarbonate concentration 32–3,
    33
arterial oxygen tension 35
arthropathy, cystic fibrosis 92
asbestos
  amosite (brown) 156
  chrysotile (white) 156

crocidolite (blue) 156, 158
  tremolite 156
asbestos bodies 157
asbestos-related lung cancer 132,
    158
asbestos-related lung
    disease 156–9, *157–9*
asbestosis 157
aspergilloma 3, 193
aspergillosis 80, *81*, 82
Aspergillus fumigatus 61, 65,
    80, *81*
  in asthma 104
aspiration pneumonia 55, 146
asterixis 16
asthma 98–114
  acute severe 112–14
    immediate management 113
    investigations 113
    treatment monitoring 113–14
  aetiology 98–100
    environmental factors 99
    indoor environment 99
    occupational environment 100
    outdoor environment 99–100
  clinical features 101–2
    morning dipping 101, 103
  cough variant 101
  definition 98
  diagnosis 102, **113**
  exercise-induced 101, 106–7
  genetic susceptibility 99
  investigations 102–4
    hypersensitivity tests 103–4,
      104
    lung function tests 102–3
  management 104–12, *105*
    anti-inflammatory
      drugs 108–9
    bronchodilators 107–8
    inhalers 110–12, *110–12*
    patient education 104–6
    SMART regimen 107
  occupational 151–4
    causes **152**
    diagnosis 152–3, *153*

Respiratory Medicine Lecture Notes, Eighth Edition. Stephen J. Bourke and Graham P. Burns.
© 2011 John Wiley & Sons, Ltd. Published 2011 by John Wiley & Sons, Ltd.

asthma (*Continued*)
    management 153–4
    pathogenesis and
        pathology 100–1, *100*
    prevalence 98
atelectasis *21*
    chest X-ray 37–8, *40, 41*
    rolled 158
atopy 99
auscultation 20
azathioprine 194
azodicarbonamide **152**

Bactec radiometric system 72
Bacteroides spp. 177
base excess **32**
BCG vaccination 76
beclometasone 108
β_2-agonists
    asthma 107
    intravenous 113
bicarbonate 32–3, **32**, *33*
    actual 32
    standard 33
biliary cirrhosis, cystic fibrosis 89
biopsy
    percutaneous needle 134, *135*
    pleural 175
    radiologically guided 175
    transbronchial 142, *143*
bird fancier's lung 146
bleomycin, lung fibrosis 142
blue bloaters 118, *119*
BODE index 120
Boerhaave's syndrome 177
bone cysts, sarcoidosis 149
breath sounds 20
breathing
    bronchial 20
    character of 16
    Cheyne-Stokes 190
    control of 12
breathlessness *see* dyspnoea
bronchial arteries 3
bronchial breathing 20
bronchial carcinoma, cavitation 39
bronchial obstruction 79, 85
bronchial thermoplasty 109
bronchial tree 1–2, *2*
bronchiectasis 3, 78–84
    aetiology 79–82, **80**, *81, 82*
    clinical features 82–3
    investigations 83, *83*
    pathogenesis 78–9, *79*
    treatment 83–4
bronchioles 1
    respiratory 1
    terminal 1

bronchiolitis, obliterative 145, 154
bronchiolitis obliterans
        syndrome 194
bronchitis
    chronic 115–16
    coalworker's 155
    eosinophilic 101
bronchoalveolar lavage 142–3
    sarcoidosis 149
bronchodilators
    asthma 107–8
    bronchiectasis 84
    COPD 121–2
    cystic fibrosis 94
    intravenous 113
bronchopneumonia 54, 59, 118
bronchopulmonary
        sequestration 85
bronchorrhoea 14
bronchoscopy 104
    lung cancer 135
budesonide 108
bullectomy 126
bupropion 121
Burkholderia cenocepacia 193
Burkholderia cepacia 89
    cepacia syndrome 89, *91*
Burkholderia pseudomallei 55
byssinosis 154

Candida albicans 61, 65
Caplan's syndrome 146, 155
carbon dioxide 8
    arterial content 11
    carriage by blood 9, *9*
    partial pressure *see* PCO$_2$
carbon monoxide transfer
        factor 28, 31–2, *31*
    single-breath method 31, *31*
    transfer coefficient 31–2
carcinoid tumour 140
cardiac output, ARDS 183
caseating granuloma 72
cavitation 39, *41*
cefuroxime, pneumonia 58
central sleep apnoea 190
cepacia syndrome 89, *91*
cephalosporins, pneumonia 58
chemotherapy, lung cancer 139
chest
    movements 18
    shape 16, 18
chest examination 18–20, *19*
    auscultation 20
    inspection 18, *19*
    palpation 18–19, *19*
    percussion 20
chest pain 15

chest X-ray 37, *38, 39*
    abnormal features 37–42,
        40–2
    antero-posterior view 37
    bronchiectasis 83, *83*
    COPD *119*
    pleural effusion 173–4, *174*
    pneumonia 56, *57*
    pneumothorax 170, *170, 171*
    postero-anterior view 37
    pulmonary embolism 161
    tuberculosis 71, *71*
Cheyne-Stokes respiration 190
Chlamydia trachomatis 54, 60
Chlamydophila pneumoniae 54, 60
Chlamydophila psittaci 52, 55, 58,
        60, 151
chronic obstructive pulmonary
        disease *see* COPD
Churg-Strauss syndrome 167
chylothorax 175
chylous effusions 176
ciclesonide 108
ciclosporin 194
ciliary dyskinesia 80–2, *82*
ciprofloxacin
    bronchiectasis 84
    COPD 126
    cystic fibrosis 94
clarithromycin
    COPD 126
    pneumonia 58
clindamycin, *Pneumocystis
        jirovecii* 64
Clostridium difficile 58
clubbing 16–17, *17*, **18**, 83
co-amoxiclav
    bronchiectasis 84
    COPD 126
    pleural effusion 177
    pneumonia 58
co-trimoxazole, *Pneumocystis
        jirovecii* 64
coalworker's bronchitis/
        emphysema 155
coalworker's pneumoconiosis
        154–5, *155*
colistin, cystic fibrosis 94
collagen vascular disease 166
colloid pressure *180*
colophony **152**
community-acquired pneumonia
        54
    pneumococcal 58–9, *59*
compression stockings 166
computed tomography *see* CT
connective tissue diseases 145–6,
        146

consolidation *21*
  chest X-ray 38
continuous positive airway
      pressure 182
  obstructive sleep apnoea 190
COPD 115–29
  admission avoidance 128
  aetiology 117
  blue bloaters 118, *119*
  clinical features and
      progression 117–18, *118*
  definition 115
  early supported discharge 128
  emergency treatment 126–8
    antibiotics 126
    oxygen 127, *127*
    ventilatory support 127–8
  investigations 118–20
    lung function tests 118–19
    radiology 119, *119*
  management 120–6
    bronchodilators 121–2
    corticosteroids 122
    hypoxia during air travel 125–6
    oxygen therapy 124–5
    pulmonary
        rehabilitation 123–4
    smoking cessation 120–1
    tiotropium 122
  pink puffers 118, *119*
COPD Assessment Test 120
cor pulmonale 120, 124, 166
corticosteroids
  asthma 108
  COPD 122
  sarcoidosis 150
costal margin paradox 18, *19*
cotton/flax dust 154
cough 14, 16
  COPD 118
cough fracture 14
cough syncope 14
cough variant asthma 101
Coxiella burnetti 55
crackles 20, 56, 83, 142
crepitations *see* crackles
CREST syndrome 166
crico-arytenoid joint, involvement
    of 145
crico-sternal distance 18
'crow's feet' 158
cryptogenic organising
    pneumonia 144
CT 42–3, *42, 43*
  bronchiectasis 83
  lung cancer *134*
CT pulmonary angiography,
    pulmonary embolism 163, *163*

CURB-65 score 55, *56*
cyanosis 16, 17
cystic fibrosis 87–97
  basic defect 87–9, *88*
    gastrointestinal tract 88–9
    lungs 88
  bronchiectasis 82, 89
  clinical features 89–92, *90–2*
  diagnosis 92–3
    atypical cystic fibrosis 93
    DNA analysis 92–3
    newborn screening 93
    sweat testing 92
  prognosis 95–6
  treatment 93–5
    antibiotics 94
    chest physiotherapy 93–4
    mucolytic medication 94
    nutrition 95
cystic fibrosis transmembrane
    conductance regulator 87
cytomegalovirus
  HIV/AIDS 65
  immunocompromised
    patients 61

D-dimer, pulmonary embolism 163
deep vein thrombosis 160–1
denufosol 96
Dermatophagoides
    pteronyssinus 99
diabetes mellitus, cystic fibrosis 89,
    90
diaphragm, actions of 3–4, *4*
diffusing capacity 28
distal intestinal obstruction
    syndrome 90–1, *92*
DNA fingerprinting,
    tuberculosis 72
DNAse, cystic fibrosis 94
Dressler's syndrome 177
dust mites 99, 106
dusts 142, 151
  cotton/flax 154
  grain **152**
  wood **152**
dyspnoea 13–14, 55, 142
  Medical Research Council
      Dyspnoea Scale 120
  paroxysmal nocturnal 14
  pleural effusion 173
  pneumothorax 170

ECG, pulmonary embolism 161
effusion
  chylous 176
  parapneumonic 176
electrocardiogram *see* ECG

electrooculogram 189
emphysema 116–17
  centriacinar 116
  coalworker's 155
  panacinar 116
empyema 175
endobronchial ultrasound 135
endotracheal intubation 182
eosinophilia, asthma 104
eosinophilic bronchitis 101
epiglottitis 59
epoxy resins **152**
Epstein-Barr virus, HIV/AIDS 65
Epworth sleepiness score 188, **189**
erythema nodosum 148
Escherichia coli 54
ethambutol, tuberculosis **72**, 73
examination 16–20, *16*
exercise testing 103
exercise-induced asthma 101,
    106–7
extracorporeal membrane
    oxygenation 182
extrinsic allergic alveolitis 146–7,
    147
exudates 176–7

factor V Leiden gene mutation 160
farmer's lung 146
FEV_1 7, 24
  workplace challenge *153*
FEV_1/FVC ratio 24
  airway obstruction 116
  COPD 118–19
fibrosis 39
flour, and asthma **152**
flow-volume loop 26–7, *27–30*
flucloxacillin, cystic fibrosis 94
fluticasone 108
food flavourer's lung 154
forced expiratory volume *see* FEV
forced vital capacity (FVC) 24
foreign body, inhaled 79, 85
formoterol 107, 121
functional residual capacity 23
fungal infections, HIV/AIDS 65
Fusobacterium spp. 85
Fusobacterium necrophorum 85
FVC *see* forced vital capacity

gas exchange 7–12
  air distribution 7
  alveolar gas equation 11–12
  arterial CO_2 content 11
  arterial O_2 content 11
  blood gas transport 9, *9*
  PCO_2 8
  PO_2 8–9, *8*

gas exchange (*Continued*)
  respiratory quotient   8
  V/Q local differences   9–10, *9, 10*
gastroesophageal reflux   194
Goodpasture's syndrome   167
grain dusts   **152**
ground glass appearance   42, 143,
    145, 147

Haemophilus influenzae   54, 89,
    118, 126
  pneumonia   59
haemoptysis   14, **15**, 82, 89
haemothorax   175
halitosis   83
Heaf test   74
heart-lung transplant   192
helium dilution   27
herpes simplex virus, HIV/AIDS   65
high-frequency jet ventilation   182
hilar lymphadenopathy   148, *149*
history   15–16
  family   15
  general medical   15
  occupational   16
  social   15
history taking   13
HIV/AIDS
  Kaposi's sarcoma   65
  lymphoma   65
  pulmonary complications   62–6, **63**
    bacterial infections   63
    fungal infections   65
    interstitial pneumonitis   65
    Mycobacterium avium-
      intracellulare complex   65
    Mycobacterium tuberculosis   64
    pneumocystis
      pneumonia   63–4
    pulmonary hypertension   65
    viral infections   65
hoarseness   15
holly-leaf pattern   158, *158*
Homan's sign   161
Hooke's law   4
Horner's syndrome   16
hospital-acquired pneumonia   54–5
Hospital Anxiety and Depression
    questionnaire   120
human immunodeficiency virus *see*
    HIV/AIDS
hygiene hypothesis   101
hyper-resonance   20
hypercalcaemia
  lung cancer   133
  sarcoidosis   149
hypercapnia   28, 182
hyperinflation   103

hypoxaemia   166
hypoxia   103
hypoxic drive   12

ibuprofen, cystic fibrosis   95
IgE
  antagonists   109
  asthma   104
immune reconstitution
    syndromes   65–6
immunodeficiency states
  bronchiectasis   79–80
  pneumonia   61–2, **62**
  see also HIV/AIDS
immunosuppression   194
infertility, cystic fibrosis   91
infiltrates   142, 143, *145*
influenza   55
  HIV/AIDS   65
inhalers   110–12, *110–12*
  breath-actuated   110
  correct technique   122–3
  dry-powder   111, *111*
  metered-dose   110, *110*
  nebulisers   111–12, *112*
  spacer devices   110, *111*
intercostal recession   4
intercostal tube drainage   171–2,
    171
interferon-γ release assays   75–6
interstitial lung disease   142–50
  clinical presentation   142
  connective tissue diseases   145–6,
    146
  differential diagnosis   142,
    144
  extrinsic allergic alveolitis   146–7,
    147
  idiopathic pulmonary
    fibrosis   143
  investigations   142–3
  sarcoidosis   147–50, *148, 149*
interstitial pneumonia *see*
    pneumonia, interstitial
interstitial pneumonitis   65
ipratropium   107, 113, 121, 126
isocyanates   **152**
isoniazid
  adverse reactions   74
  tuberculosis   **72**, 73

jugular venous pressure   16, 17

Kaposi's sarcoma   65
Kartagener's syndrome   81, *82*
Klebsiella pneumoniae   59–60, 79,
    85
kyphoscoliosis   186, *187*

lactate dehydrogenase, pleural
    effusion   175
latex   **152**
Legionella pneumophila   52, 54, 55,
    60–1
Legionnaires' disease   60
Lemière's disease   85
leukotriene receptor
    antagonists   109
lobar pneumonia   54
lower respiratory tract
    infections   52, 54
  see also pneumonia
lungs   1–12
  air movement   3
  airway resistance   5–7, *5, 6*
  bronchial tree and alveoli   1–2,
    2, 3
  collapse *see* atelectasis
  elastic properties   4, *5*
  gas exchange   7–12
  perfusion   2–3
  physiology   3–7, *4–6*
lung abscess   84–5, *84*
lung cancer   130–41
  aetiology   130–2, *131*, **131**
  asbestosis-related   132, 157, 158
  diagnosis   132–5, *133–5*
    communication of   135–6
  growth rates   132
  mortality   *131*
  non-small-cell   136, 138–9, **138**
  palliative care   139–40
  pathology   132, *132*
  scar carcinoma   131
  small-cell carcinoma   136
  treatment   136–40, *137*
lung compliance   4, *5*
lung function tests   23–36
  arterial blood gases   32–6, **32**
  carbon monoxide transfer
    factor   28, 31
  COPD   118–19
  lung volumes   23–4, *24*
  ventilatory function   23–8
lung transplantation   192–5
  COPD   126
  indications   193, *194*
  prognosis   195
  types of operation   192–3
    bilateral lung transplant
      192–3
    heart-lung transplant   192
    living lobar
      transplantation   193
    single-lung transplant   192
lung volume   23–4, *24*
  and airway resistance   7

and site of maximal airway
resistance   7
lung volume reduction surgery   126
lymph nodes, enlargement   16
lymphoid interstitial
pneumonitis   65
lymphoma   65, 176

magnesium sulphate   108, 113
Mallory-Weiss syndrome   177
mannitol, cystic fibrosis   94
Mantoux test   74
maximal mid-expiratory flow
24–5
measles   79
meconium ileus   89
mediastinal masses   41–2, *42*
mediastinal shift   170
mediastinoscopy   149
Medical Research Council Dyspnoea
Scale   120
Meigs' syndrome   176
melanoptysis   14
mesothelioma   158–9, *159*, 176
metabolic acidosis   34
metabolic alkalosis   34–5
methacholine/histamine
provocation tests   103
methylxanthines   123
metronidazole
lung abscess   85
pleural effusion   177
miliary tuberculosis   71–2
modafinil, obstructive sleep
apnoea   190
mometasone   108
montelukast   109
Moraxella catarrhalis   84, 126
mucociliary escalator   80
mucolytics   123
muscles of respiration   3–4, *4*
function tests   28
Mycobacterium abscessus   77, 89
Mycobacterium avium-intracellulare
complex   65, 77
Mycobacterium chelonae   77
Mycobacterium kansasii   77
Mycobacterium malmoense   77
Mycobacterium tuberculosis   68, 151
see also tuberculosis
Mycobacterium xenopi   77
Mycoplasma pneumoniae   54, 55,
58, 60

nasal polyps, cystic fibrosis   92
nebulisers   111–12, *112*
necrobacillosis   85
nedocromil   109

nicotine patches   121
nitric oxide
ARDS   183
exhaled   104
nitrofurantoin, lung fibrosis   142
non-invasive ventilation   128
positive pressure   186
norepinephrine, ARDS   183

obliterative bronchiolitis   145, 154
obstructive sleep apnoea   15,
186–90, *188*
clinical features   187–9, **189**
pathogenesis   187
polysomnography   189
treatment   189–90
obstructive ventilatory defect   24, *25*
occupational history   16
occupational lung disease   151–9
asbestos-related   156–9, *157–9*
asthma   151–4
byssinosis   154
pneumoconiosis   154–5
popcorn worker's lung   154
siderosis   156
silicosis   155–6, *156*
oesophageal rupture   177
omalizumab   109
ornithosis   60
oxygen
arterial content   11
carriage by blood   9, *9*
partial pressure *see* PO_2
oxygen concentrator   125
oxygen desaturation   186, *187*
oxygen saturation   **32**, 35
ARDS   **182**
oxygen therapy
ambulatory   125
asthma   113
COPD   124–5
emergency   127, *127*
long-term   124–5
oxygen-carbon dioxide diagram   *8*
oxyhaemoglobin dissociation
curve   35

palpation   18–19, *19*
Pancoast tumour   133, *134*
pancreatic insufficiency, cystic
fibrosis   89–90
pancreatitis, pulmonary
effusion   177
Panton-Valentine leukocidin   59
para-amino salicylic acid,
tuberculosis   73
parapneumonic effusion   176
paroxysmal nocturnal dyspnoea   14

PCO_2 8, **32**
PDE-4 inhibitors   123
peak expiratory flow rate   6, 24,
26, *26*
asthma   103
peak flow diary   103
penicillins, pneumonia   58
pentamidine, *Pneumocystis*
jirovecii   64
percussion   20
percutaneous needle biopsy, lung
cancer   134, *135*
pertussis   79
pet-derived allergens   99, 106
pH   **32**
physiological shunt   3
physiotherapy
cystic fibrosis   93–4
pneumonia   83
pilocarpine iontophoresis   92
pink puffers   118, *119*
plethysmography   27
pleural biopsy   175
pleural effusion   *21*, 173–7
asbestos-related   158
causes   176
clinical features   173
exudates   176–7
investigations   173–4, *174*
pleural fluid dynamics   173, *173*
rheumatoid disease   145
transudates   176
pleural empyema   85
pleural fluid aspiration   174
pneumonia   57
pleural plaques   157–8
pleural rubs   20
pleural thickening   158
pleurectomy   172
pleurisy, asbestos-related   158
pleuritic pain   15, 55, 83
pneumothorax   170
pleurodesis   172, 176
pneumococcal pneumonia   58–9,
59
pneumoconiosis   154–5
coalworker's   154–5, *155*
Pneumocystis jirovecii   62, 63–4, *65*
pneumocystis pneumonia   61, 194
pneumonia   52–67
aspiration   55, 146
atypical pathogens   60
classification   52–4, *53*
clinical features   55–6
community-acquired   54, 58
cryptogenic organising   144
Haemophilus influenzae   59
hospital-acquired   54–5

pneumonia (*Continued*)
  immunocompromised
    patients 61–2, **62**
  interstitial
    acute 145
    desquamative 145
    idiopathic 143–5
    lymphoid 145
    usual 143
  investigation 56–7, *57*
  Klebsiella 59–60
  Legionella 52, 54, 55, 60–1
  lobar 54
  Mycoplasma 54, 55, 58, 60
  pneumococcal 58–9, *59*
  Pneumocystis jirovecii 62, 63–4,
    65
  Pseudomonas aeruginosa 60
  severity of 55, *56*
  site of infection 54
  staphylococcal 59
  treatment 57–8
pneumonitis 52
pneumothorax 4, 169–72
  clinical features 170, *170, 171*
  cystic fibrosis 89
  pathogenesis 169–70
  tension *21*, 169
  treatment 170–1
PO$_2$ 8–9, *8*, **32**
polyarteritis nodosa 167
polycythaemia 120
polysomnography 189
popcorn worker's lung 154
positive end-expiratory
    pressure 182
positron emission tomography 44
prednisolone 126
  lung transplantation 194
pregnancy, pulmonary
    embolism 164
Prevotella spp. 85
primaquine, *Pneumocystis
    jirovecii* 64
progesterone, obstructive sleep
    apnoea 190
protein C deficiency 160
protein S deficiency 160
protriptylline, obstructive sleep
    apnoea 190
Pseudomonas aeruginosa 54, 84, 89
  pneumonia 60
psittacosis 60
pulmonary angiography, pulmonary
    embolism 163
pulmonary artery 2
pulmonary embolism 160–6
  clinical features 161, *162*

deep vein thrombosis 160–1
  diagnosis 164
  investigations 161, 163–4, *163*
  pregnancy 164
  treatment 164–6
    anticoagulant therapy 164–5
    prophylaxis 165
    thrombolytic therapy 164, *164*
pulmonary fibrosis 151
  idiopathic 143
pulmonary hypertension 146,
    166–7
  cor pulmonale 120, 124, 166
  HIV/AIDS 65
  idiopathic 166–7
pulmonary infarcts, cavitation 39
pulmonary masses 38–9, *41*
  causes **41**
pulmonary oedema
  permeability 180
  pressure 179–80, *180*
pulmonary rehabilitation 123–4
pulmonary vascular disease 160–8
pulmonary vasculitis 167
pulse oximetry 35
  COPD 119
  obstructive sleep apnoea 189
pyrazinamide
  adverse reactions 74
  tuberculosis **72**, 73

radioallergosorbent testing
    (RAST) 104
radiotherapy, lung cancer 139
residual volume 24
  asthma 103
respiration *see* breathing
respiratory acidosis 34
  ARDS **182**
respiratory alkalosis 34
respiratory bronchiolitis-interstitial
    lung disease 145
respiratory failure 35–6
  type 1 11, 35
  type 2 11, 35
  see also ARDS
respiratory quotient 8
respiratory rate 16
restrictive ventilatory defect 4, 24,
    25, 28
reticular honeycomb pattern 42,
    143, *145*
rheumatoid disease 145–6, *146*
rheumatoid nodules 145–6
rheumatoid pneumoconiosis *see*
    Caplan's syndrome
rhonchi *see* wheeze
rifampicin

adverse reactions 74
  tuberculosis **72**, 73
roflumilast 123

Saccharopolyspora rectivirgula 146
salbutamol 107, 113, 121, 126
salmeterol 107, 121
sarcoidosis 147–50, *148, 149*
  acute 148
    bilateral hilar
      lymphadenopathy 148, *149*
    erythema nodosum 148
  chronic 148–50
    extrapulmonary 149
    pulmonary 148–9, *149*
  diagnosis 149–50
  ocular 149
  treatment 150
SARS 61
scalene muscles 4
severe acute respiratory syndrome
    see SARS
shrinking lungs 146
siderosis 156
signs 13, 20, *21*
silhouette sign 38
silicosis 155–6, *156*
sinusitis, cystic fibrosis 92
skin prick tests 103–4, *104*
sleep-related breathing
    disorders 185–91
  central sleep apnoea 190
  obstructive sleep apnoea
    syndrome 186–90, *188*
  oxygen desaturation 186, *187*
smoking
  and COPD 117
  and lung cancer 130
smoking cessation 120–1, 123
  pharmacotherapy 121
snoring 15
social history 15
sodium cromoglycate 108–9
spacer devices 110, *111*
spirometry 24, *25–6*
  asthma 102–3
  COPD 118
sputum production, COPD 118
staphylococcal pneumonia 59
Staphylococcus aureus 54, 79, 85,
    89, 176–7
Streptococcus milleri 177
Streptococcus pneumonia 54, 55,
    58, 61, 79, 89, 126, 176
streptokinase, pleural effusion 177
streptomycin, tuberculosis 73
stridor 14, 16
subphrenic abscess 177

sweat testing   92
Symbicort   107
symptoms   13–15, **14**
   see also individual symptoms
syndrome of inappropriate
      anti-diuretic hormone
      secretion   132
systemic lupus erythematosus
   146
systemic sclerosis
      (scleroderma)   146

tactile fremitus   18
tension pneumothorax   *21*, 169
terbutaline   107, 113, 121
tetracycline, COPD   126
theophylline   108, 123
Thermoactinomyces vulgaris   146
thoracic cage disorders   186
thoracocentesis *see* pleural fluid
      aspiration
thoracoplasty   *73*
thoracoscopy, video-assisted   142,
   175
thrombolytics, pulmonary
      embolism   165, *165*
tidal volume   23
tinzaparin   164, 166
tiotropium   107, 122
tobacco smoke, exposure to   151
tobramycin
   cystic fibrosis   94
   pneumonia   58
total lung capacity   23, 27–8

asthma   103
trachea   1
   position of   18
tracheostomy   190
transbronchial biopsy   142, *143*
transfer factor   28
transudates   176
trimethoprim, COPD   126
tuberculin testing   74–6, *75*
tuberculosis   68–77
   clinical course   68–70, *70*
      pleural effusion   177
      post-primary tuberculosis   70
      primary tuberculosis   69
   control   76
      BCG vaccination   76
      contact tracing   76
      immigrant screening   76
   diagnosis   70–2, *71*
   drug-resistant   73–4
   epidemiology   68, *69*
   HIV/AIDS   64
   immunocompromised
         patients   61
   latent   74
   miliary   71–2
   treatment   72–4, **72**
      adverse reactions   74

ultrasound   42
   endobronchial   135
   pleural effusion   174, *175*
upper respiratory tract
      infections   54

uvulopalatopharyngoplasty
   190

V/Q *see* ventilation/perfusion
      matching
varenicline   121
ventilation
   high-frequency jet   182
   inverse ratio   182
   non-invasive   128, 186
   positive pressure   186
ventilation/perfusion lung scan,
      pulmonary embolism   163–4
ventilation/perfusion
      matching   8
   local differences   9–10, *9, 10*
ventilatory function   23–8
ventilatory support, COPD
   127–8
vital capacity   24
   supine   28
vocal resonance   20

Wegener's granulomatosis   167
   cavitation   39
wheeze   14, 16, 20
whispering pectoriloquy   20
whooping cough *see* pertussis
wood dusts   **152**

xenotransplantation   195

zafirlukast   109
Ziehl-Neelsen stain   72

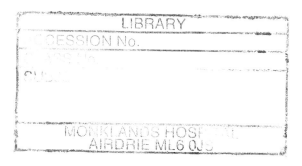

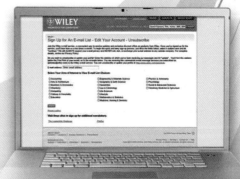
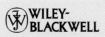